NUTRITION GUIDE FOR PHYSICIANS

NUTRITION AND HEALTH
Adrianne Bendich, PhD, FACN, Series Editor

For other titles published in this series, go to
http://www.springer.com/series/7659

Nutrition Guide for Physicians

Edited by

Ted Wilson, Ph.D
Winona State University, Department of Biology,
Winona, MN

Norman J. Temple, Ph.D
Athabasca University Center for Science, Athabasca,
Alberta, Canada

Dr. George A. Bray, M.D.
Louisiana State University, Pennington Biomedical
Research Center, Baton Rouge, LA

Marie Boyle Struble, Ph.D, R.D.
College of Saint Elizabeth, Morristown, NJ and University
of Massachusetts, Amherst, MA

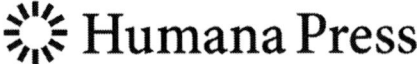 Humana Press

Editors
Ted Wilson
Department of Biology
Winona State University
Winona MN 54603
USA
ewilson@winona.edu

Norman J. Temple
Athabasca University
  Center for Science
Athabasca
AB T9S 3A3
Canada
normant@athabascau.ca

George A. Bray
Pennington Biomedical
  Research Center
Louisiana State University
6400 Perkins Rd.
Baton Rouge LA 70808
USA
brayga@pbrc.edu

Marie Boyle Struble
Department of Foods and Nutrition
College of Saint Elizabeth
Morristown, NJ 07960
USA
mstruble@cse.edu

Series Editor
Adrianne Bendich, PhD, FACN
GlaxoSmithKline Consumer Healthcare
Parsippany, NJ
USA

ISBN 978-1-60327-430-2   (hardcover)   e-ISBN 978-1-60327-431-9
ISBN 978-1-61779-409-4   (softcover)
DOI 10.1007/978-1-60327-431-9

Library of Congress Control Number: 2009939155

Dedication

To my son Dirk, may your diet become as diverse as the chapters
of this book.
Ted

To Adrian, Sharon, Philip, and Steven
Norman

To my walking buddies – Kate and McCauley – may there be many more
footprints in the sand.
Marie

To my wife Mitzi with whom I have shared so many wonderful meals.
George

Series Editor Introduction

The Nutrition and Health series of books have, as an overriding mission, to provide health professionals with texts that are considered essential because each includes (1) a synthesis of the state of the science, (2) timely, in-depth reviews by the leading researchers in their respective fields, (3) extensive, up-to-date fully annotated reference lists, (4) a detailed index, (5) relevant tables and figures, (6) identification of paradigm shifts and the consequences, (7) virtually no overlap of information between chapters, but targeted, inter-chapter referrals, (8) suggestions of areas for future research, and (9) balanced, data-driven answers to patient /health professionals questions which are based upon the totality of evidence rather than the findings of any single study.

The series volumes are developed to provide valuable in-depth information to nutrition health professionals and health providers interested in practical guidelines. Each editor has the potential to examine a chosen area with a broad perspective, both in subject matter and in the choice of chapter authors. The international perspective, especially with regard to public health initiatives, is emphasized where appropriate. The editors, whose trainings are both research and practice oriented, have the opportunity to develop a primary objective for their book, define the scope and focus, and then invite the leading authorities from around the world to be part of their initiative. The authors are encouraged to provide an overview of the field, discuss their own research, and relate the research findings to potential human health consequences. Because each book is developed de novo, the chapters are coordinated so that the resulting volume imparts greater knowledge than the sum of the information contained in the individual chapters.

"Nutrition Guide for Physicians," edited by Ted Wilson, Ph.D., Norman J. Temple, Ph.D., George A. Bray, M.D., and Marie B. Struble, Ph.D., R.D., is a very welcome addition to the Nutrition and Health series and exemplifies the series goals. This volume is especially timely as the number of research papers and meta-analyses in the clinical nutrition arena increases every year and clients and patients are very much interested in dietary components for disease prevention. Certainly, the obesity epidemic remains a major concern especially as the comorbidities, such as the metabolic syndrome, type 2 diabetes, hypertension, and hyperlipidemia, are seen even in young children. The editors have made great efforts to provide health professionals with the most up-to-date and comprehensive volume that high-lights the key, well-accepted nutrition information available to date. The edi-tors have combined their broad backgrounds in research as well as clinical practice to help the reader better understand the relevant science without the details of complex discussions of in vitro and laboratory animal studies. This comprehensive volume begins with chapters that examine the effects of macro- and micronutrients, fiber, alcohol, and other dietary components on human health and disease prevention. As an example, clear definitions and distinctions are made concerning the types of fats, and their negative and positive health aspects. An excellent explanation concerning the possi-ble reason for disparity between study findings is provided in the positing of insightful questions such as: Were all serum measurements made within hours or weeks following dietary changes? An important chapter on sugars and artificial sweeteners is included that describes the different sweeteners (nutritive and non-nutritive) that are currently available and the differences in national regulations concerning their use in different countries. Defini-tions are provided for the numerous types of vegetable-based diets that are often discussed with health professionals.

Unique to this volume, there are in-depth chapters that explain the devel-opment of the dietary recommendations and how these are translated into information on food labels. Chapters concerning the growing interest in organic foods and food safety are included. The importance of taste to food consumption is examined and the anatomy and physiology of taste are reviewed. There is an extensive analysis of the recommendations by nations on the contents of a healthy diet and suggestions for physicians and other health professionals in helping patients reach the goal of understand-ing the value of consuming a healthy diet. A separate chapter reviews the importance of certain dietary supplements containing essential vitamins and minerals and provides perspective concerning dietary supplements with less scientific data to support their claims.

The next section of the volume examines the role of nutrition in health during the life stages. The chapter on pregnancy includes preconception through lactation and postpartum. Guidelines for weight gain and consump-tion of essential nutrients and other dietary components that could impact pregnancy outcomes are included; there is a review of the dietary guid-ance during high-risk pregnancies including gestational diabetes, multiple pregnancies, and hypertension. The chapter on infancy includes a detailed description of the nutritive and other beneficial components of breast milk, but reminds us that "human milk is neither perfect nor a complete food." Childhood is a time of rapid growth and nutritional status determines the capability of reaching a child's full growth potential. Discussions about food allergies and sensitivities and deficiencies, including iron deficiency, are also included in this chapter. The chapter on adolescence and young adults examines the development of eating disorders including obesity, anorexia, bulimia, and binge eating. Healthy aging is particularly relevant as the population is growing older. By 2030 one out of every five people in the USA will be 65 years of age or older. Lifestyle changes and changes in body functions (sight, hearing, taste, digestion, bone, and muscle, etc.) can affect food choices and vice versa. This sensitive chapter provides a wealth of important advice to health professionals.

The next section contains informative chapters that look at the major diseases that have effects on and are affected by digestion and metabolism. Before examining the disease states, there is a helpful chapter that describes the major methods of nutritional assessment and how the information can be combined with the physical and laboratory biochemical examination of the patient to provide a better picture of their health status. This type of comprehensive medical examination is particularly important in the assessment of patients with eating disorders, and there is a comprehensive chapter that includes a description of these disorders. Several chapters examine the effects of obesity and its comorbidities including insulin resistance, cardiovascular complications, lipid disorders, hypertension, and hormonal imbalances. Separate chapters review the pathophysiology of the metabolic syndrome, type 1 and type 2 diabetes, hypertension, and hyperlipidemia, and relate these to the mechanisms behind the alterations in metabolism that increase chronic disease risk. Practice guidelines and tools for obesity management including up-to-date information on medical nutrition therapy and surgical obesity treatments and their implications for improving human health and reducing obesity-related diseases are tabulated for the reader. The additional chapters on coronary heart disease and blood pressure contain valuable information about salt intake, plant stanols and sterols, homocysteine, antioxidants, and review the major clinical trials that showed the power of diet to beneficially affect cardiovascular outcomes: the DASH study and the Trial of Hypertension Prevention.

Gastrointestinal disorders and disorders of the liver and pancreas are discussed in separate chapters that include malabsorption diseases, GERD, ulcers, constipation, diarrhea, diverticulosis, food allergies, cirrhosis, nonalcoholic fatty liver disease, and acute as well as chronic diseases including cancers of these organ systems. Chronic kidney disease and bone diseases and the effects of nutritional status on these diseases as well as the effects of the diseases on nutritional status are explored in separate chapters. The importance of calcium, phosphorus, vitamin D, and parathyroid hormone to both kidney and bone health becomes apparent after reading these chapters. There is a final chapter in this section that examines the effects of the most prevalent genetically inherited metabolic disorders. The key to successful treatment is neonatal genetic screening and appropriate, immediate changes in diet to help prevent the early devastating effects of the genetic defects.

The final chapters provide guidance on the potential for dietary changes to affect disease manifestation and progression. Specific syndromes in females, including premenstrual syndrome and polycystic ovarian disease, are often linked to dietary factors including obesity and eating disorders. The female athlete triad can result in amenorrhea and premature osteoporosis, whereas heavy menstrual bleeding is associated with iron-deficiency anemia. Health providers who have read this volume will be sensitized to the importance of nutritional monitoring for the overall health of their female patients who may be affected by these disabilities.

Diets can contain factors that both increase and decrease the risk of cancer. Charcoal-broiled meats contain polycyclic aromatic hydrocarbons and other molecules that are formed during the cooking process: these are known carcinogens. Alcohol is classified as a human carcinogen. In contrast, fruits and vegetables contain essential nutrients and phytochemicals that can reduce the formation of cancerous cells. Extensive tables of foods and their components are included in this chapter.

Food allergies, insensitivities, and intolerances can result in avoidances of food groups and may cause severe morbidity and even mortality (peanut allergy). Examples of the most common diagnostic tests and treatments are provided for the reader. Similarly, there are numerous well-described drug–nutrient interactions that have medically relevant effects for the patient. These are included in a separate comprehensive chapter.

Drs Wilson, Temple, Bray, and Struble are internationally recognized leaders in the fields of human nutrition including obesity research and clinical outcomes. These editors are proven excellent communicators and they have worked tirelessly to develop a book that is destined to be the benchmark in the field because of its extensive covering of the most important aspects of clinical nutrition including complex interactions between diet, health, and disease. The editors have chosen 45 of the most well-recognized and respected authors from around the world to contribute the 35 informative chapters in the volume. Hallmarks of all of the chapters include complete definitions of terms with the abbreviations fully defined for the reader and consistent use of terms between chapters. Key features of this comprehensive volume include the informative key points and keywords that are at the beginning of each chapter and suggested readings as well as bibliography at the end of each chapter. The editors have added three key appendices including a detailed table of major conversions used in nutrient calculations, suggested sources of reliable nutrition information on the web, and a copy of the dietary reference intake tables from the US Institute of Medicine. The volume also contains more than 60 detailed tables and informative figures, an extensive, detailed index, and more than 550 up-to-date references that provide the reader with excellent sources of worthwhile information about the role of diet, exercise, food intake, nutritional value of foods, human physiology, and pathophysiology of the diet-related morbidities and comorbidities.

In conclusion, "Nutrition Guide for Physicians," edited by Ted Wilson, Ph.D., Norman J. Temple, Ph.D., George A. Bray, M.D., and Marie B. Struble, Ph.D., R.D., provides health professionals in many areas of research and practice with the most up-to-date, well-referenced volume on the importance of diet to affect human health. This volume will serve the reader as the benchmark in this complex area of interrelationships between food and body weight, the central nervous system, endocrine organs, the GI tract, and the functioning of all other organ systems in the human body. Moreover, the interactions between obesity, genetic factors, and the numerous comorbidities are clearly delineated so that practitioners can better understand the complexities of these interactions. The editors are applauded for their efforts to develop this volume with their firm conviction that "nutrition serves as an essential weapon for all doctors in the battle against disease and for the enhancement of human health." This excellent text is a very welcome addition to the Nutrition and Health series.

Adrianne Bendich, Ph.D., FACN

Preface

It has often been pointed out that there is a near absence of nutrition education during medical school. If this deficiency is corrected during postgraduate medical training, it often owes more to accident than design, or perhaps to the personal interests of individual physicians. As a result most physicians presently in practice have gaping holes in their knowledge of nutrition *(1, 2)*. Correcting this deficiency is the motivation for writing this book.

Many advances took place in our understanding of basic nutrition during the 20th century. Since the 1970s there has been a flood of research studies on the role of diet in such chronic diseases as heart disease and cancer. Today, we have a vastly greater understanding of the role of diet in causing chronic diseases of lifestyle. We know, for example, that the risk of developing cancer, heart disease, and type 2 diabetes is affected by such foods as whole grain cereals, fruits, and vegetables. What we still do not understand is why it is that taking a vitamin supplement pill is not always a perfect substitute for eating these foods.

We can point to a great many examples of how dietary change can have a profound effect on health, especially for the risk of chronic diseases. Here is one recent example. Poland went through a severe economic and political crisis during the 1980s and into the 1990s. One of the results of this was a sharp decrease in availability of animal products which meant that people had much less saturated fat in their diets. This was followed by a 40% drop in mortality from cardiovascular disease during the period 1990–2002 *(3)*. Other contributing factors were an increase in consumption of fruits and vegetables and a decrease in smoking.

The views expressed in this book are interpretations by the authors of each chapter on their areas of specialization. Some readers may disagree with the opinions presented, but in nutrition, differences of opinion are often unavoidable because nutrition is an ever-changing science that lives and breathes debate and controversy.

Many ideas regarding nutrition that are widely accepted today may be discredited in coming years. The following quote illustrates this dilemma. Drummond and Wilbraham published a seminal publication entitled *The Englishman's Food* in 1939. Jack Drummond was a major nutrition authority in the 1920s and the 1930s. It would be foolhardy to believe that we can be any more accurate today in our predictions than they were over 70 years ago.

So much precise research has been done in the laboratory and so many precise surveys have been made that we know all we need to know about the food requirements of the people. . . .The position is perfectly clear-cut [with respect to Britain].

Nevertheless, over the last three decades an enormous amount of evidence has accumulated that convincingly demonstrates that nutrition serves as an essential weapon for all doctors in the battle against disease and for the enhancement of human health. To paraphrase Churchill, advances in the field of nutrition science in recent years represent "not the beginning of the end but, perhaps, the end of the beginning." In the opinion of the editors we are ready to help physicians move their patients from the hors d'oeuvres to the main course.

Cultural change at a global, national, and regional level means that our nutrition habits and our interpretation of them will change as time marches on. As the musician George Bernard Shaw said. . ."Everything I eat has been proved by some doctor or other to be a deadly poison, and everything I don't eat has been proved to be indispensable for life. But I go marching on." His comments are a reflection of the continued confusion in the public and among health professionals about what to eat and how much to eat. A simple walk through the self-help section of a book store will confirm the existence of many differing opinions of what "preventative or ideal nutrition" is all about. Some opinions verge on quackery and others are built upon solid facts. Physicians need the best possible interpretation of nutrition to provide the best advice to their patients.

In the words of Confucius: "The essence of knowledge is that, having acquired it, one must apply it." But, ironically, despite overwhelming evidence that nutrition has such enormous potential to improve human health – at modest cost – there is still a chasm between nutrition knowledge and its full exploitation for human betterment. There is also an important chasm between evaluating the strength of the supporting science and understanding its true meaning. Once the true meaning of nutrition is understood, the next hurdle is to bring dietary change to the public and the physicians who provide health care to the public.

As gatekeepers to the nutritional health of their patients, it is important that physicians have access to up-to-date nutrition resources – such as this handbook – as well as the nutrition expertise of a registered dietitian. This practical handbook is organized in three sections. Chapters 1–16 discusses general nutrition concepts and the roles and current recommendations for the macronutrients and micronutrients for optimal health. Next we address the special issues of vegetarianism, recommendations for alcoholic and non-alcoholic beverage consumption, food safety, food labeling, and the use of dietary supplements. We also illustrate useful approaches for persuading patients to make healthful behavior changes. Chapters 17–21 addresses the nutrient requirements and special nutrition-related issues for people across all stages of the life span – from pregnancy and infancy through the adolescent years to the older adult years. Chapters 22–38 summarizes the nutritional management of chronic conditions frequently seen in clinical practice – always emphasizing the therapeutic role of nutrition in the treatment and prevention of eating disorders, obesity, diabetes, coronary heart disease, hypertension, GI disorders, liver and pancreatic disease, chronic kidney disease, osteoporosis, inherited metabolic disorders, food allergies and intolerances, and cancer.

Nutrition Guide for Physicians endeavors to address the needs of those who would most benefit from up-to-date information on recent advances in the field of nutrition. Accordingly, our book contains chapters by experts in a diverse range of nutritional areas. Our aim is to present a succinct overview of recent thinking and discoveries that have the greatest capacity of physicians to improve nutritional human health.

Ted Wilson
Norman J. Temple
George A. Bray
Marie Boyle Struble

REFERENCES

1. Temple NJ. Survey of nutrition knowledge of Canadian physicians. J Am Coll Nutr 1999; 18:26–29.
2. Vetter ML, Herring SJ, Sood M, Shah NR, Kalet AL. What do resident physicians know about nutrition? An evaluation of attitudes, self-perceived proficiency and knowledge. J Am Coll Nutr 2008; 27:287–298.
3. Zatonski WA, Willett W. Changes in dietary fat and declining coronary heart disease in Poland: population based study. BMJ 2005; 331:187–188.

Contents

Contributors

KELLY C. ALLISON, PHD • *Center for Eating and Weight Disorders, University of Pennsylvania School of Medicine, Philadelphia, PA*

ASIMA R. ANWAR, BSC • *Recreation and Parks Department, Mississauga, Ontario, Canada*

LAURA A.G. ARMAS, MD • *Osteoporosis Research Center, Creighton University, Omaha, NE*

BRUNO BORSARI, PHD • *Department of Biology, Winona State University, Winona, MN*

ALICE N. BRAKO, BVM, MA, MPH, CHES • *Department of Biology, Winona State University, Winona, MN*

GEORGE A. BRAY, MD • *Pennington Biomedical Research Center, Baton Rouge, LA*

BRIDGET A. CASSADY, BSC • *Department of Foods and Nutrition, Purdue University, West Lafayette, IN*

CATHERINE M. CHAMPAGNE, PHD, RD • *Pennington Biomedical Research Center, Baton Rouge, LA*

CINDY D. DAVIS, PHD • *Division of Cancer Prevention, National Cancer Institute, Rockville, MD*

LUANNE DIGUGLIELMO, MS, RD, CSR • *Dietetic Internship Program, College of Saint Elizabeth, Morristown, NJ*

KIYAH J. DUFFEY, PHD • *School of Public Health, University of North Carolina at Chapel Hill, Chapel Hill, NC*

GIANNA FERRETTI, PHD • *Istituto di Biochimica, Università Politecnica delle Marche, Ancona, Italy*

KATE FIREOVID, MS, RD • *Department of Biology and Nutrition, University of Wisconsin – La Crosse, La Crosse, WI*

JENNIFER J. FRANCIS, MPH, RD • *Dietetics Program, Southern Maine Community College, South Portland, ME*

MARION J. FRANZ, MS, RD, CDE • *Nutrition Concepts by Franz, Inc., Minneapolis, MN*

JAMES K. FRIEL, PHD • *Dept Human Nutritional Sciences and Pediatrics, University of Manitoba, Winnipeg, Canada*

KAREN M. GIBSON, MS, RD, CD, CSSD • *Department of Nutrition and Dietetics, Viterbo University, La Crosse, WI*

DAVID HARSHA, PHD • *Pennington Biomedical Research Center, Baton Rouge, LA*

ROBERT P. HEANEY, MD • *Osteoporosis Research Center, Creighton University, Omaha, NE*

DAVID R. JACOBS, JR, PHD • *Division of Epidemiology, University of Minnesota, Minneapolis, MN*

GARVAN C. KANE, MD, PHD • *Division of Cardiovascular Disease, Department of Internal Medicine, Mayo Clinic, Rochester, MN*

CAROL J. KLITZKE, MS, RD • *Department of Nutrition and Dietetics, Viterbo University, La Crosse, WI*

JENNIFER C. LOVEJOY, PHD • *Free and Clear, Inc. and University of Washington, School of Public Health, Seattle, WA*

MARGARET A. MAHER, PHD, RD • *Department of Biology and Nutrition, University of Wisconsin – La Crosse, La Crosse, WI*

RICHARD D. MATTES, MPH, PHD, RD • *Department of Foods and Nutrition, Purdue University, West Lafayette, IN*

CLAIRE MCENVOY, SRD, MPHIL • *Nutrition and Metabolism Group, Centre for Clinical and Population Science, Belfast, UK*

JOHN A. MILNER, PHD • *Division of Cancer Prevention, National Cancer Institute, Rockville, MD*

DAVIDE NERI, PHD • *Dipartimento di Scienze Ambientali e delle Produzioni Vegetali, Università Politecnica delle Marche, Ancona, Italy*

ROMAN E. PERRI, MD • *Division of Gastroenterology and Hepatology, Vanderbilt University Medical Center, Nashville TN*

BARRY M. POPKIN, PHD • *School of Public Health, University of North Carolina at Chapel Hill, Chapel Hill, NC*

KAREN A. RAFFERTY, RD • *Osteoporosis Research Center, Creighton University, Omaha, NE*

KATHY ROBERTS, MS, RD • *College of Saint Elizabeth, Morristown, NJ*

JACKI M. RORABAUGH • *Department of Biology, Winona State University, Winona, MN*

ELEANOR SCHLENKER, PHD, RD • *Dept Human Nutrition, Foods and Exercise, Virginia Polytechnic Institute and State University, Blacksburg, VA*

SCOTT SEGAL, PHD • *Department of Biology, Winona State University, Winona, MN*

JOANNE SLAVIN, PHD, RD • *Department of Food and Nutritional Sciences, University of Minnesota, Minneapolis, MN*

JOANNE M. SPAHN, MS, RD, FADA • *Director, Evidence Analysis Library Division, Center for Nutrition Policy and Promotion, U.S. Department of Agriculture*

MARIE BOYLE STRUBLE, PHD, RD • *Department of Foods and Nutrition, College of Saint Elizabeth, Morristown, NJ*

NORMAN J. TEMPLE, PHD • *Centre for Science, Athabasca University, Athabasca, Alberta*

TED WILSON, PHD • *Department of Biology, Winona State University, Winona, MN*

JAYNE V. WOODSIDE, PHD • *Nutrition and Metabolism Group, Centre for Clinical and Population Science, Belfast, UK*

1 Fat: The Good, the Bad, and the Ugly

Jennifer C. Lovejoy

Key Points

- A certain amount of dietary fat, particularly the essential n–3 and n–6 fatty acids, is necessary for normal physiological function.
- The major types of dietary fats are saturated fats (largely from animal products) and mono- and polyunsaturated fats (found in vegetable and some animal sources).
- Fat is the most calorically dense macronutrient (9 kcal/g)
- High-fat diets have been shown to contribute to excess energy intake and obesity.
- Both total dietary fat and various types of fatty acids have been associated with cardiovascular and metabolic risk factors. In general, saturated fats and *trans* fats have an adverse effect on health risk factors, while n–3 polyunsaturated fatty acids have beneficial effects on multiple risk factors.

   Key Words: Dietary fat; polyunsaturated fat; monounsaturated fat; saturated fat; *trans* fatty acids; n–3 fatty acid; n–6 fatty acid

1. INTRODUCTION

Although in recent years public health and medical authorities have highlighted many of the "bad" health effects of dietary fats, some fat intake is actually essential to normal physiological function. For example, fat is a critical component of cell membranes and is necessary for steroid hormone synthesis. Consuming some dietary fat is also important for adequate absorption of fat-soluble vitamins (vitamins A, E, D, K, and carotenoids) from food. Furthermore, certain n–3 and n–6 polyunsaturated fatty acids are designated as essential fatty acids, meaning the body cannot synthesize them de novo and they must be consumed in the diet. Therefore, if dietary fat intake is too severely limited, it can result in physiological dysfunction and clinical

From: *Nutrition and Health: Nutrition Guide for Physicians*
Edited by: T. Wilson et al. (eds.), DOI 10.1007/978-1-60327-431-9_1,
© Humana Press, a part of Springer Science+Business Media, LLC 2010

pathology. In particular, very low fat diets are not recommended for young children, who require higher levels of fat than do adults as a concentrated source of calories for growth.

Although some dietary fat is necessary for health, in developed countries the biggest problem is too much dietary fat rather than too little. Although it is commonly pointed out that Americans have reduced their percentage of calories from fat over the last three decades, what is often unrecognized is the fact that actual fat consumption (i.e., grams of fat per day) has remained quite high since the 1960s. The reduction in fat percentage is due to the fact that total calorie intake has increased rather than that fat intake has decreased. In fact, according to the USDA, consumption of added fats from processed foods and cooking oils increased by 63% from 1970 to 2005, reaching ~86 pounds per person (vs. 33 pounds per person in 1970).

The current dietary guidelines for Americans recommend consumption of 20–35% of calories from fat, with less than 10% of calories from saturated fat (1). The guidelines go on to point out, however, that individuals who consume fat at the higher end of this range may have difficulty limiting saturated fat and avoiding excess calorie intake. The latter is an issue in part because fat is the most energy-dense macronutrient: 9 kcal/g, compared with 4 kcal/g for carbohydrate and protein. Excess dietary fat consumption is a concern because considerable research suggests that too much dietary fat can lead to obesity, inflammation, and increased chronic disease risk as discussed below.

In addition to limiting total dietary fat intake to a healthy range, attention to the type of fat consumed is also very important. Dietary lipids include triglycerides, sterols, and phospholipids. Triglycerides are the most abundant type of dietary lipid and, as such, much of the emphasis regarding dietary fat and health relates to the triglyceride fatty acid composition (i.e., whether the fatty acid is saturated, monounsaturated, or polyunsaturated). Although sterols and phospholipids comprise a small proportion of total dietary lipids, some of these compounds (e.g., cholesterol) are also quite important.

2. TYPES OF DIETARY FAT AND THEIR FOOD SOURCES

2.1. Saturated Fats

Saturated fatty acid molecules contain no double bonds (i.e., they are "saturated" with hydrogen atoms) and saturated fats are typically solid at room temperature. Dietary saturated fats come primarily from animal sources (meats, dairy, egg yolks), although certain plant oils such as coconut and palm oil are also rich in them. According to the USDA, the primary sources of saturated fats in the American diet are cheese, beef, milk, and oils.

2.2. Monounsaturated Fatty Acids (MUFA)

MUFA are fatty acids that contain one double bond and are typically liquid at room temperature, although they may solidify at refrigerator temperatures. MUFA are found in highest concentration in olive and canola oils, nuts, seeds, and avocados. Although meats contain some MUFA, they typically occur in lower amounts than saturated fatty acids.

2.3. Polyunsaturated Fatty Acids (PUFA)

PUFA contain two or more double bonds and are liquid at both room temperature and at cooler temperatures. PUFA are highly susceptible to oxidation and rancidity because of their double bonds, and thus should be stored under conditions of low light and heat and expiration dates strictly followed. Like MUFA, PUFA are also found primarily in plant foods. In the Western diet the primary sources of PUFA are plant oils such as soybean, sunflower, corn, and safflower oil.

2.4. Essential Fatty Acids and the n–6 and n–3 Families

There are two PUFA that are considered "essential" because they cannot be synthesized in the body: linoleic acid (an n–6 fatty acid) and alpha-linolenic (ALA; an n–3 fatty acid). In general, longer chain n–6 and n–3 fatty acids can be synthesized from the two essential fatty acids. For example, the long-chain n–6 fatty acid arachidonic acid (AA), which impacts inflammation and immune function, can be synthesized from linoleic acid. Due to genetic variation in enzyme function, many individuals have limited ability to synthesize the important long-chain n–3 fatty acids eicosapentaenoic acid (EPA) and docosahexaenoic acid (DHA) from ALA. Thus, some nutritionists consider EPA and DHA to be "conditionally essential."

n–6 fatty acids, including the essential linoleic acid, are found in high amounts in the common plant oils mentioned previously (sunflower, safflower, corn, and soybean oil). n–3 fatty acids can be found in both plant and animal foods. The essential n–3 fatty acid ALA is found in flaxseeds, pumpkin seeds, walnuts, and canola oil, while EPA and DHA are found in cold-water marine fish (salmon, sardines, mackerel, herring, tuna).

The balance of n–3 and n–6 intake is also important for health. Typical Western diets tend to be much higher in n–6 than n–3 fatty acids. Ideally, n–6 and n–3 PUFA should be consumed in a ratio of no more than 3:1. But because of excess consumption of high n–6 plant oils, most Western diets range from 10–20 to 1, considerably higher than the healthy range. Thus, to optimize n–3 to n–6 balance, individuals should focus on increasing n–3 PUFA intake while limiting excessive n–6 intake.

2.5. Trans Fats

The carbon chains of unsaturated fatty acids can occur in either a *cis* or a *trans* conformation (shape). Most naturally occurring unsaturated fatty acids occur in the *cis* form. Although *trans* fatty acids are a minor constituent of cow's milk and some meats, the vast majority of *trans* fatty acids in the diet come from the processing of foods, particularly the hydrogenation of oils. According to the USDA, most of the *trans* fat in the American diet comes from processed baked goods (cakes, cookies, crackers, pies, etc.) with a significant amount coming from margarine consumption.

2.6. Sterols

Cholesterol is the best-known dietary sterol. Cholesterol is a major structural component of cell membranes and is an important precursor for vitamin D and the steroid hormones: sex hormones, glucocorticoids, and mineralocorticoids. Cholesterol is found only in animal foods (meats, eggs, and dairy). In dairy products, the cholesterol is found in the butterfat portion, therefore non-fat or low-fat dairy products have substantially less cholesterol than full-fat dairy products.

In addition to cholesterol, in recent years considerable focus has been placed on plant sterols (phytosterols), which inhibit the absorption of cholesterol from the intestine and thus may reduce serum cholesterol and cardiovascular risk. Although phytosterols are poorly absorbed from whole plants, the food industry has found ways to incorporate significant amounts of these sterols into foods such as margarines, which are marketed as cholesterol-lowering products.

3. DIETARY FAT EFFECTS ON HEALTH

3.1. Obesity

3.1.1. ROLE OF TOTAL DIETARY FAT

Many studies demonstrate a positive relationship between dietary fat and obesity. A meta-analysis of ~100 randomized clinical trials demonstrated that higher fat intake is associated with higher body weight. Another meta-analysis of 28 dietary intervention trials found that reducing fat intake by 10% caused a weight loss of ~3 kg in 6 months *(2)*. For this reason, low-fat, energy-restricted diets remain the cornerstone of dietary therapy for weight loss.

High-fat diets may contribute to obesity in several ways *(3)*. First, because fat has more than twice the calories of protein or carbohydrate, it is easy to passively overconsume calories when eating high-fat foods. Second, contrary to popular belief, fat is not as satiating as protein or carbohydrate, again potentially leading to overconsumption of calories. Lastly, fat is more efficiently absorbed from the intestine than other macronutrients and produces smaller increases in postprandial energy expenditure, resulting in lower daily energy expenditure on high-fat diets.

Given the preponderance of evidence linking high-fat diets to obesity, the degree of controversy around low-fat vs. low-carbohydrate diets is striking. Several things continue to fuel this controversy. Some public health experts have called attention to population studies that have not observed a relationship between fat intake and obesity, and note that the effect of reducing fat intake on weight in clinical trials is small *(4)*. Although some epidemiological studies do not find a relationship between dietary fat and obesity, most large population studies (within and between countries) do find higher total fat intakes associated with greater obesity *(2, 3)*. And, while one might argue that a 7 pounds weight loss in 6 months is "small," it can be clinically significant (e.g., a 150 pound woman who loses 7 pounds has lost 5% of her body weight, an amount associated with significant medical benefits). Finally, in many of the randomized clinical trials of dietary fat reduction, weight loss was not the aim of the study and physical activity was held constant. It is likely that individuals who desire to lose weight and combine dietary fat reduction with increased physical activity will lose more weight.

A second reason for confusion about dietary fat and obesity is the popularity of very low carbohydrate weight loss diets. Although recent research suggests these diets do produce weight loss (due to calorie restriction), the question of long-term compliance, efficacy, and safety of very low carbohydrate/high-fat diets for weight loss remains unanswered and controversial.

Lastly, high-fat diets and sedentary lifestyles may be an especially bad combination for weight gain. When we eat carbohydrates and protein, oxidation is closely matched to intake. However, there is considerable individual variability in how much of consumed fat is oxidized. Smith et al. *(5)* showed that under sedentary conditions most people fail to oxidize the amount of fat eaten and increase their fat stores, while instituting a high amount of aerobic exercise during high-fat diet consumption caused people to better adjust fat oxidation to fat intake.

3.1.2. ROLE OF SPECIFIC FATTY ACIDS

Some studies have suggested that saturated fat may be more obesity promoting than unsaturated fats, and MUFA more obesity promoting than PUFA, but the results are inconsistent. Studies in animals and a few studies in humans suggest that long-chain $n–3$ PUFA have a beneficial effect on weight and fat loss, possibly because of an effect on energy expenditure.

Larger controlled trials are needed to confirm effects of various fatty acids on obesity and body composition.

3.2. Heart Disease

For many years, low-fat diets were recommended for reducing CVD. Currently, however, the American Heart Association places a larger emphasis on reducing saturated and *trans* fatty acids and replacing them with MUFA or PUFA rather than with carbohydrate or protein. This shift in emphasis has largely resulted from a number of clinical trials showing that low-fat diets can increase serum triglycerides and lower HDL-cholesterol when body weight is held constant. It should be noted, however, that in studies where low-fat diets are allowed to produce slight, natural weight loss, LDL-cholesterol is decreased and triglycerides and HDL-cholesterol are unchanged, resulting in a favorable CVD profile *(6)*.

Specific fatty acid type may be more important than total dietary fat for CVD. Both saturated and *trans* fatty acids have been shown to have adverse effects on serum lipids and CVD-related morbidity and mortality. For example, higher saturated fat intakes increase the risk of myocardial infarction anywhere from 50 to 200%, depending on an individual's genetic background *(7)*, and higher *trans* fatty acid intakes have been linked to increased myocardial infarction and sudden coronary death *(8)*.

On the positive side, a number of research studies suggest that populations that consume more dietary *n*–3 fatty acid have lower CVD risk. In addition, randomized controlled trials indicate that increasing *n*–3 fatty acid intake decreases the risk of myocardial infarction and sudden cardiac death in individuals with coronary heart disease *(9)*. As a result, the American Heart Association recommends that all non-pregnant adults eat fish, particularly oily fish, at least twice weekly. For individuals concerned about pollutants in fish or pregnant women and children who should limit intake of fish likely to be contaminated with mercury, decontaminated fish oil supplements or vegetarian (algae-derived) *n*–3 supplements are a good option. Research has shown that *n*–3 supplements also have beneficial effects on CVD risk *(10)*.

3.3. Type 2 Diabetes and Insulin Resistance

3.3.1. ROLE OF TOTAL DIETARY FAT

A number of epidemiological and clinical studies suggest that higher fat intakes are associated with type 2 diabetes and insulin resistance (see Ref. *11* for review), although this association is not consistent. For example, the multinational Mediterranean Group for the Study of Diabetes reported that individuals newly diagnosed with type 2 diabetes consume more total fat than non-diabetic controls ($\sim$30% vs. $\sim$27%). The San Luis Valley Diabetes

Study also observed that higher fat intake predicted development of type 2 diabetes: an increase in dietary fat of 40 g/day was associated with a 3.4-fold increased diabetes risk independent of obesity. In the Kaiser Permanente Women Twins Study, a 20 g/day increase in total fat was associated with a 9% higher fasting insulin level, a marker of insulin resistance, even after adjusting for obesity.

Randomized clinical trials also suggest a direct effect of increased dietary fat on insulin resistance (11). A number of studies of healthy individuals fed controlled high- and low-fat diets for periods ranging from 3 days to 4 weeks have shown that low-fat diets significantly improve insulin sensitivity, although not every trial has observed this effect. Long-term benefits on glucose and insulin have also been observed when dietary fat intake is reduced in patients with type 2 diabetes or impaired glucose tolerance.

Despite the evidence base suggesting that reducing dietary fat improves insulin sensitivity, there is considerable confusion among patients about dietary fat and diabetes risk due to the widely discussed glycemic index issue. The confusion results from the paradoxical effect of dietary macronutrients on acute postprandial glucose/insulin vs. their long-term effects on whole-body insulin sensitivity and secretion. Foods that are high in simple carbohydrates and starches typically raise postprandial glucose and insulin to a greater extent than foods that are high in fat. This fact has led some to conclude that high-carbohydrate/low-fat diets worsen insulin action. However, as discussed above, most evidence suggests that over several days to weeks low-fat diets improve whole-body insulin sensitivity. As insulin sensitivity improves, less insulin is needed to promote glucose uptake, resulting in lower fasting and 24-h insulin secretion despite carbohydrate's acute effects on postprandial insulin.

3.3.2. ROLE OF SPECIFIC FATTY ACIDS

The majority of epidemiological studies observe that high intakes of saturated fat or meat are associated with insulin resistance and type 2 diabetes (12, 13). Conversely, high PUFA (or vegetable fat) intake is associated with improved insulin sensitivity or glucose tolerance. Similar results are found in controlled feeding studies where high saturated fat intake worsens insulin sensitivity relative to high MUFA or PUFA intake (reviewed in Ref. 11). The majority of studies find a neutral effect of long-chain n–3 PUFA (EPA and DHA) on glucose and insulin, although several epidemiological and clinical studies observed that higher n–3 intakes are protective (reviewed in Ref. 14). Because the beneficial effects of EPA and DHA on CHD risk factors are strong, even in patients with impaired glucose tolerance and diabetes, there is still reason to recommend increasing EPA and DHA intake in patients with diabetes.

Interestingly, the level of total dietary fat appears to modulate the impact of specific fatty acids. For example, Ricardi and Rivellese did not observe a beneficial effect of diets high in MUFA on insulin action when total fat exceeded 38% *(15)*, and Lovejoy et al. failed to observe an adverse effect of saturated fat on insulin action when total fat was below 28% *(16)*. These results suggest that following the general guidelines of limiting total fat to <30%, while emphasizing specific reduction in saturated fat, will produce the best outcomes in terms of insulin sensitivity and diabetes.

3.4. Cancer

Despite considerable research into the effect of dietary fat on cancer, studies are conflicting and the overall data somewhat weak. A number of early epidemiological studies suggested a relationship between high dietary fat intakes and breast, colon, prostate, and pancreatic cancer. However, direct prospective studies, such as the Women's Health Initiative, have failed to observe benefits of reducing dietary fat in preventing breast or colorectal cancer. It is not known whether this is due to a true lack of effect of dietary fat on cancer or whether poor compliance with dietary recommendations may have weakened the results. Stronger evidence exists relating high saturated fat and/or meat consumption to development of a variety of cancers; however, more prospective studies are needed. For more information on nutritional influences upon cancer, the reader may wish to consult Chapter 33.

3.5. Inflammation

In recent years, it has been recognized that inflammation plays a key role in the development of a number of health conditions, including heart disease, insulin resistance, type 2 diabetes, obesity, and cancer. Because proinflammatory processes are detrimental in such a variety of chronic diseases, it could be argued that reducing excess inflammation should be a key nutritional goal.

High intakes of total dietary fat appear to be significantly proinflammatory. Acute consumption of a high-fat meal (e.g., a typical fast-food meal) results in increase in circulating inflammatory cytokines and worsens whole-body and tissue-specific oxidative stress *(17)*. Interestingly, acute adverse effects on vascular function are seen following high-fat meals even when those meals are somewhat "healthier" (e.g., vegetarian burger with fries vs. regular hamburger with fries) *(18)*, suggesting that total fat intake may be the primary culprit.

Also important for modulating inflammation is the ratio between the intake of dietary n–6 and n–3 fatty acids. As mentioned previously, in most Western countries, the ratio of n–6 to n–3 intakes is much higher than recommended. The n–6 PUFA arachidonic acid is the precursor of inflammatory eicosanoids such as prostaglandin E(2) and leukotriene B(4). Thus, excess consumption of n–6 fatty acids promotes inflammation, while consumption of long-chain n–3 fatty acids (DHA and EPA) is anti-inflammatory. In hospitalized patients, supplementation with n–3 PUFA reduces levels of C-reactive protein (CRP), a key inflammatory marker *(14)*. Similar reductions in inflammatory markers have been observed in healthy individuals *(19)* and patients with type 2 diabetes *(20)*.

4. CONCLUSIONS

Although a certain level of dietary fat is essential for healthy physiological functioning, dietary fat intakes in developed countries are much higher than ideal. Because fat is so energy-dense, high-fat foods contribute

Table 1
Benefits of Long-Chain n–3 PUFA

Improvement in...	Type of Effect[1]	Level of evidence[2]
Serum lipids	+++	IA, IIA
Heart disease	+++	IA, IIA
Hypertension	++	B
Stroke	++	IIA
Endothelial function	++	IIA
Cardiac arrhythmia	+++	IIA,B
Glycemia	+/–	IIA,B
Insulin sensitivity	+/–	IIA
Obesity	+/–	IIA, B
Rheumatoid arthritis	++	IIA,B
Depression/bipolar disorder	++	IA, IIA
Cancer and cachexia	+/–	IA,B
C-reactive protein/inflammation	+++	IIA,B
Inflammatory bowel disease	++	IIA,B
Alzheimer's dementia/cognitive decline with aging	++	B

[1]+++ = Strongly beneficial; ++ = Moderately beneficial; + = Somewhat beneficial; +/– = Neither beneficial nor harmful.
[2]IA = meta-analysis or systematic review; IIA= randomized, clinical trials; B=non-randomized trials including epidemiological studies or mechanistic/animal studies.

to excess calorie intake and, ultimately, weight gain and obesity. High-fat diets have also been associated with insulin resistance and development of type 2 diabetes, and with inflammation and oxidative stress.

Intake of specific fatty acids is also important in modulating disease risk. In general, saturated and *trans* fats are most strongly implicated in metabolic and heart disease risk, and high saturated fat/meat intakes have also been implicated in the development of certain cancers. In contrast, long-chain *n*–3 PUFA consumption has been shown to result in beneficial effects in all the conditions reviewed here, plus a number of others (Table 1). The role of MUFA consumption is somewhat less clear, as high MUFA diets appear to be beneficial for heart disease but may have adverse effects on body weight and metabolic disease.

Thus, considered collectively, the evidence suggests that the optimal dietary pattern with regard to fat intake is one that is relatively low in total fat (25–30%), with further restriction of saturated and *trans* fats, accompanied by optimization of the ratio of *n*–6 to *n*–3 fat to 2–3:1 by selective increase in *n*–3 and decrease in *n*–6 fats.

SUGGESTED FURTHER READING

Astrup A. The role of dietary fat in obesity. Semin Vasc Med 2005; 5:40–47.
Lovejoy JC. The influence of dietary fat on insulin resistance. Curr Diabetes Reports 2002; 2:435–440.
Linus Pauling Institute. Essential Fatty Acids. http://lpi.oregonstate.edu/infocenter/othernuts/omega3fa/

REFERENCES

1. U.S. Department of Agriculture. Dietary Guidelines for Americans 2005, Chapter 6: Fats. Available at www.health.gov/DietaryGuidelines/dga2005/document/default.htm. Last accessed June 15, 2008.
2. Bray GA, Popkin BM. Dietary fat intake does affect obesity. Am J Clin Nutr 1998; 68:1157–1173.
3. Astrup A. The role of dietary fat in obesity. Semin Vasc Med 2005; 5:40–47.
4. Willett WC, Leibel RL. Dietary fat is not a major determinant of body fat. Am J Med 2002; 113 Suppl 9B:47S–59S.
5. Smith SR, de Jonge L, Zachwieja JJ, et al. Concurrent physical activity increases fat oxidation during the shift to a high-fat diet. Am J Clin Nutr 2000; 72:131–138.
6. Yu-Poth S, Zhao G, Etherton T, et al. Effects of the National Cholesterol Education Programs step I and step II dietary intervention programs on cardiovascular disease risk factors: a meta-analysis. Am J Clin Nutr 1999; 69:632–646.
7. Yang Y, Ruiz-Narvaez E, Kraft P, Campos H. Effect of apolipoprotein E genotype and saturated fat intake on plasma lipids and myocardial infarction in the Central Valley of Costa Rica. Hum Biol 2007; 79:637–647.
8. Mozaffarian D, Willett WC. Trans fatty acids and cardiovascular risk: a unique cardiometabolic imprint? Curr Atheroscler Rep 2007; 9:486–493.

9. Marchioli R, Schweiger C, Tavazzi L, Valagussa F. Efficacy of n-3 polyunsaturated fatty acids after myocardial infarction: results of GISSI-Prevenzione trial. Lipids 2001; 36 Suppl:S119–S126.

10. Holub DJ, Holub BJ. Omega-3 fatty acids from fish oils and cardiovascular disease. Mol Cell Biochem 2004; 263:217–225.

11. Lovejoy JC. The influence of dietary fat on insulin resistance. Curr Diab Rep 2002; 2:435–440.

12. Van Dam RM, Willett WC, Rimm EB, Stampfer MJ, Hu FB. Dietary fat and meat intake in relation to risk of Type 2 diabetes in men. Diab Care 2002; 25:417–424.

13. Marshall JA, Bessesen DH, Hamman RF. High saturated fat and low starch and fibre are associated with hyperinsulinaemia in a non-diabetic population: the San Luis Valley Diabetes Study. Diabetologia 1997; 49(4):430–438

14. Nettleton JA, Katz R. n-3 Long-chain polyunsaturated fatty acids in Type 2 diabetes: A review. J Am Diet Assoc 2005; 105:428–440.

15. Riccardi G, Rivellese AA. Dietary treatment of the metabolic syndrome – the optimal diet. Br J Nutr 2000; 83, Suppl 1:S143–S148.

16. Lovejoy JC, Smith SR, Champagne CM, et al. Effects of diets enriched in saturated (palmitic), monounsaturated (oleic), or trans (elaidic) fatty acids on insulin sensitivity and substrate oxidation in healthy adults. Diabetes Care 2002; 25:1283–1288.

17. Devaraj S, Wang-Polagruto J, Polagruto J, Keen CL, Jialal I. High fat, energy-dense fast-food-style breakfast results in an increase in oxidative stress in metabolic syndrome. Metabolism 2008; 57:867–870.

18. Rudolph TK, Ruempler K, Schwedhelm E, et al. Acute effects of various fast-food meals on vascular function and cardiovascular disease risk markers: the Hamburg Burger trial. Am J Clin Nutr 2007; 86:334–340.

19. Schubert R, Kitz R, Beermann C, et al. Influence of low-dose polyunsaturated fatty acid supplementation on the inflammatory response of healthy adults. Nutrition 2007; 23:724–730.

20. Kabir M, Skurnik G, Naour N, et al. Treatment for 2 mo with n-3 polyunsaturated fatty acids reduces adiposity and some atherogenic factors but does not improve insulin sensitivity in women with Type 2 diabetes: a randomized, controlled study. Am J Clin Nutr 2007; 86:1670–1679.

2 Dietary Fiber: All Fibers Are Not Alike

Joanne Slavin and David R. Jacobs Jr.

Key Points

- Dietary fiber intake protects against chronic disease, especially cardiovascular disease.
- Usual dietary fiber intake is less than half of recommended levels, so most consumers need to increase consumption of high-fiber foods, such as whole grains, legumes, vegetables, and fruits.
- Fiber may have a role in the prevention and treatment of digestive disorders such as constipation. For more complicated digestive disorders, such as irritable bowel syndrome and ulcerative colitis, fiber may be helpful.
- While some health benefits of dietary fiber clearly pertain to its physical properties (e.g., colonic bulk), fiber and phytochemicals are almost impossible to separate in epidemiologic studies. Much of the health effect of fiber may be due to the phytochemicals with which it is associated. Therefore, best medical practice is to encourage fiber consumption from foods. Fiber supplements may be recommended for laxation and cholesterol lowering, but whole foods high in dietary fiber also contain phytochemicals that provide additional health benefits.

Key Words: Fiber; dietary fiber; whole grain; colon function

1. INTRODUCTION

In 2002, the Food and Nutrition Board of the National Academy of Sciences published a new set of definitions for dietary fiber *(1)*. Dietary fiber describes the nondigestible carbohydrates and lignin that are intrinsic and intact in plants while functional fiber consists of the isolated nondigestible carbohydrates that have beneficial physiological effects in humans. Total fiber is the sum of dietary fiber and functional fiber. Nondigestible means not

From: *Nutrition and Health: Nutrition Guide for Physicians*
Edited by: T. Wilson et al. (eds.), DOI 10.1007/978-1-60327-431-9_2,
© Humana Press, a part of Springer Science+Business Media, LLC 2010

digested and absorbed in the human small intestine. Fibers can be fermented in the large intestine or can pass through the digestive tract unfermented. There is no biochemical assay that reflects dietary fiber or functional fiber nutritional status, e.g., blood fiber levels cannot be measured because fiber is not absorbed. No data are available to determine an Estimated Average Requirement (EAR) and thus calculate a Recommended Dietary Allowance (RDA) for total fiber, so an adequate intake (AI) was developed instead. The AI for fiber is based on the median fiber intake level observed to achieve the lowest risk of coronary heart disease (CHD). A Tolerable Upper Intake Level (UL) was not set for either dietary fiber or functional fiber.

In addition to the compositional definition provided, dietary fiber must be a part of a plant matrix which is largely intact. Nondigestible plant carbo-hydrates in foods are usually a mixture of polysaccharides that are integral components of the plant cell wall or intercellular structure. This definition recognizes two key facts: first, that the three-dimensional plant matrix is responsible for some of the physicochemical properties attributed to dietary fiber and, second, that dietary fiber is associated with other macronutrients and phytochemicals normally found in foods which are important in the potential health effects. Cereal brans are anatomical layers of the grain con-sisting of intact cells and substantial amounts of starch and protein and are categorized as sources of dietary fiber.

Dietary Reference Intakes (DRI) for total fiber by life stage are shown in Table 1. The AIs for total fiber are based on the intake level observed to pro-tect against CHD based on epidemiological, clinical, and mechanistic data. The reduction of risk of diabetes can be used as a secondary endpoint to sup-port the recommended intake level. The relationship of fiber intake to colon cancer is the subject of ongoing investigation. The DRI panel suggested the recommended intakes of total fiber may also help ameliorate constipation and diverticular disease, provide fuel for colonic cells, reduce blood glucose and lipid levels, and provide a source of nutrient-rich foods of low energy density that could contribute to satiety, although these benefits were not used as the basis for the AI.

Although based on limited clinical data, a recommendation for children older than 2 years is to increase dietary fiber intake to an amount equal to or greater than their age plus 5 g/day and to achieve intakes of 25–35 g/day after age 20 (2). No published studies have defined desirable fiber intakes for infants and children younger than 2 years. Until there is more information about the effects of dietary fiber in the very young, a rational approach would be to introduce a variety of fruits, vegetables, and easily digested cereals as solid foods are brought into the diet. Other specific recommendations for the elderly have not been published so the DRI based on 14 g/1000 kcal should be used. All recommendations need to recognize the importance of adequate

Table 1

Dietary Reference Intakes for Total Fiber[a] by Life Stage Group – (g/day)

Life Stage Group	AI	
	Males[b]	Females
0–6 mo	ND[c]	ND
7–12 mo	ND	ND
1–3 yr	19	19
4–8 yr	25	25
9–13 yr	31	26
14–18 yr	38	26
19–30 yr	38	25
31–50 yr	38	25
51–70 yr	30	21
>70 yr	30	21
Pregnancy		
<18 yr		29
19–50 yr		28
Lactation		
<18 yr		29
19–50 yr		29

[a]Total fiber is the combination of dietary fiber (the edible, nondigestible carbohydrate and lignin components in plant foods) and functional fiber (which refers to isolated, extracted, or synthetic fiber that has proven health benefits).

[b]AI = adequate intake. If sufficient scientific evidence is not available to establish an Estimated Average Requirement (EAR), and thus calculate a Recommended Dietary Allowance (RDA), an AI is usually developed. For healthy breastfed infants, the AI is the mean intake. The AI for other life stage and gender groups is believed to cover the needs of all healthy individuals in the group, but a lack of data or uncertainty in the data prevents being able to specify with confidence the percentage of individuals covered by this intake.

[c]Not determined.

fluid intake, and caution should be used when recommending fiber to those with gastrointestinal diseases, including constipation. Patients should expect increased intestinal gas as the digestive tract adjusts to higher fiber intake.

Dietary fiber intake continues to be at less than recommended levels in the United States, with usual intakes averaging only 15 g/day (1). Many popular American foods contain little dietary fiber. Servings of commonly consumed grains, fruits, and vegetables contain from 1 to 3 g of dietary *(3)*. Legumes and high-fiber bread and cereal products supply more dietary fiber, but are not commonly consumed.

2. DEFINITION AND SOURCES OF DIETARY FIBER

A variety of definitions of dietary fiber exist *(4)*. Some are based primarily upon analytical methods used to isolate and quantify fiber whereas others are physiologically based. Dietary fiber is primarily the storage and cell wall polysaccharides of plants that cannot be hydrolyzed by human digestive enzymes. Lignin, which is a complex molecule of polyphenyl-propane units and present only in small amounts in the human diet, is also usually included as a component of dietary fiber. For labeling the dietary fiber content of food products within the United States, fiber is defined as the material isolated by analytical methods approved by the Association of Official Analytical Chemists *(4)*. A variety of low molecular carbohydrates, that are being developed and increasingly used in food processing, are not digested by human digestive enzymes (sugar alcohols such as sorbitol and mannitol, polydextroses, and various fructo- and galacto-oligosaccharides). These small polymers and oligosaccharides are not measured by the AOAC-approved methods for dietary fiber, but methods specific for each material are being approved by AOAC to measure these compounds *(4)*.

Resistant starch (the sum of starch and starch-degradation products not digested in the small intestine) reaches the large intestine and functions like dietary fiber there. Legumes are a primary source of resistant starch, with as much as 35% of legume starch escaping digestion. Small amounts of resistant starch are produced by processing and baking of cereal and grain products.

Dietary fiber includes plant nonstarch polysaccharides (e.g., cellulose, pectin, gums, hemicellulose, beta-glucans, and fiber contained in oat and wheat bran), plant carbohydrates that are not recovered by alcohol precipitation (e.g., inulin, oligosaccharides, and fructans), lignin, and some resistant starch. Potential functional fibers include isolated, nondigestible plant (e.g., resistant starch, pectin, and gums), animal (e.g., chitin and chitosan), or commercially produced (e.g., resistant starch, polydextrose, inulin, and indigestible dextrins) carbohydrates *(1)*.

3. BENEFITS OF ADEQUATE FIBER INTAKE

3.1. Cardiovascular Disease

There is consistent and strong data for the protection afforded by fiber against CHD. This relationship is the basis of the DRI recommendations for dietary fiber *(1)*. The committee used epidemiologic, cohort studies that estimated dietary fiber intake from food frequencies and followed subjects prospectively until CHD was detected. Fiber intake levels found to be protective against CHD were then used to determine an adequate intake (AI) of dietary fiber. Traditionally, nutrient requirements are established by determining an Estimated Average Requirement (EAR) and then calculating a Recommended Dietary Allowance (RDA). When sufficient evidence is not available to establish an EAR, an AI is usually developed.

There is much confusion regarding which components of fiber are most protective against CHD. The DRI committee concluded that fiber from cereals seems most protective. Additionally, certain functional fiber, particularly those that are soluble and viscous may alter biomarkers of interest in CHD. Viscous fibers lower blood cholesterol levels, specifically that fraction transported by low-density lipoproteins (LDL). Meta-analysis by Brown et al. *(5)* showed that daily intake of 2–10 g of soluble fiber significantly lowered serum total cholesterol and LDL-cholesterol concentrations. Three fibers, namely beta-glucan in oats and barley and psyllium husk, have been sufficiently studied for the FDA to authorize health claims that the soluble fibers in these foods in specified amounts can reduce the risk of heart disease.

Fibers also affect blood pressure (BP) and C-reactive protein (CRP), additional biomarkers linked to risk of CHD. Fiber intake was inversely associated with CRP in the National Health and Nutrition Examination Survey 1999–2000 (NHANES) *(6)*. A meta-analysis of randomized placebo-controlled trials found that fiber intake was linked to lower BP *(7)*. Reductions in BP tended to be larger in older subjects and in hypertensive populations.

3.2. Weight Control

The effects of dietary fiber on hunger, satiety, energy intake, and body weight have been reviewed *(8)*. The majority of studies with controlled energy intake reported an increase in postmeal satiety and a decrease in subsequent hunger with increased fiber intake. With ad libitum energy intake, the average effect across all the studies indicates that an additional 14 g of fiber per day results in a 10% decrease in energy intake and a weight loss of over 1.9 kg through about 17 weeks of intervention *(9)*. Additionally, the effects of increasing fiber were reported to be even more impressive in obese individuals. This group concluded that increasing the population mean dietary fiber intake from the current average of about 15 g/day to 25–30 g/day would be beneficial and may help reduce the prevalence of obesity.

Traditionally, high-fiber foods have been solid foods. However, some of the newer functional fibers, such as resistant starches and oligosaccharides, can be easily added to drinks and may not alter viscosity. Few studies on the satiating effects of drinks supplemented with these soluble, nonviscous fibers have been published. Moorhead et al. *(10)* compared test lunches with 200 g of whole carrots, blended carrots, or carrot nutrients. Whole carrots and blended carrots resulted in significantly higher satiety. Ad libitum food intake for the remainder of the day decreased in this order: carrot nutrients, blended carrots, whole carrots. The researchers concluded that both fiber content and food structure are important determinants of satiety.

Foods rich in fiber tend to have a high volume and a low energy density and should promote satiety and energy balance *(11)*. However, research on the effects of different types of fiber on appetite and food intake has been inconsistent. Results differ according to the type of fiber and whether it is added as an isolated fiber supplement rather than naturally occurring in food. Short-term studies in which fiber is fed to subjects, followed by assessment of food and energy intake at subsequent meals, suggest that large amounts of total fiber are most successful at reducing subsequent energy intake.

3.3. Type 2 Diabetes

Kaline et al. *(12)* reviewed the value of dietary fiber in the prevention of type 2 diabetes. They suggest that whole grain cereal products appear especially effective in the prevention of the disease and recommend a fiber intake of at least 30 g/day. The Nurses Health Study cohort was evaluated for the relationship among whole grain, bran, and germ intake and risk of diabetes *(13)*. Associations for bran intake were similar to those for total whole grain intake, whereas no significant association was observed for germ intake after adjustment for bran. The investigators found that a 2 serving per day increment in whole grain consumption was associated with a 21% decrease in risk of type 2 diabetes after adjustment for potential confounders and BMI. This subject is explored in more detail in chapter 24 by Franz.

3.4. Cancer

3.4.1. LARGE BOWEL CANCER

Epidemiologic evidence supports the theory that dietary fiber may protect against large bowel cancer. Data collected from 20 populations in 12 countries showed that average stool weight varied from 72 to 470 g/day and was inversely related to colon cancer risk *(14)*. When results of 13 case-control studies of colorectal cancer rates and dietary practices were pooled, the authors concluded that the results provided substantive evidence that consumption of fiber-rich foods is inversely related to risk of both colon and rectal cancers *(15)*. The authors estimated that the risk of colorectal cancer in the US population could be reduced by about 31% with an average increase in fiber intake from food sources of about 13 g/day.

Intervention studies focused on colonic polyps do not support the protective properties of fiber against colon cancer *(16, 17)*. The studies found no significant effect of high-fiber intakes on the recurrence of colorectal adenomas. The European Prospective Investigation into Cancer and Nutrition (EPIC) is a prospective cohort study comparing the dietary habits of more than a half-million people in 10 countries with colorectal cancer incidence *(18)*. People who ate the most fiber (those with total fiber averaging 33 g/day) had a 25% lower incidence of colorectal cancer than those who ate the least fiber (12 g/day). The investigators estimated that populations with low average fiber consumption could reduce colorectal cancer incidence by 40% by doubling their fiber intake.

3.4.2. BREAST CANCER

Limited epidemiologic evidence has been published on fiber intake and human breast cancer risk. A pooled analysis of 12 case-control studies found that high intake of dietary fiber was associated with reduced risk *(19)*. Not all studies reported a relationship between dietary fiber intake and breast cancer incidence. A pooled analysis of eight prospective cohort studies of breast cancer found that fruit and vegetable consumption during adulthood was not significantly associated with reduced risk *(20)*. Results with other cancers are similar to colon and breast cancer in being mixed on whether fiber intake is protective. In general, results of case–control studies are more positive than results with prospective trials.

3.5. Bowel Function

Many fiber sources, including cereal brans, psyllium seed husk, methylcellulose and a mixed high-fiber diet, increase stool weight, thereby promoting normal laxation. Stool weight continues to increase as fiber intake increases *(21)*, but the added fiber tends to normalize defecation frequency to one bowel movement daily and gastrointestinal (GI) transit time to 2–4 days. The increase in stool weight is caused by the presence of the fiber, by the water that the fiber holds, and by fermentation of the fiber which increases bacteria in stool. It is a common but erroneous belief that the increased stool weight is due primarily to water. The moisture content of human stool is 70–75% and this does not change when more fiber is consumed.

Unlike blood, fecal samples have not been collected and evaluated for a large cohort of healthy subjects. Cummings et al. *(21)* conducted a meta-analysis of 11 studies in which daily fecal weight was measured accurately in 26 groups of people ($n = 2\ 06$) on controlled diets of known fiber content. Fiber intakes were significantly related to stool weight ($r = 0.84$). Stool weight varied greatly among subjects from different countries, ranging from 72 to 470 g/day. Stool weight was inversely related to colon cancer risk in this study. Spiller (22) suggested that there is a critical fecal weight of 160–200 g/day for adults, below which colon function becomes unpredictable and risk of colon cancer increases. Stool weights in Westernized populations range from 80–120 g/day so to increase stool weight to recommended levels would require an increase of about 20 g/day of effective fiber, such as that supplied by wheat bran.

Constipation and diarrhea are two extremes of abnormal bowel function. Constipation is defined as three or fewer spontaneous bowel movements per week. The longer feces remain in the large intestine, the more water is absorbed into the intestinal cells, resulting in hard feces and increased defecation difficulty. Leung (23) reviewed the literature on etiology of constipation and found essentially no evidence-based publications. He suggests that teaching on constipation is based on myths handed down from one generation to the next. Etiological factors thought to be related to constipation, dietary fiber intake, fluid intake, physical activity, drugs, sex hormones, and disease status, have not been systematically evaluated for their relationship to constipation.

Patients often relate the importance of that morning cup of coffee (24) or smoking on regular bowel habit. Gender is known to alter colonic function (25). Even on rigidly controlled diets of the same composition, there is a large variation in daily stool weight among subjects. Tucker et al. (26) examined the predictors of stool weight when completely controlled diets were fed to normal volunteers. They found that personality was a better predictor of stool weight than dietary fiber intake, with outgoing subjects more likely to produce higher stool weights.

3.6. Colon Disease

3.6.1. DIVERTICULOSIS

A high-fiber diet is standard therapy for diverticular disease of the colon (27). Formed diverticula will not be resolved by a diet adequate in fiber, but the bulk provided by such a diet will prevent the formation of additional diverticula, lower the pressure in the lumen, and reduce the chances that one of the existing diverticula will burst or become inflamed. Generally, for a patient with diverticulosis small seeds or husks that may not be fully digested in the upper GI tract are eliminated from a high-fiber diet as a precaution against having these small pieces of residue become lodged within a diverticulum. Prevention of diverticular disease with fiber is still unclear from the limited research. About 10–25% of individuals with diverticular disease will develop diverticulitis. Whether fiber is protective against that condition is not known *(28)*.

3.6.2. IRRITABLE BOWEL SYNDROME

GI motility has been related to psyche. Irritable bowel syndrome (IBS) affects about 20% of adults in the United States and Europe. IBS may disturb GI motility and reduce small intestinal absorption, resulting in an increase in water that reaches the large intestine; diarrhea may result if the large intestinal lumen cannot absorb the excess water; other disruptions to motility may cause constipation. In addition to diarrhea and constipation, symptoms of IBS include bloating, straining, urgency, feeling of incomplete evacuation, and passage of mucus *(29)*.

Individuals with inflammatory bowel disease (IBD; Crohn's disease and ulcerative colitis) may experience exudative diarrhea when nutrient absorption is diminished, which adds to the increased osmotic load from the presence of mucus, blood, and protein from the inflamed gastrointestinal tract. Dietary fiber intake may improve symptoms of patents with IBD.

4. POTENTIAL NEGATIVE EFFECTS OF DIETARY FIBER

Potential negative effects of fiber include reduced absorption of vitamins, minerals, protein, and calories. It is unlikely that healthy adults who consume fiber in amounts within the recommended ranges will have problems with nutrient absorption; however, high-fiber intakes may not be appropriate for children and the elderly.

Generally, dietary fiber in recommended amounts is thought to normalize transit time and should help when either constipation or diarrhea is present; however, case histories have reported diarrhea when excessive amounts of fiber are consumed so it is difficult to individualize fiber intake based on bowel function measures. Thus, stool consistency cannot be used as a benchmark of appropriate fiber intake. Esophageal obstruction from a hygroscopic pharmacobezoar containing glucomannan has been described *(30)*. This soluble fiber holds water and forms a highly viscous solution when dissolved in water. Glucomannan has been promoted as a diet aid since it swells in the GI tract, theoretically producing a feeling of satiety and fullness. This case illustrates potential negatives of use of highly viscous fiber supplements in patients with a history of upper GI pathologies.

Fiber is just one low-digestible carbohydrate in the diet. Sugar alcohols and resistant starch are also poorly digested and absorbed. Thus, all of the low-digestible carbohydrates may cause diarrhea and other GI symptoms, such as flatulence, bloating, and abdominal discomfort *(31)*. A large intake of sugar alcohols can cause osmotic diarrhea because water follows the undigested and unabsorbed carbohydrates into the large intestine; if time is inadequate for the intestinal cells to absorb the excess water, it will be eliminated in the feces. The dose of dietary fiber or other poorly digested carbohydrate that will have a laxative effect or contribute to other GI symptoms depends on a number of factors related to the food and the consumer. GI symptoms, although transient, may affect consumers' perception of well-being and their acceptance of food choices containing fiber and other resistant carbohydrates. Educational messages to expect some GI symptoms with increased fiber consumption and to increase fluid intake are needed.

5. CONCLUSIONS

Dietary fiber is inversely associated with risk of several chronic diseases, including obesity, cardiovascular diseases, and type 2 diabetes, although effects on cancer are uncertain. High-fiber foods and bulk laxatives may improve laxation and should be cautiously introduced in those with constipation and colonic disorders. While some health benefits of fiber clearly pertain to its physical properties (e.g., colonic bulk), fiber and the phytochemicals that it marks are almost impossible to separate in epidemiologic studies. Much of the health effect of fiber may be due to the phytochemicals with which it is associated. Therefore, the medical profession should encourage consumption of foods high in fiber, such as whole grains, legumes, fruits, and vegetables.

SUGGESTED FURTHER READING

Institute of Medicine. Dietary Reference Intakes Proposed Definition of Dietary Fiber. National Academy Press, Washington, DC, 2001; pp. 1–64.

Slavin JL. Position of the American Dietetic Association: health implications of dietary fiber. J Am Diet Assoc 2008; 108:1716–1731.

Timm DA, Slavin JL. Dietary fiber and the relationship to chronic diseases. Am J Lifestyle Med 2008; 2:233–240.

Bijkerk CJ, Muris JWM, Knottnerus JA, Hoes AW, NeWit NJ. Systematic review: the role of different types of fibre in the treatment of irritable bowel syndrome. Aliment Pharmacol Ther 2004; 19:245–251.

Leung FW. Etiologic factors of chronic constipation – review of the scientific evidence. Dig Dis Sci 2007; 52:313–316.

REFERENCES

1. Institute of Medicine. Dietary Reference Intakes: Energy, Carbohydrates, Fiber, Fat, Fatty Acids, Cholesterol, Protein and Amino Acids. The National Academies Press, Washington, DC, 2002.

2. Williams CL, Bollella M, Wynder EL. A new recommendation for dietary fiber intake in childhood. Pediatrics 1995; 96:985–988.

3. Marlett JA, Cheung T-F. Database and quick methods of assessing typical dietary fiber intakes using data for 228 commonly consumed foods. J Am Diet Assoc 1997; 97:1139–1148,1151.
4. Institute of Medicine. Dietary Reference Intakes Proposed Definition of Dietary Fiber. National Academy Press, Washington, DC, 2001; pp. 1–64.
5. Brown L, Rosner B, Willett WW, Sacks FM. Cholesterol-lowering effects of dietary fiber: a meta-analysis. Am J Clin Nutr 1999; 69:30–42.
6. Ajani UA, Ford ES, Mokdad AH. Dietary fiber and C-reactive protein: findings from National Health and Nutrition Examination Survey data. J Nutr 2004; 134: 1181–1185.
7. Streppel MT, Arends LR, van't Veer P, Grobbee DE, Geleijnse JM. Dietary fiber and blood pressure: A meta-analysis of randomized placebo-controlled trials. Arch Intern Med 2005; 165:150–156.
8. Slavin JL. Dietary fiber and body weight. Nutrition 2005; 21:411–418.
9. Howarth NC, Saltzman E, Roberts SB. Dietary fiber and weight regulation. Nutr Rev 2001; 59:129–139.
10. Moorhead AS, Welch RW, Livingstone BM, McCourt M, Burns AA, Dunne A. The effects of the fibre content and physical structure of carrots on satiety and subsequent intakes when eaten as part of a mixed meal. Br J Nutr 2006; 96:587–595.
11. Slavin JL, Green H. Fibre and satiety. Nutr Bull 2007; 32 (Suppl 1):32–42.
12. Kaline K, Bornstein SR, Bergmann A, Hauner H, Schwarz PEH. The importance and effect of dietary fiber in diabetes prevention with particular consideration of whole grain products. Horm Metab Res 2007; 39:687–693.
13. de Munter JS, Hu FB, Spiegelman D, Franz M, van Dam RM. Whole grain, bran, and germ intake and risk of type 2 diabetes: a prospective cohort study and systematic review. PLoS Med 2007; 4:e261.
14. Cummings JH, Bingham SA, Heaton KW, Eastwood MA. Fecal weight, colon cancer risk and dietary intake of nonstarch polysaccharides (dietary fiber). Gastroenterology 1992; 103:1783–1789.
15. Howe GR, Benito E, Castelleto R, et al. Dietary intake of fiber and decreased risk of cancers of the colon and rectum: Evidence from the combined analysis of 13 case-control studies. J Natl Cancer Inst 1992; 84:1887–1896.
16. Schatzkin A, Lanza E, Corle D, et al, and the Polyp Prevention Trial Study Group. Lack of effect of a low-fat, high-fiber diet on the recurrence of colorectal adenomas. N Engl J Med 2000; 342:1149–1155.
17. Alberts DS, Marinez ME, Kor DL, et al, and the Phoenix Colon Cancer Prevention Physicians' Network. Lack of effect of a high-fiber cereal supplement on the recurrence of colorectal adenomas. N Engl J Med 2000; 324:1156–1162.
18. Bingham SA, Day NE, Luben R, et al. Dietary fibre in food and protection against colorectal cancer in the European Prospective Investigation into Cancer and Nutrition (EPIC): an observational study. Lancet 2003; 361:1496–1501.
19. Howe GR, Hirohata T, Hislop TG, et al. Dietary factors and risk of breast cancer: Combined analysis of 12 case-control studies. J Natl Cancer Inst 1990; 82:561–569.
20. Smith-Warner SA, Spiegelman D, Yaun SS, et al. Intake of fruits and vegetables and risk of breast cancer: a pooled analysis of cohort studies. JAMA 2001; 285: 769–776.
21. Cummings JH. The effect of dietary fiber on fecal weight and composition. In: Spiller GA, ed. CRC Handbook of Dietary Fiber in Human Nutrition, 2nd ed. CRC Press, Boca Raton, FL, 1993, pp. 263–349.

22. Spiller GA. Suggestions for a basis on which to determine a desirable intake of dietary fibre. In: Spiller GA, ed. CRC Handbook of Dietary Fiber in Human Nutrition. CRC Press, Boca Raton, FL, 1993, pp. 351–354.

23. Leung FW. Etiologic factors of chronic constipation – review of the scientific evidence. Dig Dis Sci 2007; 52:313–316.

24. Brown SR, Cann PA, Read NW. Effect of coffee on distal colon function. Gut 1990; 31:450–453.

25. Lampe JW, Fredstrom SB, Slavin JL, Potter JD. Sex differences in colonic function: a randomized trial. Gut 1993; 34:531–536.

26. Tucker DM, Sandstead HH, Logan GM, et al. Dietary fiber and personality factors as determinants of stool output. Gastroenterology 1981; 81:879–883.

27. Eglash A, Lane CH, Schneider DM. Clinical inquiries. What is the most beneficial diet for patients with diverticulosis? J Fam Pract 2006; 55:813–815.

28. Korzenik JR. Case closed? Diverticulitis: epidemiology and fiber. J Clin Gastroenterol 2006; 40(Suppl 3):S112–S116.

29. Bijkerk CJ, Muris JWM, Knottnerus JA, Hoes AW, NeWit NJ. Systematic review: the role of different types of fibre in the treatment of irritable bowel syndrome. Aliment Pharmacol Ther 2004; 19:245–251.

30. Vanderbeek PB, Fasano C, O'Malley G, Hornstein J. Esophageal obstruction from a hygroscopic pharmacobezoar containing glucomannan. Clin Toxicol (Phila) 2007; 45:80–82.

31. Grabitske HA, Slavin JL. Low-digestible carbohydrates in practice. J Am Diet Assoc 2008; 108:1677–1681.

3 Sugar and Artificial Sweeteners: Seeking the Sweet Truth

Barry M. Popkin and Kiyah J. Duffey

Key Points

- Caloric sweetener intake has increased significantly around the world.
- There has been a shift toward intake of calorically sweetened beverages as a larger proportion of caloric sweeteners.
- Beverage calories are ingested differently from food calories. We do not reduce food intake when we consume caloric beverages; thus the universal finding that increased caloric beverage intake is linked with growing adiposity and metabolic abnormalities.
- Non-nutritive sweetener intake has grown greatly; however, the impact of this on long-term health remains to be understood.

Key Words: Sugar; beverage; body weight; high-fructose corn syrup; non-nutritive sweeteners

Over the past half-century, sweeteners have played an increasingly large role in the diets of persons in the United States and other higher-income countries. Countries worldwide, regardless of their national income, have also experienced increases in availability of caloric sweeteners. As the proportion of processed over unprocessed food consumption has grown, intake of sweeteners has increased exponentially. The most dramatic changes are observed in the shift away from water and other unsweetened beverages toward sweetened caloric beverages. However, this is not the only shift. Thousands of processed foods contain a mix of caloric sweeteners. There is a long history of scholars being particularly worried about the health impact of these added sugars as they have studied the influence of modern food processing and "westernization" on the global diet. In most cases, however, given the large number of changes in our diet, it has been very

From: *Nutrition and Health: Nutrition Guide for Physicians*
Edited by: T. Wilson et al. (eds.), DOI 10.1007/978-1-60327-431-9_3,
© Humana Press, a part of Springer Science+Business Media, LLC 2010

difficult to pinpoint exactly the association of sweeteners with observed health outcomes. A detailed discussion of these issues as they relate to sweeteners can be found in a book by Popkin *(1)* and for diet sweeteners in a paper by Mattes and Popkin *(2)*.

1. DEFINING SWEETENERS – CALORIC AND NONCALORIC

The standard definition used by researchers for caloric sweeteners includes all caloric carbohydrate sweeteners and excludes all naturally occurring sugars (which represent an important component of our energy intake). Henceforth, we use the term "caloric sweetener" instead of "added sugar" as there is such a range of non-sugar products used today; high-fructose corn syrup (HFCS) is a prime example as it is the sweetener used in all US soft drinks.

There are two major sugar crops: sugar beets and sugar cane. Sugar and syrups are also produced from the sap of certain species of maple trees, from sweet sorghum when cultivated explicitly for making syrup, and from sugar palm. Under the name sweeteners, the Food and Agricultural Organization of the United Nations includes products used for sweetening that are either derived from sugar crops, cereals, fruits, or milk, or produced by insects. This category includes a wide variety of monosaccharides (glucose and fructose) and disaccharides (sucrose and saccharose), which exist either in a crystallized state as sugar or in thick liquid form as syrups. Included in sweeteners are maple sugar and syrups, caramel, golden syrup, artificial and natural honey, maltose, glucose (a monosaccharide or simple sugar), dextrose (the biologically active form of the glucose molecule, also known as D-glucose), high-fructose corn syrup (also known as isoglucose), other types of fructose, sugar confectionery, and lactose. In the last several decades, increasingly larger quantities of cereals (primarily maize) have been used to produce sweeteners derived from starch.

Non-nutritive or diet sweeteners represent an ever-growing set of products. These are often called intense sweeteners because their sweetness is so potent – 200–700 times the sweetness of sucrose. These include the better known products:

- Aspartame – Equal and NutraSweet (when used in processed foods and beverages): This is FDA approved and is 160–200 times sweeter than sugar.
- Saccharin – Sweet 'N Low: Used in baked products and as a tabletop sweetener. The FDA approves it and it is 200–700 times sweeter than sugar.
- Sucralose – Splenda: This is used across the board and is FDA approved. It is again 600 or more times sweeter than sugar.

Then there are less common sweeteners such as Acesulfame potassium – Sunett, Sweet One; Neotame; Stevia; and Tagatose – Naturlose. These items are regulated except for Stevia, which is a natural food constituent. There are some international bodies in Europe (European Food Safety Agency) and the Joint Commission of Experts on Food Additives of the World Health Organization (WHO) and the Organization of Food and Agriculture (FAO) that have established broad acceptable daily limits for these intense noncaloric sweeteners.

Cyclamate is the only low-caloric sweetener that has been banned in some countries, such as the United States, while over 100 countries worldwide allow its use, including European countries.

Unfortunately, we are unable to present information on consumption patterns for the non-nutritive sweeteners (NNS) since contents in food of each of these items is not required and there exist no direct measurement of these NNS in the US food supply or for that matter in any country in the world.

2. CONSUMPTION PATTERNS OF SWEETENERS

2.1. Methods for Obtaining Sweetener Data

Before addressing patterns and trends of sugar and HFCS intake it is important to note how these data are obtained, as there is no clearly available method. Additional references are provided where available as we will only briefly discuss the methods here.

Global food data: Current measurements of the total food available for human consumption, called food disappearance data, are calculated by taking total food production (accounting for imports and exports) and subtracting net losses from processing and from food fed to animals. Such data are a reasonable approximation of the trends in food consumption at the national level, although they do not reflect actual consumption at the level of the individual. Comparison of food disappearance data with household and individual food intake data estimates that disappearance data measure about 20–27% more food available for consumption than is evidenced by the actual consumption levels. Furthermore, compared to nonperishable foods, perishable foods tend to be over-estimated using disappearance data because a greater proportion is lost or wasted. For foodstuffs with added sugar we expect to see a much more limited problem of misestimation due to wastage.

Foods containing HFCS: Neither comprehensive information of the types of foods and beverages containing HFCS nor direct measurements of HFCS in foods and beverages are readily available. A majority of the information on availability comes from lists compiled by individuals who have examined ingredients of foods in their homes or from organizations concerned with

HFCS-related food allergies. For further information on foods considered to contain HFCS see Duffey and Popkin *(3)*.

Sugars: Direct estimates of added sugar in individual foods were obtained from the USDA food composition table and its recipe and servings files.

Estimates of HFCS intake: Direct estimates of HFCS are not available. In 1986, a task force for the FDA produced estimates of intake of natural and added sugars, including HFCS, sucrose, and other corn sweeteners. Using these availability data for HFCS and added sugar, Walter Glinsmann and colleagues generated food-group wide estimates of the proportion of added sweetener that was HFCS *(4)*. Given their successful implementation previously *(5)*, these estimates are utilized in the following presentation of consumption trends. A more detailed discussion of this method can be found elsewhere *(3)*.

2.2. Global Trends in Availability

Food disappearance data provide a broad sense of overall patterns. Worldwide, trends indicate a large increase in caloric sweetener available for consumption (Table 1). In 2000 there were 74 more kilocalories (kcal) per capita of caloric sweetener consumed than in 1962. The percentage of calories from caloric sweetener increased considerably (a 32% increase or an additional 1.4 percentage points in the percent of energy from caloric sweeteners) and represents a 21% increase in the proportion of carbohydrates that is refined sugar. In Table 1, countries are ordered into quintiles according to their 1962 per capita GNP. Trends indicate that as GNP per capita of a country increases, all measures of caloric sweetener increase significantly, but the effect is greatest among countries in the lowest quintiles. For example, between 1962 and 2000 the caloric intake of sugar increased by 172% for countries in the lowest quintile, but only 104% for those in the highest quintile.

Using pooled 1962 and 2000 data, we found that approximately 82% of the change in caloric sweetener intake can be attributed to GNP and urbanization changes and the remaining 18% to changes in unmeasured factors, which would relate to shifts in either the behavior of the food industry or consumer behavior *(6)*.

2.3. United States per Capita Trends in Total Caloric Sweeteners

Despite a slight decline between 2000 and 2002, there has been a dramatic increase in calories from added sugars over the past 35 yr. By 2004 added sugars provided approximately 370 kcal/person/d (17% of total energy)

Table 1

World Trends in Caloric Sweetener Intake for GNP Quintiles (1962 values)
Quintiles of GNP (Using 1962 GNP Levels for Each Country)

	Quintile 1	Quintile 2	Quintile 3	Quintile 4	Quintile 5	Total
Caloric sweetener (kcal/capita/d)						
1962	90	131	257	287	402	232
2000	155	203	362	397	418	306
Total carbohydrates (kcal/capita/d)						
1962	1464	1552	1542	1627	1677	1572
2000	1690	1670	1752	1779	1693	1717
Total energy (kcal/capita/d)						
1962	2008	2090	2157	2411	2960	2322
2000	2346	2357	2716	2950	3281	2725
% Caloric sweetener of total energy						
1962	4.5	6.2	11.9	12.0	13.5	9.5
2000	6.4	8.3	13.4	13.7	12.7	10.9
% Caloric sweetener of total carbohydrates						
1962	6.2	8.5	16.8	17.7	24.4	14.6
2000	9.0	12.1	20.6	22.4	24.6	17.7
GNP (the values are calculated for 2000 price levels)						
1962	216	478	983	2817	12,234	3282
2000	435	839	2836	5915	28,142	7198
% URBAN						
1962	10.0	21.6	37.3	46.7	66.2	36.1
2000	27.7	41.3	58.7	70.0	78.0	54.9

Sources: Food and Agriculture Organization FAOSTAT data set for food balance data and by Popkin BM and Nielsen SJ. The sweetening of the world's diet. Obes Res 2003; 11: 1325–1332.

in the diet of the average American. Similarly, over the past 15 yr, the contribution of HFCS to energy intake has increased significantly. Between 1989 and 2000, total caloric intake from HFCS rose from 77 to 189 kcal/person/d. At its peak in 2000 HFCS represented 9% of total energy intake and 16.5% of total carbohydrate consumption among Americans 2 years and older. Although absolute levels vary, these trends were observed for all age groups with the largest rise in consumption of added sugar (217 kcal/person/d) and HFCS (172 kcal/person/d) among Americans

19–39 years old. Greater detail of overall trends and trends by age groups are provided elsewhere *(3)*.

2.4. Caloric Sweeteners in Beverages

For the most part, HFCS is the added caloric sweetener found in beverages. Numerous beverages, including fruit juices and fruit drinks, sweetened coffees and teas, and, of course, soda, are estimated to contain at least some amount of HFCS, although soda and fruit drink far surpass the others in terms of their contribution to daily energy intake [158 and 40 kcal/person/d, respectively, in 2004 (Fig. 1)]. For comparison, the next largest contributor was sports drinks, which accounted for just 3 kcal/person/d. On the other hand, beverages other than soda and fruit drink provide a sizable number of calories from added sugar in 2004. Sweetened tea, for example, was estimated to provide roughly 14 kcal/person/d, high fat milk (including chocolate milk) accounted for an additional 5 kcal/person/d (Fig. 1), and alcohol and sweetened coffee were estimated to account for an additional 3 kcal/person/d, collectively. Detailed beverage data not presented here can be found elsewhere *(3)*.

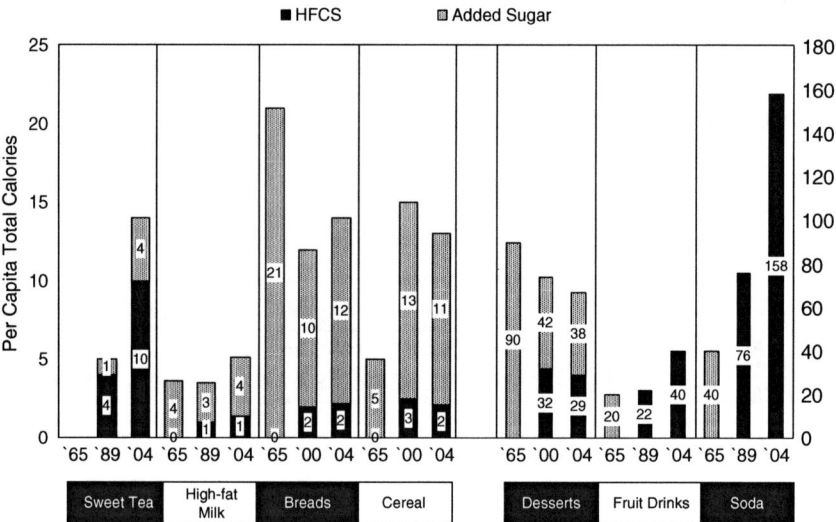

Fig. 1. Calories of HFCS and Added Sugar* from Selected Food and Beverage Groups: Highest Contributors
*Data are from Nationwide Food Consumption Survey 1965 (beverages 8 foods), Continuing Survey of Food intake in individuals 1989–91 (beverages), and National Health and Nutrition Examination Survey 1999–2000 (foods) and 2003–2004 (beverages and foods); results use survey designs to account for clustering, and are weighted to be nationally representative

2.5. Caloric Sweeteners in Foods

There is little direct evidence of the exact date on which HFCS was introduced into food processing and manufacturing. What information we do have suggests that this occurred in the mid-1990 s; thus our HFCS estimates begin in 1999.

Compared to soda and fruit drinks, foods provide considerably fewer calories from HFCS, and their contribution to calories from HFCS has remained relatively stable. In 2004, desserts (including pudding, cakes, cookies, and pies) were the largest source of calories from HFCS (29 kcal/person/d) accounting for approximately 1% of total energy (Fig. 1). The next highest contributors, ready-to-eat cereals and breads (including bread, bagels, tortillas, biscuits, and muffins), each accounted for just 2 kcal/person/d of HFCS (Fig. 1). Certain fast food groups (e.g., hamburgers and cheeseburgers) also provided a small number of calories of HFCS, although this represented an insignificant proportion of total energy intake (<1%).

Foods provide considerably more daily calories from added sugar than HFCS. Calories of added sugars obtained from snacks, cereal, salad dressing, and non-milk dairy food groups increased between 1965 and 2000 (2002 for dairy) and then leveled off or declined slightly by 2004. The opposite trend was observed for breads, with a decline in calories from added sugar between 1965 and 2000 (–11 kcal/person/d) and a small increase (+2 kcal/person/d) by 2004. Compared to all other food groups in 2004, desserts provided significantly more calories from added sugar (38 kcal/person/d) (Fig. 1). Most food groups accounted for ≤1% of total energy and <1% of total carbohydrates. The exceptions were cereal, breads, and desserts, which accounted for between 1% (cereal) and 6% (desserts) of total carbohydrates.

Figure 2 illustrates the shifts away from foods, such as desserts, toward beverages as a primary source of added sugar in the diets of Americans. In 2004 the average American obtained 66% fewer calories per day of added sugars from foods and 300% more calories from beverages over 1965. Overall beverage patterns and trends have been described in detail elsewhere *(7)*.

2.6. United States per Consumer Trends

Among consumers, caloric intake from both added sugar and HFCS are considerably greater than per capita estimates (Table 2). For example, a relatively small percent (10%) of persons report consuming sweetened tea. For them it provides an estimated 134 kcal/consumer/d of added sugar compared with an estimated per capita amount of only 14 kcal/person/d. Likewise, the values for HFCS are 95 kcal/consumer/d vs. 10 kcal/per capita/d.

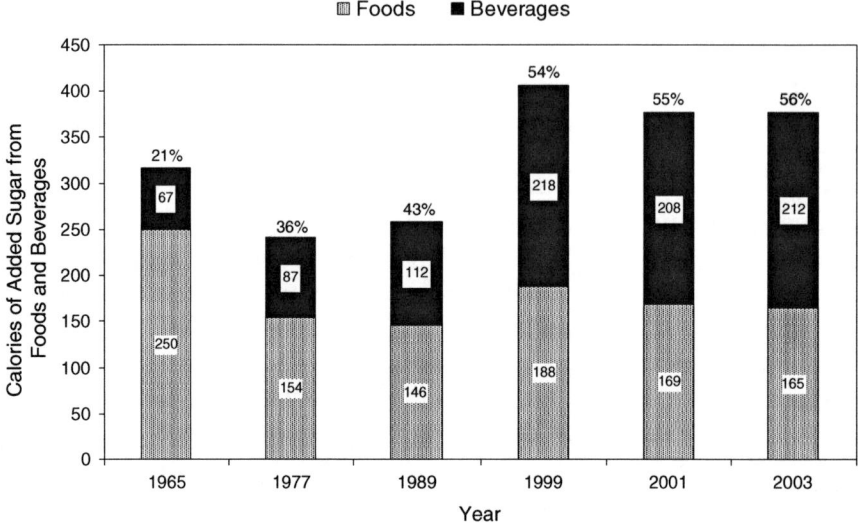

Fig. 2. The Proportion of Calories of Added Sugar* from Beverages Has Risen While
That From Food Has Dropped Significantly
*Data are from Nationwide Food Consumption Survey 1965 (beverages and foods), Continuing Survey of Food intake in individuals 1989–91 (beverages), and National Health
and Nutrition Examination Survey 1999–2000 (foods) and 2003–2004 (beverages and
foods); results use survey designs to account for clustering, and are weighted to be
nationally representative

The 24% of cereal consumers obtain 40 more calories (53 kcal/consumer/d
vs. 13 kcal/per capita/d) from added sugar compared with the per capita
estimates, and for the 46% of reported soda consumers there is a 98% difference in energy from added sugar (as HFCS). However, per consumer and
per capita estimates do not differ greatly for breads (Table 2).

3. HEALTH EFFECTS OF ADDED CALORIC SWEETENERS

Regardless of the food in which it is contained, sugar is not different from
any other calorie with respect to its effects on overall energy balance and
weight. A refined carbohydrate that is rapidly metabolized, sugar creates
some unique effects on metabolic control, in particular related to control of
blood glucose by diabetes and satiety. However, sugar obtained from beverages appears to have more far-reaching health effects.

Beverages: As Mattes, in particular, has shown, we find little or no dietary
compensation when a beverage is consumed, regardless of its protein, fat, or
carbohydrate content *(8)*. Since two thirds of all caloric sweeteners in the
United States and a large proportion of caloric sweeteners in other countries

Table 2
Per Capita, Percent Consuming, and Per Consumer Estimates of Top Six
Foods and Beverages Contributing to Added Sugar and HFCS Intake, Among
Americans ≥2 Years

	Added Sugar			HFCS	
	Per Capita (kcal)	Percent Consuming‡	Per Consumer (kcal)	Per Capita (kcal)	Per Consumer (kcal)
Soft Drinks					
1965	40.3	24	167.0	–	–
1977	51.4§	30	180.6§	–	–
1989–1991	73.5 §	34	224.2 §	51.9	158.3
1999–2000	153.5§	50	309.8 §	108.3 §	218.7§
2003–2004	158.1	46	312.7	111.6	220.8
Fruit Drink					
1965	20.1	16	128.7	–	–
1977	191	14	139.1§	–	–
1989–1991	19.5	15	152.1§	13.8	107.4
1999–2000	37.7§	20	191.2§	26.6 §	135.0§
2003–2004	40.3	20	181.6	28.5	138.2)
Sweet Tea					
1965	n/a	n/a	n/a	–	–
1977	7.3	5	137.7	–	–
1989–1991	4.6§	6	91.5§	3.3	64.6
1999–2000	12.2§	9	134.6§	8.6§	95.0§
2003–2004	13.5	10	134.4	9.5	94.9
Desserts					
1965	90.0	65	139.0	–	–
1977	55.1§	49	118.5§	–	–
1989–1991	49.1§	45	121.3	–	–
1999–2000	73.8§	55	134.0	31.5	57.2
2003–2004	67.3	57	118.7	28.7	50.7
Cereal					
1965	5.2	26	19.9	–	–
1977	6.7§	27	26.1§	–	–
1989–1991	11.0§	28	40.9§	–	–
1999–2000	15.2§	26	58.9§	2.5	9.7
2003–2004	12.8§	24	53.1	2.1§	8.8

(*Continued*)

Table 2
(Continued)

	Added Sugar			HFCS	
	Per Capita (kcal)	Percent Consuming[‡]	Per Consumer (kcal)	Per Capita (kcal)	Per Consumer (kcal)
Breads					
1965	20.6	92	22.3	–	–
1977	14.8[§]	85	17.5[§]	–	–
1989–1991	12.3[§]	79	16.1[§]	–	–
1999–2000	12.1	75	2.0	2.6	
2003–2004	13.5	76	17.8	2.2	2.9

Data are from Nationwide Food Consumption Survey 1965 ($n=13,549$) and 1977 ($n=29,553$), Continuing Survey of Food Intake in Individuals 89–91 ($n=14,689$), and National Health and Nutrition Examination Survey 1999–2000 ($n=8173$) and 2003–2004 ($n=8275$).

[‡] The same values for percent consuming each food and beverage groups are applicable for HFCS, data are not repeated in the HFCS column.

[§] Means are statistically different from the previous year using student's t-test, $p<0.01$.
Source: Duffey and Popkin *(3)*

come from beverages, consumption of these calorically sweetened beverages results in added calories and enhanced positive energy balance. This, in turn, can increase the likelihood of becoming obese and also affects directly (as well as via obesity) the likelihood of being diabetic or developing an array of other CVD-linked metabolic parameters. Several convincing reviews have been written on this topic *(9, 10)*. When studies have been funded by the beverage industry, the results turn significantly in their favor *(11)*.

The animal and human literature behind this set of assertions is quite diffuse. Beginning with a series of early studies, Mattes and his colleagues began to show the minimal compensation that occurs when humans are fed caloric beverages in terms of reduction of food intake *(12)*. Other early scholars found similar results, and dozens of later studies, including some smaller trials and carefully controlled experimental designs, have also replicated these findings.

Noncaloric intense sweeteners: There have been several visible studies that suggest that consumption of diet soft drinks are linked with increased risk of the metabolic syndrome *(13, 14)*. In one intriguing animal study, conducted by respected colleagues, it was found that feeding rats diet sweeteners was linked with enhanced caloric intake. This suggests some type of biological effect *(15)*.

There are, however, many unresolved issues related to the effects of diet sweeteners. One is their effects on long-term dietary behavior. Is there some homeostatic or other control which is adversely affected by diet sweeteners, as might be suggested by the study by Swithers and Terry mentioned above *(15)*. Or is it the case, as we are presently examining, that those who consume diet beverages may shift their food intake to compensate for the reduced calories in their beverages (unpublished work)? This topic is certainly deserving of further research *(2)*.

HFCS – why it is used: HFCS is interesting for many reasons. The driving force behind the development of HFCS related partly to difficulty in getting sucrose in a liquid form for commercial application. In addition, sugar is unstable in acid solutions. In other words, there is a food science contribution of HFCS. For baked goods, it reduces crystallization, for yoghurt it controls moisture and regulates tartness, for beverages it is critical to stability in acidic beverages, and for cereal products it slows spoilage and extends freshness. Further, its production is subsidized. Federal subsidies for corn farmers played a key role in enhancing its use, with a majority of US farm policies focused on promoting increased production of inexpensive corn.

Role of HFCS in health: From a health and obesity perspective specifically, there are many key issues to understand. HFCS is both sweeter and cheaper than most other sweeteners, though recent increases in corn price might affect this. It is used in most beverages and it is hypothesized by some scholars to be linked with an increase in the intensity of the sweetness of soft drinks and other caloric beverages *(5)*.

All beverages have direct effects on obesity and diabetes. However, aside from the lack of caloric compensation when beverages are consumed, the question is, are there uniquely negative impacts of HFCS on human health? Early speculation was that HFCS might bypass satiety mechanisms and reduce fullness signals. Bray and colleagues speculated that the digestion, absorption, and metabolism of fructose differ from that of glucose *(5)*. Furthermore, Bray felt that fructose, unlike glucose, did not stimulate insulin secretion or enhance leptin production. Since insulin and leptin act as key afferent signals in the regulation of food intake and body weight, this suggests that dietary fructose may contribute to increased energy intake and weight gain. Also, he speculated that calorically sweetened beverages may be sweeter and enhance caloric over-consumption; he provided evidence for this assertion *(5)*. Subsequent research by Havel in particular seems to show that the differences in digestion, absorption, and metabolism of HFCS did not negatively affect appetite control. The actual mechanisms were not clarified in this study; however, he does find that consumption of HFCS did not lead to increased caloric intake compared to other sugars *(16)*. A second study found similar effects *(17)*.

There is emerging research that points to other potentially adverse health effects of HFCS. Consumption appears related to an increase in uric acid *(18, 19)*. Johnson and his colleagues proposed that the epidemic of the metabolic syndrome is due in part to fructose-induced hyperuricemia that reduces endothelial nitrous oxide levels and induces insulin resistance *(20)*. Fructose-induced hyperuricemia results in endothelial dysfunction and insulin resistance and might be a novel causal mechanism of the metabolic syndrome.

4. DISCUSSION

Globally, there has been a significant increase in consumption of caloric sweeteners. The health effects of these sugars are seen most clearly in consumption of calorically sweetened beverages. There is a growing literature that points to an emerging consensus that intake of caloric beverages is not compensated by reduced food intake. Subsequent weight gains are significant when caloric beverage intake is increased or remains high for any length of time. Furthermore, studies have linked intake of these same beverages with diabetes and the metabolic syndrome.

The consumption of caloric sweeteners in food, which represents a diminished proportional share of caloric sweeteners but not necessarily one that has declined in absolute terms, has been much less studied and understood. One mechanism which remains to be studied and understood relates to the long-term effects of sugar intake on sweetness preferences and needs. Do we habituate to caloric sweetener levels so that we need to increase our intake of sweetened foods and beverages?

HFCS provides the food manufacturing sector with many advantages; unfortunately its future is clouded with potentially adverse effects on kidney and heart health. Much more work needs to be done to fully understand the effects of increased uric acid secretion linked with HFCS consumption.

In general, it is surprising that such an important component of our diet as NNS remain unmeasured in terms of intake and unstudied in terms of health effects. We do not address the effects of NNS on health here as there is a very limited literature. The major concern has been the effects of cyclamates and aspartame on health. However, what about the total effect of NNS on habit formation? Do we overcompensate with increased food intake when we consume these products? Why are these products linked in some studies with the metabolic syndrome? Mattes and Popkin are preparing a review of some of these issues; however, their general conclusion is that there is a major gap in our literature as it relates to NNS and health *(2)*.

SUGGESTED FURTHER READING

Mattes RD, Popkin, BM. Intended and Unintended Effects of Sweeteners on Energy Balance. Chapel Hill, North Carolina, 2008.

Duffey KJ, Popkin BM. High-fructose corn syrup: Is this what's for dinner? Am J Clin Nutr 2008; 88:1722S–1732S.

Mourao DM, Bressan J, Campbell WW, Mattes RD. Effects of food form on appetite and energy intake in lean and obese young adults. Int J Obes 2007; 31:1688–1695.

Vartanian LR, Schwartz MB, Brownell KD. Effects of soft drink consumption on nutrition and health: a systematic review and meta-analysis. Am J Public Health 2007; 97:667–675.

REFERENCES

1. Popkin BM. The World Is Fat-The Fads, Trends, Policies, and Products that are Fattening the Human Race. Avery-Penguin Group, New York, 2008.
2. Mattes RD, Popkin B. Intended and Unintended Effects of Sweeteners on Energy Balance. Chapel Hill, North Carolina, 2008. (under revise and resubmit status, AJCN).
3. Duffey KJ, Popkin BM. High-fructose corn syrup: Is this what's for dinner? Am J Clin Nutr 2008; 88:1722S–1732S.
4. Glinsmann W, Irausquin, H, Park, Y. Evaluation of health aspects of sugars contained in carbohydrate sweeteners: Report of Sugars Task Force. J Nutr 1986; 116:S1–216.
5. Bray GA, Nielsen SJ, Popkin BM. Consumption of high-fructose corn syrup in beverages may play a role in the epidemic of obesity. Am J Clin Nutr 2004; 79:537–543.
6. Popkin B, Drewnowski A. Dietary fats and the nutrition transition: New trends in the global diet. Nutr Rev 1997; 55:31–43.
7. Duffey K, Popkin BM. Shifts in patterns and consumption of beverages between 1965 and 2002. Obesity 2007; 15:2739–2747.
8. Mourao DM, Bressan J, Campbell WW, Mattes RD. Effects of food form on appetite and energy intake in lean and obese young adults. Int J Obes 2007; 31:1688–1695.
9. Vartanian LR, Schwartz MB, Brownell KD. Effects of soft drink consumption on nutrition and health: a systematic review and meta-analysis. Am J Public Health 2007; 97:667–675.
10. Malik VS, Schulze MB, Hu FB. Intake of sugar-sweetened beverages and weight gain: a systematic review. Am J Clin Nutr 2006; 84:274–288.
11. Lesser LI, Ebbeling CB, Goozner M, Wypij D, Ludwig DS. Relationship between funding source and conclusion among nutrition-related scientific articles. PLoS Med 2007; 4:e5.
12. DiMeglio D, Mattes R. Liquid versus solid carbohydrate: effects on food intake and body weight. Int J Obes 2000; 24:794–800.
13. Lutsey PL, Steffen LM, Stevens J. Dietary intake and the development of the metabolic syndrome: The Atherosclerosis Risk in Communities Study. Circulation 2008; 117: 754–761.
14. Dhingra R, Sullivan L, Jacques PF, et al. Soft drink consumption and risk of developing cardiometabolic risk factors and the metabolic syndrome in middle-aged adults in the community. Circulation 2007; 116:480–488.
15. Swithers SED, Terry L. A role for sweet taste: Caloric predictive relations in energy regulation by rats. Behav Neurosci 2008; 122:161–173.
16. Stanhope KL, PJ Havel. Endocrine and metabolic effects of consuming beverages sweetened glucose, fructose, sucrose, or HFCS. Am J Clin Nutr 2008; 87:1194–1203.

17. Soenen S, Westerterp-Plantenga MS. No differences in satiety or energy intake after high-fructose corn syrup, sucrose, or milk preloads. Am J Clin Nutr 2007; 86: 1586–1594.
18. Nakagawa T, Hu H, Zharikov S, et al. A causal role for uric acid in fructose-induced metabolic syndrome. Am J Physiol Renal Physiol 2006; 290:F625–631.
19. Nakagawa T, Tuttle KR, Short RA, Johnson RJ. Hypothesis: fructose-induced hyperuricemia as a causal mechanism for the epidemic of the metabolic syndrome. Nature Clin Practice Nephrol 2005; 1:80–86.
20. Johnson RJ, Segal MS, Sautin Y, et al. Potential role of sugar (fructose) in the epidemic of hypertension, obesity and the metabolic syndrome, diabetes, kidney disease, and cardiovascular disease. Am J Clin Nutr 2007; 86: 899–906.

4 The Vitamins and Minerals: A Functional Approach

Marie Boyle Struble

Key Points

- Vitamins and minerals are essential micronutrients required throughout all stages of the life span.
- Vitamins are organic compounds required by the body for numerous metabolic reactions in small amounts (microgram or milligram quantities).
- Minerals are inorganic compounds; major minerals are found in the body in quantities greater than 5 g; trace minerals are found in amounts less than 5 g.
- Neither vitamins nor minerals supply calories to the diet.
- Abnormally high intakes of one or more vitamins or minerals may adversely affect the absorption and balance of other vitamins and minerals.

Key Words: Vitamins; minerals; deficiency diseases; toxicity; antioxidants; dietary reference intakes; food sources of nutrients

1. INTRODUCTION

About a century ago, scientists ushered in a new era in the science of nutrition – the discovery of vitamins *(1)*. They quickly realized that these substances, found in minute amounts in foods, were just as essential to health as fats, carbohydrates, and proteins. Knowledge of the vital roles played by vitamins quickly advanced, and today life threatening vitamin deficiencies are rare in developed countries such as the United States and Canada. Still, the vitamin and mineral research that has been conducted during the past decade or so has marked the beginning of yet another chapter in the annals of nutrition.

Vitamins fall into two categories: water-soluble and fat-soluble. To date, scientists have identified 13 vitamins (listed in Table 1), each with its own

From: *Nutrition and Health: Nutrition Guide for Physicians*
Edited by: T. Wilson et al. (eds.), DOI 10.1007/978-1-60327-431-9_4,
© Humana Press, a part of Springer Science+Business Media, LLC 2010

Table 1
The Vitamins and Minerals

Water-Soluble Vitamins	**The Major Minerals**
Thiamin	Calcium
Riboflavin	Phosphorus
Niacin	Magnesium
Vitamin B_6	Sodium
Folate	Chloride
Vitamin B_{12}	Potassium
Pantothenic acid	Sulfur
Biotin	**The Trace Minerals**
Vitamin C	Iodine
Fat-Soluble Vitamins	Iron
Vitamin A	Zinc
Vitamin D	Copper
Vitamin E	Fluoride
Vitamin K	Selenium
	Chromium
	Molybdenum
	Manganese

unique roles to play. The nine water-soluble vitamins – eight B vitamins and vitamin C – are excreted by the body if blood levels rise too high. As a result, these vitamins rarely reach toxic levels in the body. In contrast, because the four fat-soluble vitamins – A, D, E, and K – are stored in the liver and in body fat, it is possible for megadoses of fat-soluble vitamins to build up to toxic levels and cause toxicities.

Of the minerals important in human nutrition, most have diverse functions and work with enzymes to facilitate chemical reactions. Also, like the vitamins, most minerals are required in the diet in very small amounts. The *major* minerals occur in relatively large quantities in the body and are needed in the daily diet in relatively large amounts – on the order of a gram or so each. The *trace* minerals occur in the body in minute quantities and are needed in smaller amounts in the daily diet. Table 1 lists the major and trace minerals.

Eating patterns that exclude entire food groups or fail to include the minimum number of servings from each group may lead to vitamin or mineral deficiencies over time. This chapter discusses the vitamins and minerals known to be important in human nutrition and provides information about food sources and human requirements. The discussions about the vitamins and minerals are organized according to the biological roles these substances play in the body.

2. THE ANTIOXIDANT NUTRIENTS

Some chemical reactions that occur in the body involve the use of oxygen. Although these reactions are essential to the body's ability to function, they also lead to the creation of highly toxic free radical compounds. Environmental pollutants, such as cigarette smoke and ozone, also prompt the formation of free radicals. Left unchecked, these compounds can cause severe cell injury and ultimately may contribute to the development of chronic diseases such as cancer and heart disease.

Fortunately, the body has a built-in defense system to protect against potential damage from free radicals. That *defense* system makes use of the antioxidant nutrients: vitamin C, vitamin E, and the carotenoid called β-carotene (see Table 2). In addition, the body manufactures certain enzymes, one of which contains the mineral selenium, that help to fight free radicals.

2.1. Vitamin C

The antioxidants all work in one way or another to squelch free radicals before they injure the body. Vitamin C helps stop free radicals in their tracks, working with vitamin E to block damaging chain reactions that appear to promote heart disease and cancer. In addition, vitamin C is a powerful scavenger of environmental air pollutants.

Vitamin C also has other roles. It is required for the production and maintenance of collagen, needed for the body's connective tissue, including bones, teeth, skin, and tendons. Vitamin C also boosts the body's ability to fight infection. Vitamin C is most famous for its long-standing notoriety as a cure for the common cold. Despite the popularity of vitamin C as a cold remedy, however, many carefully controlled studies have shown that it plays an insignificant role – if any at all – in preventing colds. Table 2 lists sources of vitamin C-rich foods. Deficiencies arise in infants who are not given a source of vitamin C, as well as in children and older adults who do not consume adequate amounts of fruits and vegetables.

2.2. Vitamin E

Vitamin E is widespread in the food supply, and deficiencies are rare. The link between vitamin E and heart disease and other chronic diseases is an area of active scientific research. Because vitamin E performs a key role as an antioxidant in the body, scientists suspect that it is involved in protecting

Table 2
A Guide to the Vitamins and Minerals with Antioxidant Function

Vitamin	Best Sources	Chief Roles	Deficiency Symptoms	Toxicity Symptoms
Vitamin C (water-soluble) DRI adult: Men: 90 mg/d Women: 75 mg/d UL adult: 2,000 mg/d	Citrus fruits, cabbage-type vegetables (Brussels sprouts, cauliflower, broccoli), tomatoes, potatoes, bell peppers, lettuce, cantaloupe, strawberries, mangoes, papayas	Antioxidant; restores vitamin E to its active form; synthesizes collagen (helps heal wounds, maintains bone and teeth, strengthens blood vessel walls); strengthens resistance to infection; helps body absorb iron	Scurvy: anemia, depression, frequent infections, bleeding gums, loosened teeth, pinpoint hemorrhages, muscle degeneration, rough skin, bone fragility, poor wound healing, hysteria	Nausea, abdominal cramps, diarrhea, headache, fatigue, insomnia; hot flashes; increased risk for kidney stones
Vitamin E (fat-soluble) DRI adult: 15 mg/d UL adult: 1,000 mg/d	Vegetable oils, green leafy vegetables, wheat germ, whole grain products, liver, egg yolks, salad dressings, mayonnaise, margarine, nuts, seeds	Antioxidant (protects fat-soluble vitamins and polyunsaturated fats); stabilizes cell membranes	Weakness, breakage of red blood cells, anemia, hemorrhaging	May increase bleeding (blood clotting time)

	Best Sources	Chief Roles	Deficiency Symptoms	Toxicity Symptoms
β-Carotene (fat-soluble precursor of vitamin A) DRI: not determined	Broccoli, spinach, other dark leafy greens, deep-orange fruits and vegetables (cantaloupe, apricots, peaches, squash, carrots, sweet potatoes, pumpkin)	Antioxidant	Not known	Yellowing of skin (not harmful)
Mineral Selenium (trace mineral) DRI adult: 55 µg/d UL adult: 400 µg/d	Seafood, meats, whole grains, vegetables (depending on soil conditions)	Part of an enzyme system that helps protect body compounds from oxidation; works with vitamin E; regulates thyroid hormone	Fragile red blood cells, cataracts, growth failure, heart damage	Nausea, abdominal pain; brittleness of nails and hair; liver and nerve damage

the membranes of the lungs, heart, brain, and other organs against damage from pollutants and other environmental hazards. Scientists also believe that the vitamin E residing in the fatty cell membranes that surround cells acts as a scavenger of free radicals that enter the area *(2)*. When vitamin E is absent, the free radicals can attack the cell and start a chemical chain reaction that damages the cell membrane, and ultimately causing it to break down completely. For more than a decade, research suggested that vitamin E may protect against heart disease because it can thwart the free radicals that might otherwise damage the walls of blood vessels and contribute to coronary artery disease *(3)*. However, except for persons with low levels of vitamin E in their blood, recent evidence is inconclusive and does not support the notion that taking routine vitamin E supplements will help prevent chronic heart disease *(4)*.

Vitamin E toxicity appears to be rare, occurring only in people who take extremely high doses. Suspected symptoms include alteration of the body's blood-clotting mechanisms and interference with the function of vitamin K. Table 2 lists food sources of vitamin E.

2.3. The Vitamin A Precursor: β-Carotene

β-Carotene is a member of the carotenoid family of pigments. The carotenoids possess antioxidant properties and work with vitamins C and E in the body to protect against free radical damage that leads to diseases of the respiratory tract, such as lung cancer, as well as other chronic conditions. Certain carotenoids with antioxidant properties, found in dark-green leafy vegetables such as spinach, kale, collard greens, and Swiss chard, may help prevent age-related macular degeneration, as well as lower the risk of cataracts *(5)*.

The best known function of vitamin A relates to vision; when vitamin A is deficient, vision is impaired. Specifically, the eye has difficulty adapting to changing light levels. For a person deficient in vitamin A, a flash of bright light at night (after the eye has adapted to darkness) is followed by a prolonged spell of night blindness. Because night blindness is easy to diagnose, it aids in the diagnosis of vitamin A deficiency. The vitamin also helps to maintain healthy epithelial tissue, and is involved in the production of sperm, the normal development of fetuses, the immune response, hearing, taste, and growth.

Vitamin A toxicity is not nearly as widespread as deficiency. Nevertheless, it can also lead to severe health consequences, including joint pain, dryness of skin, hair loss, irritability, fatigue, headaches, weakness, nausea, and liver damage. Table 2 lists food sources of β-carotene and vitamin A.

2.4. Selenium

Selenium is a trace mineral found in the soil in varying amounts. Selenium functions as part of an antioxidant enzyme system that defends the body by preventing the formation of free radicals. Selenium can also substitute for vitamin E in some of that vitamin's antioxidant activities. Research is currently underway to investigate a possible role for selenium in protecting against the development of some forms of cancer *(6)*. A deficiency of selenium is associated with Keshan heart disease prevalent in some areas of China with selenium-poor soil *(6)*. Refer to Table 2 for a brief description of selenium and common food sources of this mineral.

3. NUTRIENTS FOR HEALTHY BLOOD

Many vitamins and minerals serve blood-related functions in the body (see Table 3). Folate and vitamin B_{12} assist with the formation of new blood cells. Vitamin B_6, zinc, copper, and iron are associated with hemoglobin. Vitamin K is needed for blood clotting.

3.1. Folate

Folate (also called folic acid or folacin) is a coenzyme with many functions in the body. It is particularly important in the synthesis of DNA and the formation of red blood cells. A folate deficiency creates misshapen red blood cells that are unable to carry sufficient oxygen to the body's other cells, thereby causing a macrocytic anemia. Thus, folate deficiency results in a generalized malaise with many symptoms, including fatigue, diarrhea, irritability, forgetfulness, lack of appetite, and headache. Folate deficiency may also elevate a person's risk for certain cancers – notably cervical cancer in women and colon cancer *(7)*. Folate plays a crucial role in a healthy pregnancy. A strong body of evidence indicates that consuming a generous amount of folate reduces the risk of bearing a baby with a neural tube defect. Sources of folate in foods are listed in Table 3. Because high levels of blood folate can mask a true vitamin B_{12} deficiency, total folate intake should not exceed 1 mg daily *(8)*.

3.2. Vitamin B_{12}

Vitamin B_{12} maintains the myelin sheaths that surround and protect nerve fibers. The nutrient also works closely with folate, enabling it to manufacture red blood cells. A deficiency of vitamin B_{12} causes the same sort of anemia as seen in people with a folate deficiency, characterized by large, immature red blood cells. Other problems resulting from a B_{12} deficiency include a creeping paralysis of the nerves and muscles that can cause permanent

Table 3
A Guide to the Vitamins and Minerals for Healthy Blood

Vitamin	Best Sources	Chief Roles	Deficiency Symptoms	Toxicity Symptoms
Folate (water-soluble) DRI adult: 400 µg/d UL adult: 1,000 µg/d	Green leafy vegetables, liver, legumes, seeds, citrus fruits, melons, enriched breads and grain products	Red blood cell formation; protein metabolism; new cell division	Anemia, heartburn, diarrhea, smooth red tongue, depression, poor growth, neural tube defects; increased risk of heart disease, stroke, and certain cancers	Diarrhea, insomnia, irritability; may mask a vitamin B_{12} deficiency
Vitamin B_{12} (water-soluble) DRI adult: 2.4 µg/d	Animal products: meat, fish, poultry, shellfish, milk, cheese, eggs; fortified cereals	Helps maintain nerve cells; red blood cell formation; synthesis of genetic material	Anemia, smooth red tongue, fatigue, nerve degeneration progressing to paralysis	None reported
Vitamin B_6 (water-soluble) DRI adult (19–50 yr): 1.3 mg/d UL adult: 100 mg/d	Meat, poultry, fish, shellfish, legumes, fruits, soy products, whole grain products, green leafy vegetables	Protein and fat metabolism; formation of antibodies and red blood cells; helps convert tryptophan to niacin	Nervous disorders, skin rash, muscle weakness, anemia, convulsions, kidney stones	Depression, fatigue, irritability, headaches, numbness, damage to nerves, difficulty walking

	Best Sources	Chief Roles	Deficiency Symptoms	Toxicity Symptoms
Vitamin K (fat-soluble) DRI adult: Men: 120 µg/d Women: 90 µg/d	Bacterial synthesis in digestive tract, liver, green leafy and cabbage-type vegetables, soybeans, milk, vegetable oils	Synthesis of proteins for blood clotting and bone mineralization	Hemorrhage, decreased calcium in bones	Interference with anticlotting medication; synthetic forms may cause jaundice
Mineral Iron (trace mineral) DRI adult: Men: 8 mg/d Women (19–50 yr): 18 mg/d Women (>50 yr): 8 mg/d UL adult: 45 mg/d	Red meats, fish, poultry, shellfish, eggs, legumes, dried fruits, fortified cereals	Hemoglobin formation; part of myoglobin; energy utilization	Anemia: weakness, pallor, headaches, reduced immunity, inability to concentrate, cold intolerance	Iron overload: infections, liver injury, acidosis, shock

(Continued)

Table 3
(Continued)

Mineral	Best Sources	Chief Roles	Deficiency Symptoms	Toxicity Symptoms
Zinc (trace mineral) DRI adult: Men: 11 mg/d Women: 8 mg/d UL adult: 40 mg/d	Protein-containing foods: meats, fish, shellfish, poultry, grains, vegetables	Part of insulin and many enzymes; involved in making genetic material and proteins, immunity, vitamin A transport, taste, wound healing, making sperm, fetal development	Growth failure in children, delayed development of sexual organs, loss of taste, poor wound healing	Fever, nausea, vomiting, diarrhea, kidney failure
Copper (trace mineral) DRI adult: 900 µg/d UL adult: 10,000 µg/d	Meats, seafood, nuts, drinking water	Helps make hemoglobin; part of several enzymes	Anemia, bone changes (rare in human beings)	Nausea, vomiting, diarrhea

nerve damage if left untreated. Table 3 lists food sources of the vitamin – found exclusively in animal foods. Strict vegetarians need to find alternative sources of the nutrient, such as vitamin B_{12}-fortified soy beverages, fortified cereals, or B_{12} supplements.

People who inherit a genetic defect that leaves the body unable to make intrinsic factor in the stomach are unable to absorb and make use of vitamin B_{12} and are at risk of vitamin B_{12} deficiency unless they get B_{12} injections. Other people likely to experience a deficiency are the estimated 20% of seniors in their sixties and 40% of those in their eighties that develop atrophic gastritis which in turn hampers the body's ability to use the vitamin. Vitamin B_{12} deficiency resulting from atrophic gastritis appears to be easily treated with B_{12} supplements or injections (9).

3.3. Vitamin B_6

Like the other B vitamins, vitamin B_6 functions as a coenzyme and is an indispensable cog in the body's machinery. For example, vitamin B_6 helps make hemoglobin for red blood cells. It also plays many roles in protein metabolism. In fact, a person's requirement for vitamin B_6 is proportional to protein intakes. Because the vitamin performs this and so many other tasks, a deficiency causes a multitude of symptoms, including weakness, irritability, and insomnia. Low levels of vitamin B_6 may also weaken the body's immune response and increase a person's risk of heart disease. Vitamin B_6 is found in meats, vegetables, and whole grain cereals, and true vitamin B_6 deficiencies are rare – occurring in some people who eat inadequate diets and whose nutrient needs are higher than usual because of pregnancy, alcohol abuse, some diseases, use of certain prescription drugs, and other unusual circumstances.

3.4. Vitamin K

The key function of vitamin K is its role in the blood-clotting system of the body. It is essential for the synthesis of at least 4 of the 13 proteins involved, along with calcium, in making the blood clot. Many foods supply ample amounts of the vitamin; particular standouts are green leafy vegetables and members of the cabbage family.

Vitamin K toxicity is rare, but it can occur when supplemental doses are taken. In particular, adults who must pay attention to the amount of vitamin K in their diet are those who take anticoagulant drugs designed to prevent a clot from causing a stroke or heart attack. People taking such medications are advised to keep their consumption of vitamin K fairly constant from day to day because large fluctuations can limit the effectiveness of the anticlotting drugs (10).

3.5. Iron

Iron is bound into the protein hemoglobin in the red blood cells, and it helps transport oxygen and thus permits the release of energy from fuels to do the cells' work. When the iron supply is too low, iron-deficiency anemia occurs, characterized by weakness, tiredness, apathy, headaches, increased sensitivity to cold, and a paleness that reflects the reduction in the number and size of the red blood cells.

People must select foods carefully to obtain enough iron, because it is present in such small quantities in most foods. The best meat sources are red meats, poultry, fish, oysters, and clams. Among the grains, whole grains and enriched and fortified breads and cereals are best, and dried beans are a good source. Foods in the milk group are notoriously poor iron sources.

Large amounts of iron can be toxic to the body. Iron overload is a condition in which the body absorbs excessive amounts of iron. Researchers are currently investigating a possible link between excess iron stores in the body and increased risk of chronic conditions such as heart disease. In a 3-year study of 2,000 healthy men, researchers in Finland found that the risk of heart attack was twice as great for men with the highest levels of stored iron in their bodies (11). Although iron is a vital nutrient in the body, it can also act as a powerful oxidizing agent in reactions that produce free radicals.

3.6. Zinc

Zinc is found in every cell of the body and plays a major role along with more than 50 enzymes that regulate cell multiplication and growth; normal metabolism of protein, carbohydrate, fat, and alcohol; and the disposal of damaging free radicals. Zinc is associated with the hormone insulin, which regulates the body's fuel supply. It is involved in the utilization of vitamin A, taste perception, thyroid function, wound healing, the synthesis of sperm, and the development of sexual organs and bone. More recently, zinc has become known for its role in promoting a healthy immune system (12).

Zinc deficiency can cause night blindness, hair loss, poor appetite, susceptibility to infection, delayed healings of cuts or abrasions, decreased taste and smell sensitivity, and poor growth in children. Because zinc is lost from the body daily in much the same way as protein is, it must be replenished daily. Zinc is a relatively nontoxic element. However, it can be toxic if consumed in large enough quantities. Consumption of high levels of zinc can cause a host of symptoms, including vomiting, diarrhea, fever, and exhaustion (13). Excess supplemental zinc can cause imbalances of both copper and iron in the body. Zinc is highest in foods of high protein content, such as shellfish and meats. As a rule of thumb, two servings a day of animal protein will provide most of the zinc a healthy person needs. Whole grain products are also good sources.

3.7. Copper

This trace mineral has important roles in a variety of metabolic and physiological processes. For example, copper is involved in making red blood cells, manufacturing collagen, healing wounds, and maintaining the sheaths around nerve fibers. Refer to Table 3 for common food sources of copper.

4. NUTRIENTS FOR HEALTHY BONES

Bones are made up of a complex matrix of living tissue based on the protein collagen, into which the crystals of the bone minerals – principally calcium and phosphorus – are deposited. The principal determinant of bone health is *peak bone mass*. Besides calcium, several other vitamins and minerals are needed for the growth and maintenance of a healthy skeleton (see Table 4). Vitamin D directs a large bone-making and bone-maintenance team composed of several nutrients and other compounds, including vitamins C and K; hormones; the protein collagen; and the minerals calcium, phosphorus, magnesium, and fluoride.

4.1. Vitamin D

Vitamin D's special role in bone health involves assisting in the absorption of dietary calcium and helping to make calcium and phosphorus available in the blood that bathes the bones, so that these minerals can be deposited as the bones harden. Because the body can make vitamin D from a cholesterol compound with the help of sunlight, people can meet their needs for the nutrient either via sun exposure or through diet. Five to fifteen minutes of sun exposure to the face, hands, and arms on a clear, summer day two to three times per week may be sufficient for maintenance of vitamin D status for most healthy people *(14)*. Dark-skinned people require longer exposure to sunlight than light-skinned people since the pigments of dark skin reduce vitamin D synthesis. However, from November through February, people who live north of latitude 40° (from northern Pennsylvania to northern California), are not exposed to enough ultraviolet rays from the sun to synthesize adequate vitamin D *(15)*. The same holds true for housebound or institutionalized elderly people, who not only get outside less often than younger people but also tend to be much less efficient at producing vitamin D via the skin/sun synthesis pathway *(16)*. For these people, eating vitamin D-rich foods, such as fortified milk, fatty fish (including sardines, herring, mackerel, and salmon), eggs, and some fortified cereals, is particularly

Table 4
A Guide to the Vitamins and Minerals for Healthy Bones

Vitamin	Best Sources	Chief Roles	Deficiency Symptoms	Toxicity Symptoms
Vitamin D (fat-soluble) DRI adult: 5 μg/d 51–70 yr: 10 μg/d >70 yr: 15 μg/d UL adult: 50 μg/d (1.25 IU) Vitamin K See Table 3	Self-synthesis with sunlight; fortified milk, fortified margarine, eggs, liver, fish	Calcium and phosphorus metabolism (bone and tooth formation); aids body's absorption of calcium	Rickets in children; osteomalacia in adults; abnormal growth, joint pain, soft bones	Deposits of calcium in soft tissues (kidneys, liver, heart), mental retardation, abnormal bone growth
Vitamin A DRI (adult): Men: 900 μg RAE/d Women: 700 μg RAE/d	*Vitamin A:* fortified milk and margarine, cream, cheese, butter, eggs, liver β-Carotene: broccoli, spinach, other dark leafy greens, deep-orange fruits and vegetables (cantaloupe, apricots, peaches, squash, carrots, sweet potatoes, pumpkin)	Vision; growth and repair of body tissues; maintenance of mucous membranes; reproduction; bone and tooth formation; immunity; hormone synthesis; antioxidant (in the form of β-carotene only)	Night blindness, rough skin, susceptibility to infection, impaired bone growth, abnormal tooth and jaw alignment, eye problems leading to blindness, impaired growth	Blurred vision, irritability, loss of appetite, increased activity of bone-dismantling cells causing reduced bone density and bone pain, dry skin, rashes, liver disease, birth defects β-Carotene: harmless yellowing of skin

Mineral	Best Sources	Chief Roles	Deficiency Symptoms	Toxicity Symptoms
Calcium (major mineral) DRI adult: 1,000 mg/d >50 yr: 1,200 mg/d UL adult: 2,500 mg/d	Milk and milk products, small fish (with bones), tofu, certain green vegetables, legumes, fortified juices	Principal mineral of bones and teeth; involved in muscle contraction and relaxation, nerve function, blood clotting, blood pressure	Stunted growth in children; bone loss (osteoporosis) in adults	Excess calcium is usually excreted except in hormonal imbalance states
Phosphorus (major mineral) DRI adult: 700 mg/d UL adult: 4,000 mg/d	Meat, poultry, fish, dairy products, soft drinks, processed foods	Part of every cell; mineralization of bones and teeth; involved in buffer systems that maintain acid–base balance; used in energy metabolism	Muscle weakness and bone pain (rarely seen)	May cause calcium excretion; calcium deposits in soft tissues (e.g., kidneys)

(Continued)

Table 4
(Continued)

Mineral	Best Sources	Chief Roles	Deficiency Symptoms	Toxicity Symptoms
Magnesium (major mineral) DRI adult: Men (19–30 yr): 400 mg/d Men (>31 yr): 420 mg/d Women (19–30 yr): 310 mg/d Women (>31 yr): 320 mg/d UL adult: 350 mg/d from nonfood sources	Nuts, legumes, whole grains, dark-green vegetables, seafoods, chocolate, cocoa	Involved in bone mineralization, protein synthesis, enzyme action, normal muscular contraction, nerve transmission	Weakness, confusion, depressed pancreatic hormone secretion, growth failure, hallucinations, muscle spasms	Excess intakes (from overuse of laxatives) has caused low blood pressure, lack of coordination, coma, and death
Fluoride (trace mineral) DRI adult: Men: 4 mg/d Women: 3 mg/d UL adult: 10 mg/d	Drinking water (if fluoridated or naturally contains fluorine), tea, seafood	Formation of bones and teeth; helps make teeth resistant to decay	Susceptibility to tooth decay	Fluorosis (discoloration of teeth); nausea, vomiting, diarrhea

important (see Table 4). Children who fail to get enough vitamin D characteristically develop bowed legs, which are often the most obvious sign of the deficiency disease rickets. In adults, vitamin D deficiency causes osteomalacia.

Although vitamin D deficiency depresses calcium absorption, resulting in low blood calcium levels and abnormal bone development, an excess of vitamin D does just the opposite. It increases calcium absorption, causing abnormally high concentration of the mineral in the blood, which then tends to be deposited in the soft tissues. This is especially likely to happen in the kidneys, resulting in the formation of calcium-containing stones called *kidney stones*.

4.2. Vitamin K

Accumulating evidence also supports an active role for vitamin K in the maintenance of bone health. Vitamin K works in conjunction with vitamin D to synthesize a bone protein that helps to regulate the calcium levels in the blood. Low levels of vitamin K in the blood have been associated with low bone-mineral density, and researchers have noted a lower risk of hip fracture in older women who have high intakes of vitamin K than in those who have low intakes *(17)*.

4.3. Calcium

Calcium is the most abundant mineral in the body. Ninety-nine percent of the body's calcium is found in the bones which support and protect the body's soft tissues. Bones also provide calcium to the body fluids whenever the supply runs low. Although only about 1% of the body's calcium is in its fluids, circulating calcium is required for the transmission of nerve impulses, is essential for muscle contraction, appears to be essential for the integrity of cell membranes, and is involved in the maintenance of normal blood pressure. Calcium must also be present if blood clotting is to occur, and it is a cofactor for several enzymes. A calcium deficit during the growing years and in adulthood contributes to osteoporosis.

Calcium appears almost exclusively in three classes of foods: milk and milk products; green vegetables such as broccoli, kale, bok choy, collards, and turnip greens; and a few fish and shellfish. Milk and milk products typically contain the most bioavailable calcium per serving.

4.4. Phosphorus

Phosphorus is second to calcium in mineral abundance in the body. About 85% of it is found combined with calcium in the crystals of the bones and teeth as calcium phosphate, the chief compound that gives them strength and rigidity. Phosphorus is also a part of DNA and RNA, the genetic code material present in every cell. Phosphorus is thus necessary for all growth.

Phosphorus plays many key roles in the cells' use of energy nutrients. Many enzymes and the B vitamins become active only when a phosphate group is attached. The B vitamins play a major role in energy metabolism, as discussed later in this chapter. Phospholipids contain phosphorus as part of their structure. They help to transport other lipids in the blood; they also form part of the structure of cell membranes, where they affect the transport of nutrients and wastes into and out of the cells. Table 4 lists food sources of phosphorus. High intakes can interfere with calcium absorption.

4.5. Magnesium

Magnesium helps to relax muscles after contraction and promotes resistance to tooth decay by helping to hold calcium in tooth enamel. Magnesium also acts in all the cells of the muscles, heart, liver, and other soft tissues, where it forms part of the protein-making machinery and is necessary for the release of energy. A deficiency of magnesium may be related to sudden death from heart failure and to high blood pressure (18). A dietary deficiency of magnesium is not likely but may occur as a result of vomiting, diarrhea, alcohol abuse, or protein malnutrition. Good food sources are listed in Table 4.

4.6. Fluoride

Only a trace of fluoride occurs in the human body, but studies have demonstrated that for people who live where diets are high in fluoride, the crystalline deposits in their teeth and bones are larger and more perfectly formed than in people who live where diets are low in fluoride. It not only protects children's teeth from decay but also makes the bones of older people resistant to adult bone loss and osteoporosis. Thus, its continuous presence in body fluids is desirable. Drinking water is the usual source of fluoride. Many community water supplies are fluoridated as a public health measure. Where fluoride is lacking in the water supply, the incidence of dental decay is very high.

5. VITAMINS, MINERALS, AND ENERGY METABOLISM

Many vitamins and minerals are essential for energy metabolism, as described in the following sections.

5.1. Thiamin

One of the B vitamins, thiamin, acts primarily as a coenzyme in reactions that release energy from carbohydrates. Thiamin also plays a crucial role in processes involving the nerves. It is so vital to the functioning of the entire body that a deficiency affects the nerves, muscles, heart, and other organs. A severe deficiency, called beriberi, causes extreme wasting and loss of muscle tissue, swelling all over the body, enlargement of the heart, irregular heartbeat, and paralysis. Ultimately, the victim dies from heart failure. A mild thiamin deficiency, in contrast, often mimics other conditions and typically manifests itself as vague, general symptoms such as stomachaches, headaches, fatigue, restlessness, sleep disturbances, chest pains, fevers, personality changes (aggressiveness and hostility), and neurosis. Thiamin is found in a variety of meats, legumes, fruits, and vegetables, as well as in all enriched and whole grain products (see Table 5).

5.2. Riboflavin

Like thiamin, the B vitamin riboflavin acts as a coenzyme in energy-releasing reactions. It also helps to prepare fatty acids and amino acids for breakdown. Deficiencies of the vitamin, which are rare, are characterized by severe skin problems, including painful cracks at the corners of the mouth; a red, swollen tongue; and teary or bloodshot eyes.

Milk and dairy products contribute a good deal of the riboflavin in many people's diets. Meats are another good source, as are dark-green vegetables such as broccoli. Leafy green vegetables and whole grain or enriched bread and cereal products also supply a generous amount of riboflavin in most people's diets.

5.3. Niacin

Like thiamin and riboflavin, the B vitamin niacin is part of a coenzyme that is vital to producing energy. Without niacin to form this coenzyme, energy-yielding reactions come to a halt. Over time, a deficiency leads to the disease pellagra, characterized by diarrhea, dermatitis, and, in severe cases, dementia – a progressive mental deterioration resulting in delirium, mania or depression, and eventually death. Milk, eggs, meat, poultry, and fish contribute the bulk of the niacin equivalents consumed by most people, followed by enriched breads and cereals.

Diet aside, in recent years, niacin has been increasingly used as a drug-like supplement to help lower cholesterol. Doses ranging from 10 to 15 times the RDA have been shown to reduce LDL-cholesterol and raise HDL-cholesterol *(19)*. The hitch, however, is that such high doses of niacin can

Table 5
A Guide to the Vitamins and Minerals for Energy Metabolism

Vitamin	Best Sources	Chief Roles	Deficiency Symptoms	Toxicity Symptoms
Thiamin (water-soluble) DRI adult: Men: 1.2 mg/d Women: 1.1 mg/d	Meat, pork, liver, fish, poultry, whole grain and enriched breads, cereals and grain products, nuts, legumes	Helps enzymes release energy from carbohydrate; supports normal appetite and nervous system function	Beriberi: edema, heart irregularity, mental confusion, muscle weakness, apathy, impaired growth	None reported
Riboflavin (water-soluble) DRI adult: Men: 1.3 mg/d Women: 1.1 mg/d	Milk, leafy green vegetables, yogurt, cottage cheese, liver, meat, whole grain or enriched breads, cereals and grain products	Helps enzymes release energy from carbohydrate, fat, and protein; also promotes healthy skin and normal vision	Eye problems, skin disorders around nose and mouth, magenta tongue, hypersensitivity to light	None reported
Niacin (water-soluble) DRI adult: Men: 16 mg NE/d Women: 14 mg NE/d UL adult: 35 mg/d	Meat, eggs, poultry, fish, milk, whole grain and enriched breads, cereals and grain products, nuts, legumes, peanuts	Helps enzymes release energy from energy nutrients; promotes health of skin, nerves, and digestive system	Pellagra: flaky skin rash on parts exposed to sun, loss of appetite, dizziness, weakness, irritability, fatigue, mental confusion, indigestion, delirium	Flushing, nausea, headaches, cramps, ulcer irritation, heartburn, abnormal liver function, rapid heartbeat with doses above 500 mg/d

	Best Sources	Chief Roles	Deficiency Symptoms	Toxicity Symptoms
Vitamin B$_6$ *See* Table 3				
Folate *See* Table 3				
Vitamin B$_{12}$ *See* Table 3				
Biotin (water-soluble) DRI adult: 30 µg/d	Widespread in foods	Coenzyme in energy metabolism; fat synthesis	Loss of appetite, nausea, depression, muscle pain	None reported
Mineral Iron *See* Table 3	*Best Sources*	*Chief Roles*	*Deficiency Symptoms*	*Toxicity Symptoms*
Zinc *See* Table 3				
Iodine (trace mineral) DRI adult: 150 µg/d UL adult: 1,100 µg/d	Iodized salt, seafood, bread	Part of thyroxine, which regulates metabolism	Goiter, cretinism	Depressed thyroid activity

(Continued)

Table 5
(Continued)

Mineral	Best Sources	Chief Roles	Deficiency Symptoms	Toxicity Symptoms
Chromium (trace mineral) DRI adult: Men (19–50 yr): 35 μg/d Women (19–50 yr): 25 μg/d UL adult: 1,100 μg/d	Meats, unrefined foods, vegetable oils	Associated with insulin needed for release of energy from glucose	Abnormal glucose metabolism	Occupational exposures damage skin and kidneys

lead to side effects such as nausea, flushing of the skin, rash, fatigue, and liver damage.

5.4. Iodine

Iodine occurs in the body in an infinitesimal quantity, but its principal role in human nutrition is well known. It is part of the thyroid hormones, which regulate body temperature, metabolic rate, reproduction, and growth. Iodine deficiency causes goiter, a condition estimated to affect 200 million people worldwide. In addition to causing sluggishness and weight gain, an iodine deficiency can have serious effects on fetal development. Severe thyroid undersecretion by a woman during pregnancy causes the extreme and irreversible mental and physical retardation of the child known as cretinism.

The amount of iodine in foods reflects the amount present in the soil in which plants are grown or on which animals graze. Soil iodine is greatest along the coastal regions. Although most consumers have access to fruits and vegetables grown in coastal areas rich in iodine, it is important of using iodized salt to maintain an adequate iodine intake.

5.5. Chromium

This is a trace mineral involved in carbohydrate metabolism. It works closely with insulin to help the cells take up glucose and break it down for energy *(20)*. Good food sources of chromium include dark chocolate, nuts, mushrooms, asparagus, and whole grains.

6. MINERALS AND FLUID BALANCE

Sodium is the chief cation needed to maintain fluid volume outside cells; potassium is the chief cation inside the cells. Chloride is the major negatively charged ion in the fluids outside the cells, where it is found mostly in association with sodium. Many factors in addition to the intake of sodium and chloride work together to keep the fluid volume fairly constant inside and outside of cells (see Table 6).

Sodium is part of sodium chloride, ordinary table salt, a food seasoning and preservative. The recommended daily sodium intake is set at 1,500 mg for young adults, 1,300 mg for adults aged 51–70, and 1,200 mg for older adults. Because average sodium intakes are about 3,300 mg/d, substantially higher than recommended, the *Dietary Guidelines for Americans* recommends consuming little sodium and salt and staying below the upper limit of 2,300 mg/d of sodium (approximately one teaspoon of salt). The use of highly salted foods can contribute to hypertension in those who are genetically susceptible.

Table 6
A Guide to the Minerals for Fluid and Electrolyte Balance

Mineral	Best Sources	Chief Roles	Deficiency Symptoms	Excess/Toxicity Symptoms
Sodium (major mineral) DRI adult (19–50 yr): 1,500 mg/d UL adult: 2,300 mg/d	Salt, soy sauce; processed foods such as cured, canned, pickled, and many boxed foods	Helps maintain normal fluid and acid–base balance; nerve impulse transmission	Muscle cramps, mental apathy, loss of appetite	High blood pressure
Chloride (major mineral) DRI adult (19–50 yr): 2,300 mg/d UL adult: 3,600 mg/d	Salt, soy sauce; processed foods	Part of hydrochloric acid found in the stomach, necessary for proper digestion, fluid balance	Growth failure in children, muscle cramps, mental apathy, loss of appetite	Normally harmless (the gas chlorine is a poison but evaporates from water); vomiting
Potassium (major mineral) DRI adult: 4,700 mg/d	All whole foods: meats, milk, fruits, vegetables, grains, legumes	Facilitates many reactions, including protein synthesis, fluid balance, nerve transmission, and contraction of muscles	Muscle weakness, paralysis, confusion; can cause death; accompanies dehydration	Causes muscular weakness; triggers vomiting; if given into a vein, can stop the heart
Phosphorus See Table 4				

Potassium is critical to maintaining the heartbeat. The sudden deaths that occur during fasting, severe diarrhea, or severe vomiting are thought to be due to heart failure caused by potassium loss. As the principal cation inside cells, potassium plays a major role in maintaining water balance and cell integrity.

The relationship of potassium and sodium in maintaining the blood pressure is not entirely clear *(21)*. Abundant evidence supports the simple view that the two minerals have opposite effects. In any case, it is clear that increasing the potassium in the diet can promote sodium excretion under most circumstances and thereby lower the blood pressure *(22)*. Whole foods of all kinds, including fruits, vegetables, grains, meats, fish, and poultry, are among the richest sources of potassium.

Chloride accompanies sodium in the fluids outside the cells. Because it can move freely across membranes, it is also found inside the cells in association with potassium. In the blood, chloride helps in maintaining the acid–base balance. In the stomach, the chloride ion is part of hydrochloric acid, which is needed for protein digestion. Nearly all dietary chloride comes from sodium chloride.

SUGGESTED FURTHER READING

Institute of Medicine. Dietary Reference Intakes: The Essential Guide to Nutrient Requirements. National Academies Press, Washington, DC, 2006.

Shils ME, Shike M, Ross AC, Caballero B, Cousins RJ. Modern Nutrition in Health and Disease, 10th ed, Lippincott, Williams & Wilkins, Philadelphia, 2006.

Bowman BA, Russell RM. Present Knowledge in Nutrition, 9th ed. International Life Sciences Institute, Washington, DC, 2006.

www.nal.usda.gov/fnic Search USDA's Food and Nutrition Information Center for individual vitamins, food composition, and vitamin and mineral-related topics.

www.eatright.org The American Dietetic Association's site, with position papers on vitamin supplements, mineral topics, functional foods, and many resources.

REFERENCES

1. This Chapter is adapted from: Boyle M. The vitamins, minerals, and water: A functional approach. In: Boyle M, Long S. Personal Nutrition, 7th ed. Wadsworth/Cengage Learning, Belmont, CA, 2009, pp. 200–257.
2. Kris-Etherton PM, Lichtenstein AH, Howard BV, Steinberg D, Witztum JL. Nutrition Committee of the American Heart Association Council on Nutrition, Physical Activity, and Metabolism. Antioxidant vitamin supplements and cardiovascular disease. Circulation 2004; 110:637–641.
3. Goran Bjelakovic G, Nikolova D, Gluud LL, Simonetti RG, Gluud C. Mortality in randomized trials of antioxidant supplements for primary and secondary prevention: Systematic review and meta-analysis. JAMA 2007; 297:842–857.
4. Miller ER, Pastor-Barriuso R, Dalal D, Riemersma RA, Appel LJ, Guallar E. Meta-analysis: High dosage vitamin E supplementation may increase all-cause mortality. Ann Intern Med 2005; 142:37–46.

5. (a) Age Related Eye Disease Research Group. A randomized, placebo-controlled clinical trial of high dose supplementation with vitamins C and E, beta carotene, and zinc for age-related macular degeneration and vision loss, AREDS Report No. 8. Arch Ophthalmol 2001; 119:1417–1436; (b) As ref. 5a. AREDS Report No. 9. ibid. 1439–1452.

6. Food and Nutrition Board. Institute of Medicine. Dietary Reference Intakes for Vitamin C, Vitamin E, Selenium, and Carotenoids. National Academy Press, Washington, DC, 2000.

7. Rampersaud G, Bailey L, Kauwell G. Relationship of folate to colorectal and cervical cancer: Review and recommendations for practitioners. J Am Diet Assoc 2002; 102:1273–1282.

8. Food and Nutrition Board. Institute of Medicine. Dietary Reference Intakes for Thiamin, Riboflavin, Niacin, Vitamin B_6, Folate, Vitamin B_{12}, Pantothenic Acid, Biotin, and Choline. National Academy Press, Washington, DC, 1998.

9. Stabler SP, Allen RH. Vitamin B_{12} deficiency as a worldwide problem. Ann Rev Nutr 2004; 24:299–326

10. Johnson MA. Influence of vitamin K on anticoagulant therapy depends on vitamin K status and the source and chemical forms of vitamin K. Nutr Rev 2005; 63:91–100.

11. Klipstein-Grobusch K, Dietary iron and risk of myocardial infarction in the Rotterdam Study. Am J Epidemiol 1999; 149:421–428.

12. Walker CF, Black RE. Zinc and the risk for infectious disease. Ann Rev Nutr 2004; 24:255–275.

13. King JC, Cousins, RJ. Zinc. In: Shils ME, Shike M, Ross AC, Caballaro B, Cousins RJ, (eds.): Modern Nutrition in Health and Disease, 10th ed. Lippincott, Williams & Wilkins, Philadelphia, 2006.

14. Holick MF. Sunlight and vitamin D for bone health and prevention of autoimmune diseases, cancers, and cardiovascular disease. Am J Clin Nutr 2004; 80:1678S–1688S.

15. Holick MF. Vitamin D. In: Shils ME, Shike M, Ross AC, Caballaro B, Cousins RJ, (eds.): Modern Nutrition in Health and Disease, 10th ed. Lippincott, Williams & Wilkins, Philadelphia, 2006.

16. Holick MF. High prevalence of vitamin D inadequacy and implications for health. Mayo Clin Proc 2006; 81:353–373.

17. Cockayne S, Adamson J, Lanham-New S, Shearer MJ, Gilbody S, Torgerson DJ. Vitamin K and the prevention of fractures: Systematic review and meta-analysis of randomized control trials. Arch Intern Med 2006; 166:1256–1261.

18. Jee SH, Miller ER, Guallar E. The effect of magnesium supplementation on blood pressure: A meta-analysis of randomized clinical trials. Am J Hyperten 2002; 15:691–696.

19. Canner PL. Benefits of niacin in patients with versus without the metabolic syndrome and healed myocardial infarction (from the Coronary Drug Project). Am J Cardiol 2006; 97:477–479.

20. Stoecker BJ. Chromium. In Shils ME, Shike M, Ross AC, Caballaro B, Cousins RJ, eds. Modern Nutrition in Health and Disease, 10th ed. Lippincott, Williams & Wilkins, Philadelphia, 2006.

21. Androque HJ, Madias NE. Sodium and potassium in the pathogenesis of hypertension. N Engl J Med 2007; 356:1966–1978.

22. Standing Committee on the Scientific Evaluation of Dietary Reference Intakes, Food and Nutrition Board, Institute of Medicine. Dietary Reference Intakes: Water, Potassium, Sodium, Chloride, and Sulfate. National Academy Press, Washington, DC, 2004, pp. 4–26.

5 Dietary Reference Intakes: Cutting Through the Confusion

*Jennifer J. Francis
and Carol J. Klitzke*

Key Points

- The dietary reference intakes (DRIs) are a set of reference values for nutrients for assessing and planning diets for individuals and groups.
- The DRIs include values for
  - o Estimated average requirement (EAR)
  - o Recommended dietary allowance (RDA)
  - o Adequate intake (AI)
  - o Tolerable upper intake level (UL)
- The purpose of the DRI is to describe a nutrient intake that will promote health and prevent or delay chronic diet-related diseases.
- The DRIs form the scientific foundation for federal food programs, including nutrition labeling, requirements for school meals, and design of supplemental food packages for the Women, Infants, and Children Program.
- The Dietary Guidelines for Americans and MyPyramid translate the DRI into recommendations and guides for consumer food selection.

Key Words: Dietary reference intakes; recommended dietary allowances; deficiency; toxicity; energy balance; MyPyramid

1. INTRODUCTION

The dietary reference intakes (DRIs) include four nutrient reference values created by the Institute of Medicine to be used for assessing and planning diets of individuals and groups. These values reflect the optimal amount

From: *Nutrition and Health: Nutrition Guide for Physicians*
Edited by: T. Wilson et al. (eds.), DOI 10.1007/978-1-60327-431-9_5,
© Humana Press, a part of Springer Science+Business Media, LLC 2010

of select nutrients needed to promote health, prevent disease, and avoid overconsumption. The DRI replaces the recommended dietary allowances (RDA), in use since 1941 in the United States, and the recommended nutrient intakes (RNI) in Canada. The DRI was first published in a series of reports between 1997 and 2005, and in 2006 a definitive summary and practitioner's guide was issued *(1)*. The Netherlands, Japan, and South Korea adapted the concept of the DRI for use in their countries *(2–4)*.

2. THE DIETARY REFERENCE INTAKES

The DRI consists of four sets of values: Estimated average requirement (EAR), recommended dietary allowance (RDA), adequate intake (AI), and tolerable upper intake level (UL). DRIs are provided for 12 life stage groups, based on age and gender, with additional categories for pregnant and lactating women. Additionally, there are separate recommendations for the estimated energy requirement (EER) and acceptable macronutrient distribution ranges (AMDR).

2.1. Estimated Average Requirement

The EAR represents the average daily intake that is likely to meet the nutritional requirements of approximately half of the healthy individuals in a group. Nutrient needs vary from individual to individual. The EAR is set at the point which would meet or exceed the nutrient needs for half of the individuals in a group, but falls short for the half of the group with higher than average requirements. As such, it is not to be used as a recommendation or goal for nutrient intake for individuals. Rather, it is used as a tool for statistical analysis of adequacy and for setting the RDA, as described below. It is important to note that when determining the EAR for nutrients, requirements were based on indicators of adequacy, such as urinary excretion, tissue saturation, and blood levels, rather than merely the amount required to prevent deficiency disease.

2.2. Recommended Dietary Allowance

The RDA is set at a level which exceeds the nutrient needs of nearly all healthy individuals in a population. When the requirement for a nutrient in a population follows a normal distribution pattern, the RDA is based on the EAR plus two standard deviations. If the distribution is skewed, the RDA is set at a level between the 97th and 98th percentile for the nutrient requirement. By this definition, the RDA will exceed the nutrient requirements for most people in the population; therefore, intakes below the RDA do not necessarily denote a deficiency. However, the RDA can serve as a goal or recommendation for the nutrient intake of individuals.

2.3. Adequate Intake

When there is insufficient scientific evidence to set an EAR, no RDA can be determined. In such cases, an AI is set based on the levels of nutrients consumed by apparently healthy individuals. The AI, though a less exact measure than the RDA, is assumed to be adequate for nearly all healthy individuals in a population. Like the RDA, the AI can serve as a goal or recommendation for the nutrient intake of individuals.

2.4. Tolerable Upper Intake Level

The UL represents the highest average level of nutrient intake that poses no risk of adverse health effects. Intakes above the UL increase risk of toxicity.

2.5. Estimated Energy Requirement

The EER represents the average intake of energy necessary to maintain energy balance for healthy individuals. Values for EER are calculated using equations that take into consideration age, gender, weight, height, and physical activity. Although EER may be calculated for four different activity levels (sedentary, low active, active, and very active), optimal health is consistent with "active" level or higher of physical activity. Like the EAR, the EER represents the average estimated need for individuals. This is done, rather making a generous recommendation, in order to avoid intakes that are excessive for most individuals.

2.6. Acceptable Macronutrient Distribution Ranges

The AMDR represents the range of healthful intakes for carbohydrate, fat, and protein, expressed as a percentage of total energy intake. These ranges were set at amounts determined to reduce the risk of chronic diseases, such as obesity, heart disease, diabetes, and cancer, while providing adequate nutrients. Additional recommendations are given for cholesterol, trans fats, saturated fats, and added sugar.

3. LIMITS AND USES OF THE DRI

3.1. Limits

Careful use of the DRI as a tool for diet assessment and planning must take several limiting factors into consideration. First, the DRI applies to healthy individuals; it is not intended for people who are malnourished or who have disease conditions that alter nutrient needs. Second, the values represent average intakes. The intakes of individuals vary from day to day, and minor deviations from the DRI are not cause for concern. Third, the DRI represents recommended intake of nutrients from food rather than from supplements. The whole food package delivers a mix of nutrients and non-nutrients that are consistent with health. Attempting to meet the DRI recommendations through use of supplements rather than food is likely to result in a loss of balance in the diet. Fourth, the DRIs should be considered a benchmark against which to assess adequacy, not a minimum requirement. Lastly, it must be understood that the true nutrient needs of any one individual cannot be known, and, therefore, comparing intake to the DRI should be only one part of the assessment process.

3.2. Statistical Analysis

Because of the statistical basis used to develop the DRI, it is possible to use statistical equations to calculate the probability that an individual's diet is inadequate, adequate, or excessive in a particular nutrient. The *Dietary Reference Intakes, the Essential Guide to Nutrient Requirements (1)* explains these assessment techniques.

3.3. General Guidelines for Diet Assessment of Individuals

For general purposes, the following guidelines may apply.

- For nutrient intakes below an established EAR, the probability of adequacy is less than 50%, so intake likely needs to be increased.
- For nutrient intakes between the established EAR and the RDA, intake probably needs to be increased.
- For nutrient intakes at or above the RDA or AI, intake is likely to be adequate, as long as it reflects long-term intake.
- For nutrient intakes below the AI, it cannot be said with confidence that intake is deficient; however, intake should probably be increased to the level of the AI in order to ensure adequacy.
- For intakes below the UL, there is little or no risk of adverse effects.
- For intakes above the UL, there is increased risk for adverse effects, so intake should be decreased.
- For energy nutrients, intakes between the lower and upper levels set by the AMDR are acceptable. Intakes below or above the AMDR probably need to be adjusted.

• The EER is not an appropriate tool for nutrition assessment. Body mass index (BMI) is a better tool for assessing energy intake over the long term.

In sum, intakes above the RDA or AI, and below the UL are most likely to be adequate without risk of adverse effects. Appendix C presents a simplified table of DRI values (RDA and AI).

4. DRI AND THE CONSUMER

The DRI forms the scientific basis for public policy, including nutrition labeling, fortification of foods, menu-planning requirements for school meals, and composition of supplemental food packages given to low-income women participating in the Women, Infants, and Children Program *(5)*.

Because of the complexity of the DRI, *The Dietary Guidelines for Americans 2005* was created and published by the US Department of Health and Human Services and the US Department of Agriculture (USDA). It provides dietary guidance in the form of recommendations to promote health and reduce the risk of chronic disease. The Dietary Guidelines Advisory Committee used the DRI when creating the Guidelines *(6)*.

MyPyramid (the new version of the Food Guide Pyramid) is a graphic representation of the advice provided by the Dietary Guidelines. This is further described in Chapter 11. The DRI is used as a basis for comparison to ensure that the intake patterns recommended by MyPyramid are nutritionally adequate. Population-weighted averages of typical food choices from the MyPyramid food groups provide nutrient intakes at or above the DRI recommendations for nearly all nutrients *(6)*.

Individuals who use MyPyramid to guide their food choices and the Dietary Guidelines to inform their dietary habits are likely to consume adequate nutrients over the long term.

5. SUMMARY

The DRI replaces and expands upon the RDAs used in the United States and the RNIs used in Canada. The four sets of DRI reference values can be used to assess and plan the diets of individuals and groups. For individuals, the EAR can be used to statistically assess the probability that the diet is adequate in particular nutrients over the long term. For general consumer purposes a diet that provides nutrients above the RDA or AI and below the UL is likely to provide adequate nutrients without risk of adverse effects. A diet chosen in accordance with MyPyramid can provide nutrients within those limits.

SUGGESTED FURTHER READING

Institute of Medicine. Dietary Reference Intakes: The Essential Guide to Nutrient Requirements. National Academies Press, Washington, DC, 2006.

Barr SI, Murphy SP, Agurs-Collins TD, Poos MI. Planning diets for individuals using the Dietary Reference Intakes. Nutr Rev 2003; 61:352–360.

Barr SI, Murphy SP, Poos MI. Interpreting and using the Dietary Reference Intakes in dietary assessment of individuals and groups. J Am Diet Assoc 2002; 102:780–788.

Murphy, SP, Guenther PM, Kretsch MJ. Using the Dietary Reference Intakes to assess the intakes of groups: pitfalls to avoid. J Am Diet Assoc 2006; 106:1550–1553.

Murphy SP, Barr SI. Challenges in using the Dietary Reference Intakes to plan diets for groups. Nutr Rev 2005; 63:267–271.

REFERENCES

1. Institute of Medicine. Dietary Reference Intakes: The Essential Guide to Nutrient Requirements. National Academies Press, Washington, DC, 2006.
2. Paik HY. Dietary Reference Intakes for Koreans (KDRIs). Asia Pac J Clin Nutr 2008; 17(S2):416–419.
3. Sasaki S. Dietary Reference Intakes (DRIs) in Japan. Asia Pac J Clin Nutr 2008; 17(S2):420–444.
4. Spaaji CJK. New dietary reference intakes in the Netherlands for energy, proteins, fats, and digestible carbohydrates. Eur J Clin Nutr 2004; 58:191–194.
5. Committee on Use of Dietary Reference Intakes in Nutrition Labeling, Institute of Medicine. Dietary Reference Intakes: Guiding Principles for Nutrition Labeling and Fortification. Nutr Rev 2004; 62:73–79.
6. U.S. Department of Health and Human Services and U.S. Department of Agriculture. Dietary Guidelines for Americans, 2005. 6th ed. Government Printing Office, Washington, DC, 2005.

6 Food Labels and Sources of Nutrients: Sorting the Wheat from the Chaff

Karen M. Gibson, Norman J. Temple, and Asima R. Anwar

Key Points

- Food labels provide the information needed to guide the selection of foods that will help individuals meet nutrition and health goals.
- This chapter explains how to best utilize the information contained on food labels.
- The chapter lists the major nutrients provided by the food groups and by various foods.
- The chapter also lists major food sources of various nutrients.

Key Words: Nutrition labeling; daily value; health claims; food sources of select nutrients

1. THE NUTRITION FACTS LABEL

Many consumers read food labels to help them make healthy choices. But labels are only useful if one knows how to use them. Unfortunately, the ease of comprehension leaves much to be desired. Regulations require that nutritionally important nutrients or food components found in a food must be listed on the Nutrition Facts Label *(1, 2)*. A typical Nutrition Facts Label is shown in Fig. 1. The label addresses nutrients that are associated with certain chronic diseases or with nutrient deficiencies. By law, a food label must contain the following information:

- List of ingredients arranged in descending order by weight (main ingredient first).

From: *Nutrition and Health: Nutrition Guide for Physicians*
Edited by: T. Wilson et al. (eds.), DOI 10.1007/978-1-60327-431-9_6,
© Humana Press, a part of Springer Science+Business Media, LLC 2010

Nutrition Facts

Serving Size 1 cup (228g)
Servings Per Container 2

Amount Per Serving

Calories 250   Calories from Fat 110

                                                        % Daily Value*

Total Fat 12g	**18%**
Saturated Fat 3g	**15%**
Trans Fat 3g	
Cholesterol 30mg	**10%**
Sodium 470mg	**20%**
Potassium 700mg	**20%**
Total Carbohydrate 31g	**10%**
Dietary Fiber 0g	**0%**
Sugars 5g	
Protein 5g	

Vitamin A	4%
Vitamin C	2%
Calcium	20%
Iron	4%

* Percent Daily Values are based on a 2,000 calorie diet.
Your Daily Values may be higher or lower depending on
your calorie needs.

		Calories:	2,000	2,500
Total Fat	Less than		65g	80g
Sat Fat	Less than		20g	25g
Cholesterol	Less than		300mg	300mg
Sodium	Less than		2,400mg	2,400mg
Total Carbohydrate			300g	375g
Dietary Fiber			25g	30g

Fig. 1. Sample nutrition facts label.

- Serving size (using a standardized serving size), plus the number of servings per container.
- Amount per serving of the following: total calories, fat, total fat, saturated fat, trans fat, cholesterol, sodium, total carbohydrate, dietary fiber, sugars, protein, vitamins A and C, calcium, and iron. However, if the food has a negligible amount of a particular food component, then it may be omitted from the label.
- The sugars listed on the label include naturally occurring sugars (like those in fruit and milk) as well as those added to a food or drink. Check the ingredient list for specifics on added sugars.
- Other information may be included but this is optional unless the product is making a claim regarding that particular nutrient.

A key number is the serving size. This is stated in familiar units, such as cups or pieces, followed by the metric amount, such as the number of grams. In general, serving sizes are standardized to make it easier to compare similar foods. For example, the serving size for all ice creams is half a cup and all beverages are 8 oz. It is important to be aware that the serving size indicated on a food label may not represent the amount a person actually eats on one occasion. In addition, the serving sizes on food labels are not always the same as those of the USDA Food Guide or the diabetic exchange plan. A serving of rice on a food label is one cup, whereas in the USDA Food Guide and exchange list, it is half a cup.

When looking at the serving size, consumers need to compare the serving size listed with the amount of the food that they will actually eat. In the sample label above, for example, one serving of this food equals one cup. But if the consumer eats the whole package (i.e., two cups), that obviously doubles the calories and other nutrient amounts. [Note: In this chapter we use the word calories for consistency with actual food labels. However, in the rest of this book, calories are abbreviated as kcal.]

Another feature of food labels is the use of Daily Values (DVs). DVs are shown on the sample label (right and bottom of Fig. 1). They reflect dietary recommendations for nutrients and dietary components that have important relationships with health. The DV indicates how much of a nutrient that should be obtained in the daily diet. The DVs cover cholesterol, sodium, and potassium as well as the macronutrients that are sources of energy, namely carbohydrate (including fiber) and fat. A %DV for protein is only listed if the food is meant for use by infants or children. Not all nutrients have a %DV listed. Reference DVs for trans fat and sugars have not been established. Amounts are shown based on a 2,000 and a 2,500 calorie diet. A 2,000 calorie diet is considered about right for sedentary younger women, active older women, and sedentary older men. A 2,500 calorie diet is considered about right for many men, teenage boys, and active younger women.

The DVs are based on the following allowances:

Total fat: maximum of 30% of calories
Saturated fat: maximum of 10% of calories
Carbohydrates: minimum of 60% of calories
Protein: 10% of calories
Fiber: 12.5 g of fiber per 1,000 calories
Cholesterol: maximum of 300 mg
Sodium: maximum of 2,400 mg

Food labels list the amount of a nutrient in a serving of the food as a percentage of its DV (Fig. 1). In other words, the DV for a nutrient represents the percentage contribution one serving of the food makes to the daily diet for that nutrient based on current recommendations for healthful diets. The * used after the heading "%Daily Value" refers to the footnote located at the bottom of the Nutrition Facts Label. This reminds the consumer that the %DVs listed on the label are based on a 2,000 calorie diet only. A lower DV

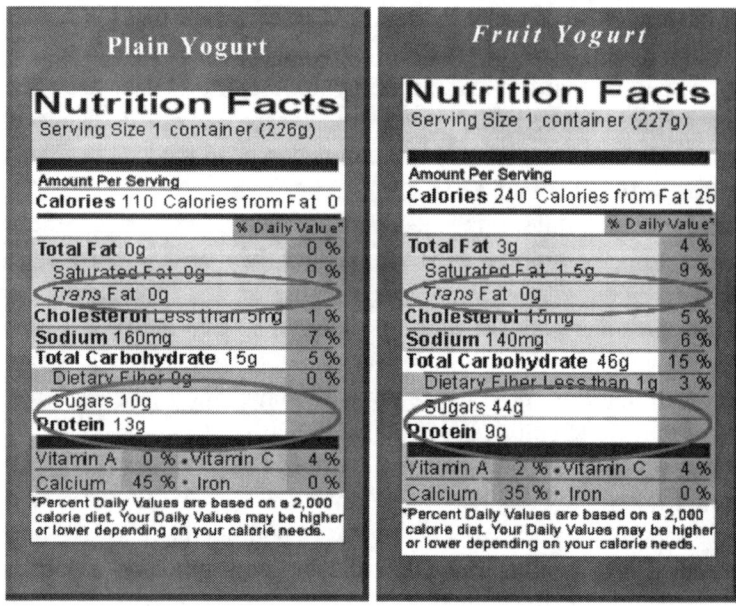

Fig. 2. Labels from containers of yogurt.

is desirable for total fat, saturated fat, cholesterol, and sodium; a DV of 5% or less is a good indicator. A higher DV is desirable for total carbohydrates, dietary fiber, iron, calcium, vitamins A and C, and other vitamins and minerals that may be listed, with 10% or more representing a good source, while a DV of 20% is considered high.

The above explanation for DVs may seem rather confusing. However, DVs are very easy to use in practice. The "%Daily Value" helps consumers easily see whether a food contributes a little or a lot of a nutrient.

2. USING THE NUTRITION FACTS LABEL

Lets now put the above information to use. Fig. 2 shows the labels from two containers of yogurt. For this purpose we will assume that the subject, Harry, is an active man. This means his energy intake is around 2,500 calories. Which is the healthier choice for Harry?

In each case the whole container is one serving. Examination of the labels reveals the following notable facts:

- The fruit yogurt has 3 g of fat. Half of this (1.5 g) is saturated fat. This represents 9% of the DV in a 2,000 calorie diet. As Harry's energy intake is higher, the percentage in his case will be lower. If Harry has concerns about his blood cholesterol, then the plain yogurt is preferable.

- The plain yogurt has a much lower energy content (110 vs. 240 calories). This is because it contains much less fat and sugar. If Harry is watching his weight, then this is an important consideration.
- Being a milk product, yogurt is a rich source of calcium. We see that both types of yogurt have a high percentage for this nutrient.
- Sodium is a vital number to look at as many processed foods contain excessive amounts. The plain yogurt contains 160 mg. This is similar to the amount in a cup of milk.
- The plain yogurt contains more protein (13 vs. 9 g). This is of little importance as protein excess or deficiency is seldom a problem. Appendix III informs us that Harry's recommended intake (RDA) is 56 g, an amount that is readily obtainable from the diet.
- The supermarket customer might be tempted to buy the yogurt marked "Fruit Yogurt" in large letters on the front of the container, making the assumption that it contains significant amounts of fruit. The container might even have large colored images of fruits. But a closer inspection of the Nutrition Facts Label reveals that this yogurt has no more vitamin C and barely any more fiber than the plain yogurt.

Let's now summarize the key rules for reading labels:

- Read the list of ingredients. Always remember that the large print on the front of the container may be misleading.
- Learning all the rules is ideal. But most people do not have the inclination for that. The next best thing is to focus on four key numbers: calories, sodium, saturated fat, and fiber. Start by figuring out reasonable targets for each of these. For Harry, in the above example, he may be well motivated to keep himself healthy and will set his targets at 2,500 calories, 1,800 mg sodium, 20 g saturated fat, and 32 g fiber.
- For each food determine these four values. This must be based on the amount actually eaten. The food can then be evaluated based on either the actual amounts or the percentages. As a simple litmus test, if the numbers for these four values are consistent with a healthy diet, then everything else will probably fall into place.

Lastly, we will look at how the calorie content of food is calculated. Fat contains 9 calories/g, while carbohydrate and protein each have 4. So fruit yogurt has 27 calories as fat (3 times 9), 184 as carbohydrate (46 times 4), and 36 as protein (9 times 4). This adds up to 257 calories. The discrepancies with the numbers on the label are because of rounding errors. Knowing how to make these calculations can be useful. For example, examination of a food label followed by a quick calculation may reveal, for example, that half the energy in a cake comes from fat.

While reading food labels can obviously be very informative, many people may wish to know the total nutrient and energy content of their diet. Appendix II gives web sites that allow this to be done at no cost.

3. MAJOR NUTRIENT CONTRIBUTIONS OF THE FOOD GROUPS AND OF VARIOUS FOODS

Below is listed the major nutrient(s) found in each of the food groups.

Fruit: vitamins A and C, folate, potassium, and fiber.

Vegetables: vitamins A, C, E, and K, folate, magnesium, potassium, and fiber.

Grains: folate, niacin, riboflavin, thiamin, iron, magnesium, selenium, and fiber.

Meat, fish, poultry, and eggs: protein, niacin, thiamin, vitamins B_6 and B_{12}, iron, magnesium, potassium, and zinc.

Legumes and nuts: protein, folate, thiamin, vitamin E, iron, magnesium, potassium, zinc, and fiber.

Milk, yogurt, and cheese: protein, riboflavin, vitamin B_{12}, calcium, magnesium, and potassium. In addition, vitamins A and D are present if the food is fortified.

Oils: vitamin E and polyunsaturated fats. Vegetable oils, such as corn oil, sunflower oil, and most brands of soft margarine, are rich sources of n–6 polyunsaturated fats. Oils rich in n–3 polyunsaturated fats include flaxseed oil (a rich source), followed by soybean oil and then canola oil.

4. FOOD SOURCES OF SELECT NUTRIENTS

4.1. Lipids

Polyunsaturated fat: *See* above information on oils. The n–3 fats in plant oils are mainly linolenic acid. Rich source of n–3 fats include fatty fish, such as sardines, mackerel, salmon, trout, and herring. Fish oils are particularly rich in the long-chain n–3 fats (DHA and EPA).

Saturated fat: most animal fats including whole milk, cream, butter and cheese; fatty cuts of beef and pork, poultry and lamb products, tropical oils including palm, palm kernel, and coconut oils.

Trans fat: hard margarine (made with hydrogenated oils), deep-fried foods, cakes, cookies, donuts, pastry, crackers, snack chips, and imitation cheese. Some meat and dairy products are minor sources.

Cholesterol: eggs, liver, milk products (if high in fat), meat, poultry, and shellfish.

4.2. Dietary Fiber

Whole grain products such as barley, oats, oat bran, and rye; fruits, legumes, seeds and husks, and vegetables.

4.3. Vitamins

Folate: dark green vegetables, dry beans, peas and lentils, enriched grain products, fortified cereals, liver, orange juice, and wheat germ.

Vitamin A: liver, dark green and deep orange or rich yellow vegetables and fruits (broccoli, apricots, cantaloupe, carrots, squash, sweet potatoes, pumpkin), and fortified foods such as milk and milk products, butter, and eggs.

Vitamin B_6: bananas, fish (most), liver, meat, nuts and seeds, potatoes and sweet potatoes, poultry, and whole grain and fortified cereals.

Vitamin B_{12}: eggs, fish and shellfish, fortified cereals, meat, milk and milk products, and organ meats.

Vitamin C: citrus fruits, dark green vegetables (such as bell peppers, broccoli, cabbage, Brussels sprouts and cauliflower), cantaloupe, strawberries, tomatoes, potatoes, papayas, and mangoes.

Vitamin D: egg yolk, fortified cereals, fortified milk, liver, and fatty fish.

Vitamin E: margarine, nuts and seeds, peanuts and peanut butter, vegetable oils, wheat germ, and whole grain and fortified cereals.

Vitamin K: broccoli, Brussels sprouts, cabbage, leafy green vegetables, mayonnaise, and soybean.

4.4. Minerals

Calcium: milk and milk products, some brands of tofu, corn tortillas, some nuts such as almonds, greens such as bok choy, mustard, and turnip greens, and broccoli.

Iodine: iodized salt, saltwater fish, and shellfish.

Iron: meats, fish, and poultry; eggs, legumes, whole grains, and enriched or fortified breads and cereals. Dark green leafy vegetables and dried fruits contribute some iron.

Magnesium: cocoa and chocolate, most dark green vegetables, dry beans, peas, and lentils, fish, nuts and seeds, peanuts and peanut butter, and whole grains.

Sodium: foods prepared in brine such as pickles, olives, and sauerkraut; salty or smoked meats such as lunch meats, corned, or chipped beef, ham, hot dogs, sausage; salty or smoked fish, canned and instant soups, condiments such as bouillon cubes, MSG, mustard, catsup, and sauces such as soy, teriyaki, Worcestershire, and barbeque.

Zinc: dry beans, peas, lentils, meat, poultry, seeds, shellfish, whole grain, and fortified cereals.

5. HEALTH CLAIMS

Certain health claims may be stated on food labels. These are authorized by the Food and Drug Administration (FDA) and are meant to inform shoppers that certain foods, nutrients, or ingredients – as part of an overall healthy diet – may reduce the risk of a specific disease. The FDA authorizes these types of health claims based on an extensive review of the scientific literature. Certain health claims can also be made as a result of a successful notification to the FDA of a health claim based on an "authoritative statement" from a scientific body of the U.S. government or the National Academy of Sciences. The science behind some health claims is stronger than for others. For example, the link between heart disease risk and saturated fat and cholesterol is solid, according to the FDA. The agency therefore allows the following statement: "Diets low in saturated fat and cholesterol may reduce the risk of heart disease." In comparison, the evidence relating folic acid, vitamin B6, and vitamin B12 to reduced risk of cardiovascular disease is still emerging. Therefore, the language allowed by the FDA is such: "As part of a well-balanced diet that is low in saturated fat and cholesterol, folic acid, vitamin B6 and vitamin B12 may reduce the risk of vascular disease."

There are currently 12 approved health claims for food labels and these are listed below:

- Calcium and osteoporosis
- Sodium and hypertension
- Dietary fat and cancer
- Dietary saturated fat and cholesterol and risk of coronary heart disease (CHD)
- Fiber-containing grain products, fruit, and vegetables and cancer
- Fruits, vegetables, and grain products that contain fiber, particularly soluble fiber, and risk of CHD
- Fruits and vegetables and cancer
- Folate and neural tube defects
- Dietary noncariogenic carbohydrate sweeteners and dental caries
- Soluble fiber from certain foods and risk of CHD
- Soy protein and risk of CHD
- Plant sterol/stanol esters and risk of CHD

Health Claims Authorized Based on an Authoritative Statement by Federal Scientific Bodies:

- Whole grain food and risk of CHD and certain cancers
- Potassium and the risk of high blood pressure and stroke
- Fluoridated water and reduced risk of dental caries
- Saturated fat, cholesterol, and *trans* fat, and reduced risk of CHD

If we go back to the example used above with Harry and the yogurt containers, both items may use the health claim "foods high in calcium, along with a healthy diet and regular exercise, may help reduce the incidence of osteoporosis."

In addition to "health claims," food labels may also contain nutrient content claims. These words now have strict definitions as listed below:

- Free: synonyms include "zero," "no," "without," "negligible source of"
- Low: synonyms include "little," "few" (for calories), "contain a small amount of"
- Reduced/less: synonyms include "lower" ("fewer" for calories)

SUGGESTED FURTHER READING

This website from the FDA provides an explanation on how to understand and use the Nutrition Facts Label. http://www.cfsan.fda.gov/~dms/foodlab.html

Taylor CL, Wilkening VL. How the nutrition food label was developed, part 1: The nutrition facts panel. J Am Diet Assoc 2008; 108:437–442.

Taylor CL, Wilkening VL. How the nutrition food label was developed, part 2: The purpose and promise of nutrition claims. J Am Diet Assoc 2008; 108:618–623.

This website provides much information about the composition of foods and the sources of nutrients. http://www.nutritiondata.com operated by NutritionData

A Canadian website can be found by doing a Google search for "nutrient value of some common foods". This provides detailed information on the nutrition content of large numbers of foods.

REFERENCES

1. Taylor CL, Wilkening VL. How the nutrition food label was developed, part 1: The nutrition facts panel. J Am Diet Assoc 2008; 108:437–442.
2. Taylor CL, Wilkening VL. How the nutrition food label was developed, part 2: The purpose and promise of nutrition claims. J Am Diet Assoc 2008; 108:618–623.

7 Vegetarian and Vegan Diets: Weighing the Claims

Claire McEvoy and Jayne V. Woodside

Key Points

- 1–10% of the population in developed countries are thought to be vegetarian, with higher numbers among women.
- Vegetarian and vegan diets are heterogeneous in nature, which makes provision of dietary recommendations difficult.
- Populations following vegetarian diets have potential health benefits including reduced risk of coronary heart disease and obesity.
- Very restrictive or unbalanced vegetarian diets can result in nutrient deficiencies, particularly iron, calcium, zinc, and vitamins B_{12} and D.
- Carefully planned vegetarian and vegan diets can provide adequate nutrition for all stages of life.

Key Words: Vegetarian diets; vegan diet; Mediterranean diet; health benefits; plant-based diets; nutrient deficiencies; plant proteins

1. INTRODUCTION

Vegetarian diets are becoming increasingly popular in developed countries. While no reliable prevalence data for vegetarian populations exists, results of polls and surveys have reported population prevalence of between 1 and 10% in the European Union, United States, and Canada *(1)*. A recent study in the United States reported that 2.8% of respondents never ate meat, poultry, fish, or seafood, although 4–10% would classify themselves as vegetarian *(2)*. Vegetarian diets are often heterogeneous in nature, involving a wide range of dietary practices. These are summarized in Table 1. Even within classifications of dietary practices there can be a high level of variability depending on the individual dietary restriction(s). Vegetarian or

From: *Nutrition and Health: Nutrition Guide for Physicians*
Edited by: T. Wilson et al. (eds.), DOI 10.1007/978-1-60327-431-9_7,
© Humana Press, a part of Springer Science+Business Media, LLC 2010

Table 1
Classification of Vegetarian and Vegan Diets

Vegetarian Diet	Description
Semi- or demi-	Excludes red meat. May exclude poultry. Fish is usually eaten
Piscatarian	Excludes red meat and poultry but includes fish and possibly shellfish
Lacto-ovo-	Excludes all meat, poultry, and fish. Milk, milk products, and eggs are usually eaten
Vegan	Consumes no foods of animal origin. Emphasis on plant foods, grains, legumes, nuts, seeds, and vegetable oils
Raw food	An extreme form of veganism with the emphasis on organic, home-grown, or wild foods in their raw or natural state. Usually comprises 80% by weight raw plants. Periods of fasting and laxative use may be practiced
Fruitarian	An extreme form of veganism, which excludes all foods of animal origin and also living plants. Diet is mainly raw: 70–80% fruit with small amounts of beans, bread, tofu, nuts, and seeds
Macrobiotic	This extreme diet progresses through 10 levels becoming increasingly restrictive. It is based on 50–60% whole grain, 25–30% fruit and vegetables (fruits can also be restricted), 5–10% beans and sea vegetables, and restricted beverages. Fish may be eaten initially 2–3 times per week. Foods may be gradually eliminated through the 10 levels. At the final level only cereal (brown rice) is eaten

vegan diets may be practiced for a variety of reasons, including health, cultural, philosophical, religious, and ecological beliefs, or simply because of taste preferences. This chapter will discuss vegetarian and vegan diets and their contribution to human health.

2. HEALTH BENEFITS OF VEGETARIAN DIETS

There has been renewed interest in the proposed benefit of plant-based diets in reducing the risk of chronic diseases such as cardiovascular disease (CVD), cancer, and type 2 diabetes. Mediterranean-style diets are associated with a reduced risk of CVD; this occurs through modification of known risk factors, including blood pressure, body mass index (BMI), insulin resistance, and lipid profiles. The Mediterranean diet is characterized by a moderate/low intake of red meat and an increased intake of monounsaturated fat, fresh fruit, vegetables, legumes, nuts, dietary fiber, and oily fish. Balanced vegetarian diets also tend to be rich in complex carbohydrate, dietary fiber, n–6 fatty acids, folic acid, vitamins C and E, and magnesium. However, in contrast to a Mediterranean or omnivorous diet, vegetarian diets (particularly vegan diets) tend to be lower in protein, n–3 fatty acids, vitamins A and B_{12}, zinc, and calcium; this is due to the absence of red meat, animal protein, and/or dairy products.

Epidemiological evidence suggests that vegetarians have a relatively low mortality rate compared to the general Western population (3–5). Much of this evidence comes from studies where different populations have been compared. However, we must at this point inject a note of caution. These studies have investigated health-conscious populations such as Seventh Day Adventists. Such populations not only have a high prevalence of vegetarianism but also generally have numerous other lifestyle differences from the general population, including consuming little alcohol, having low rates of smoking, and possibly having increased levels of physical activity. These confounding factors make it difficult for epidemiologists to disentangle the role of vegetarianism from the other factors. Another line of research is prospective cohort studies, i.e., comparing vegetarians vs. omnivores within the same population and tracking the development of disease. In addition to nutritional differences, vegetarians typically have lifestyle differences from omnivores, making it extremely difficult to make definitive conclusions regarding the relationship between a vegetarian diet and risk of disease. The above problems apply to studies on the relationship between vegetarianism and specific diseases, such as CVD and cancer.

2.1. Vegetarian Diets and Cardiovascular Disease (CVD)

Several epidemiological studies have reported that vegetarians have a reduced risk of CVD when compared to omnivores. In particular, they have a lower risk of coronary heart disease (CHD). Generally, the lowest risk is seen in those eating fish but not meat. These findings may be explained, in part, by the observed differences in lipid profiles, blood pressure, and weight measures.

2.1.1. VEGETARIAN DIET AND SERUM LIPIDS

Vegetarians generally have lower serum levels of total cholesterol, low-density lipoprotein (LDL)-cholesterol, and triglycerides when compared to omnivores. This can be explained, to a large extent, by the fact that vegetarian diets, particularly vegan diets, tend to be lower in saturated fat and trans fat and higher in dietary fiber compared to omnivorous diets *(6)*.

Nuts are consumed more frequently in vegetarian diets and they are inversely correlated with CHD risk. Nuts, especially almonds and hazelnuts, are high in monounsaturated fat and have produced appreciable reductions in LDL-cholesterol. This topic is also discussed in Chapter 1.

2.1.2. VEGETARIAN DIETS AND BLOOD PRESSURE

Vegetarian diets appear to reduce blood pressure which is associated with risk of CVD (i.e., both CHD and stroke) *(5, 6)*. Nonvegetarians prescribed vegetarian diets demonstrate lower blood pressure in both normotensive and hypertensive subjects. Furthermore, the prevalence of hypertension appears to be lower in vegetarian populations, especially vegans *(7)*.

Important findings came from the Dietary Approaches to Stop Hypertension (DASH) study. The DASH diet had a significant lowering effect on blood pressure, independent of sodium intake, in both hypertensive and normotensive adults *(8)*. The DASH diet is largely plant based, high in nuts, allows plenty of low-fat milk, recommends fish/chicken rather than red meat, and is low in saturated fat, cholesterol, and refined carbohydrates. The diet is therefore similar to a varied vegetarian diet.

2.2. Vegetarian Diets and Obesity

Vegetarians, and particularly vegans, have lower body weights than the general population, with a low prevalence of obesity *(6, 9, 10)*. BMI is on average 1–2 kg/m^2 less in vegetarians and vegans compared with nonvegetarians *(6, 9, 10)*. Actual nutrient intakes in vegetarian diets are discussed in more detail later in this chapter.

2.3. Cancer

It is widely recognized that diet is one of the most important avoidable causes of cancer after smoking. It has been suggested that approximately one third of cancer deaths can be avoided by changes in diet *(11)*. There is little scientific evidence evaluating whole dietary approaches in the prevention of cancer, therefore limited recommendations advocating vegetarian diets can be made. However, there is some good evidence for a protective effect of some dietary components that are more likely to be consumed in greater frequency within a vegetarian diet. Fruit and vegetable intake have been found to be protective for certain cancers, particularly for mouth, esophageal, larynx, lung, gastric, and possibly prostate cancer *(11, 12)*. It is currently recommended that diets should include 400 g of total fruit and vegetables per day, which equates to about 4 or 5 servings *(11, 12)*.

Additionally, there is a growing body of evidence demonstrating a very direct and positive relationship between red and processed meat consumption and colon cancer risk. A recent meta-analysis concluded that the risk of colorectal cancer increased 24% for each daily increase of 120 g of red meat and 36% for each daily increase of 30 g of processed meat *(13)*. Preliminary results of the European Prospective Investigation Cancer and Nutrition (EPIC), involving approximately 520,000 adults in 10 European countries, recorded 1,329 incident cases of colorectal cancer. The investigators observed a 35% higher risk of colorectal cancer when >160 g/d of red meat is consumed compared with 20 g/d *(14)*. A significant negative association between dietary fiber and colorectal cancer risk was also observed.

2.4. Type 2 Diabetes

Clinical studies investigating the impact of vegan/vegetarian diets in people with type 2 diabetes have shown significant reductions in fasting blood sugar, cholesterol, and triglyceride levels *(15)*. Epidemiological studies have supported the hypothesis that vegetarian diets protect against type 2 diabetes. The Seventh Day Adventist study in the United States reported a significantly reduced incidence of diabetes in vegetarians compared with nonvegetarians *(4)*. Additionally, data from the prospective Health Professionals follow-up study in 42,500 men over 12 yr reported that frequent consumption of processed meat was associated with a 46% increase in the risk of type 2 diabetes *(16)*. However, these important findings are confounded by significant weight loss in the intervention group throughout the diet period, in addition to increased exercise and lifestyle modifications in some cases.

2.5. Bone Health

Adequate calcium intake is important for optimal bone mineral density. This is achievable for vegetarians consuming dairy products but may be more difficult for vegans. There is surprisingly little information regarding long-term bone health of vegans although there is some suggestion that bone mineral density may be reduced especially in those following macrobiotic diets. However, bone quality is also important for fracture prevention. There is a growing body of evidence suggesting that a diet high in fruit and vegetables and low in animal protein can reduce the renal acid load and therefore reduce calcium loss and bone resorption *(17)*.

3. NUTRIENT DEFICIENCIES IN VEGETARIAN DIETS

Carefully planned vegetarian and vegan diets can provide adequate nutrients for optimum health *(18)*. Evidence suggests that infants and children can be successfully reared on vegan and vegetarian diets *(19, 20)*. However, all dietary practices, including nonvegetarian diets, can be deleterious for health if essential nutrients are not consumed according to individual needs. Therefore, it is essential that vegetarian and vegan diets contain a balance of nutrients from a wide variety of foods. If the diet becomes more restrictive, the risk of nutritional deficiencies increases. This is particularly the case for infants and children, and for women who are pregnant, lactating, or menstruating. Nutrients most likely to be deficient in unbalanced or very restrictive vegetarian diets are energy, protein, calcium, iron, zinc, vitamins D and B_{12}, and n–3 fatty acids. These are discussed in more detail below.

3.1. Energy

Energy intakes are comparable in vegetarian and nonvegetarians *(21)*. However, energy intake may be of concern in vegan infants and children, particularly those following macrobiotic or raw food diets. The growth rates of vegetarian children have been found to be similar to nonvegetarian children *(21)*. However, vegan children can show a tendency for smaller stature when compared to a reference population; height measurements may still reside within normal limits and catch-up growth usually occurs by the age of 10 yr *(20)*. In a UK study, vegan children, both boys and girls, were found to be slightly lighter than a reference population *(21)*. This may, of course, be advantageous. Failure to thrive in infants and children has been observed in extremely restrictive diets, such as fruitarian diets, and these diets are not recommended for children. Furthermore, protein-energy malnutrition and nutrient deficiencies have been reported in infants and children fed inappropriate vegetarian diets *(21)*. The vegan diet is bulky, owing to increased amounts of dietary fiber which may cause early satiety in children, thereby limiting energy intake. Frequent meals and snacks, using soy protein, and alternative fat sources can be used to increase the energy density of the diet and support growth and development in vegan children. Nut and nut butters, which are calorific, can be introduced after 3 yr *(19)*.

3.2. Protein

Protein intakes tend to be lower in vegetarian and vegan adults and children *(20, 21)*. Protein is reported as approximately 12% of energy intake, which is sufficient for nitrogen balance, *provided energy intake is adequate (21)*. Plant proteins tend to have lower biological values than animal protein and the protein is in a less utilizable form. However, when a wide range of plant protein is consumed (soy protein, textured vegetable protein, legumes, nuts, seeds, and grains), essential amino acid requirements can be adequately met. It is generally felt that there is no need for protein combining at mealtimes *(20)*. Protein requirements may be higher in vegan athletes, lactating or pregnant women, infants, and children. Infants should be breastfed exclusively for the first 6 mo or a commercial soy-based formula used. Products such as home-prepared milks, rice milk, nut, or seed milk should not be used to replace breast milk or commercial soy milk for infants under 1 yr due to differences in macronutrient and micronutrient ratio. The weaning guidelines for vegetarian infants are the same as nonvegetarian infants *(18)*. Protein requirements are therefore most likely to be met in vegan diets when adequate energy intake is consumed.

3.3. Calcium

Calcium intakes are adequate for lactovegetarians but can be lower than recommended amounts in vegan adults and children *(19, 20)*. Good sources of calcium in vegan diets are shown in Table 2, and a general discussion of calcium and bone health can be found in Chapter 30.

When calcium intake is lower, intestinal absorption is greater; adequate calcium intake for bone mass may therefore be achievable at a lower calcium intake. Additionally, high intake of protein, sodium, and caffeine increase body losses of calcium. Owing to their reduced intake of these dietary components vegans may therefore be able to conserve a higher proportion of dietary calcium intake than omnivores *(21)*. However, any advantage for calcium absorption in vegans could be offset by the high phytate and oxalate content of the vegan diet. Low oxalate green vegetables such as cabbages, spring greens, and kale have higher calcium bioavailability (49–61%) and should be consumed regularly by vegans *(18)*. For optimal calcium intake in vegetarians and vegans, the American Dietetic Association recommends a minimum of eight servings per day of bioavailable calcium foods such as those listed in Table 2 *(18)*. This requirement may be greater in teenagers and women who are lactating or pregnant.

3.4. Iron

Iron deficiency can occur as a result of inadequate intake but also because of poor absorption from the GI tract. An adequate intake of iron in vegetarians and vegans can easily be achieved, assuming their diet is balanced. However, plant sources of nonheme iron are less bioavailable than heme iron found in meat. Phytate, soy protein, and polyphenols/tannins within the plant-based diet can inhibit iron absorption. For that reason, it is

Table 2
Main Sources of Nutrients in Vegetarian/Vegan Diets *(18)*

Nutrient	Main Vegetarian Source	Amount Per Average Serving	Notes
Calcium	Green vegetables (broccoli, cabbage, collard greens, bok choy, turnip greens, kale) Fortified soy products (milk, yogurts, tofu, tempeh) Fortified cereals Dried figs *(5)* Almonds Sesame tahini	79–239 mg 92–430 mg 55–315 mg 137 mg 88 mg 128 mg	Oxalate/phytate reduces bioavailability Intestinal absorption increases when intake reduced
Iron	Cooked soybeans, tofu, tempeh Cooked legumes (lentils, chickpeas, adzuki, kidney) Dried pumpkin/ squash seeds, cashews, sunflower seeds, tahini Fortified cereal Baked potato (including skin)	2.2–6.6 mg 2.2–3.3 mg 2.1–5.2 mg 2.1–18 mg 2.3 mg	Nonheme iron absorption enhanced by ascorbic acid, small amounts of alcohol, retinol, and carotenes Inhibited by phytates, tannins/polyphenols, and soy protein
Zinc	Soybeans (cooked/roasted), tofu, fortified veggie meats Baked beans, lentils, navy beans Pumpkin/squash seeds dried, cashews, sunflower seeds toasted Fortified cereal Wheat germ Cooked peas	1.0–4.2 mg 1.8–2.3 mg 1.8–2.6 mg 0.7–15 mg 1.8 mg 1.0 mg	Phytate reduces bioavailability of zinc

Vitamin B_{12}	Fortified cereal	0.6–6.0 µg	Supplement may be
	Fortified yeast	1.5 µg	required
	Fortified soy milk	0.4–1.6 µg	
Vitamin D	Fortified cereal	0.5–1.0 µg	Supplement may be
	Fortified soymilk	0.5–1.5 µg	required
	Vegan margarines	?	
n–3 Fatty acids	Ground flax seed	1.9–2.2 g	Supplement may be
	Flaxseed oil	2.7 g	required
	Canola oil	1.3–1.6 g	
	Cooked soybeans	1.0 g	
	Walnuts	2.7 g	
	Walnut oil	1.4–1.7	

recommended that iron intakes should be 1.8 times higher in vegetarians and vegans than in nonvegetarians *(18)*. Ascorbic acid, retinol, alcohol, and carotenes can enhance the absorption of nonheme iron.

The prevalence of iron deficiency anemia is no greater in vegetarians than in omnivores, although iron stores tend to be lower, especially in women *(22)*. Women of child-bearing age are most at risk. Dietary advice should focus on encouraging a variety of nonheme iron sources (cooked legumes, fortified breads and cereals, baked potatoes, soy proteins), encouraging high intakes of ascorbic acid with meals to aid absorption, and avoiding consumption of inhibitors such as tea or coffee with meals. There is some tentative evidence that fermentation of soy proteins to produce miso and tempeh can reduce the phytate content and improve iron availability *(18)*. Additionally, iron cookware may be advocated since significant amounts of iron dissolve in food *(22)*.

3.5. Zinc

The majority of zinc in the Western diet comes together with animal protein. Legumes, whole grains, nuts, and seeds are reasonable plant-substitute sources of zinc. However, the bioavailability of zinc is reduced by high levels of supplemental calcium and by phytate, which is also found in legumes, whole grains, nuts, and seeds. Vegetarians and vegans appear to have adequate zinc status but lower serum levels than nonvegetarian counterparts *(22)*. Little is known regarding the effects of marginal zinc deficiency. Although adaptation to a low intake may occur over time, thanks to increased intestinal absorption *(22)*, good plant sources of zinc, as shown in Table 2, should be encouraged.

3.6. Vitamin B₁₂ (Cobalamin)

Vitamin B_{12} is required by the body in microgram amounts and is found only in foods of animal origin. Nutritional deficiency of this vitamin is extremely rare as the human body stores several years' worth of it. Elderly and strict vegan individuals are most at risk. Deficiency of B_{12} can cause pernicious anemia and can result in megaloblastic anemia with central nervous system demyelination if not treated early. Symptoms in infants and children include irritability, abnormal flexes, and feeding difficulties; prolonged deficiency can lead to permanent developmental disabilities (23). Diagnosing B_{12} deficiency prior to symptom development in vegetarians is difficult, usually due to a high folic acid intake masking the hematological signs of deficiency. Since folate intake is often higher in vegan diets, elevated serum methylmalonic acid, holo transcobalamin, and/or homocysteine may be more sensitive indicators of a vitamin B_{12} deficiency (23). Purported plant-based sources (tempeh, algae extracts, and sea vegetables) have been found to contain more inactive corrinoids than true B_{12} (23) and thus they are not reliable sources of B_{12}. Risk of B_{12} deficiency in vegans is increased if their diet is not supplemented with fortified products (fortified yeast extract, fortified soy products, and breakfast cereals). It is recommended that vegans include three sources of dietary B_{12} per day. If this is not achievable, a daily supplement of 5–10 µg is recommended for adults (18). Supplementation of 25–100 µg/d has been used to maintain vitamin B_{12} levels in older people. Unless the maternal diet is adequate in B_{12} breastfed infants should receive 0.4 µg/d from birth to 6 mo and 0.5 µg/d after that time (19).

3.7. Vitamin D

If a person obtains adequate exposure to sunlight and has normal liver function, the body can produce 25-hydroxyvitamin D. However, for many people, especially those in urban environments and during the winter months, dietary supplementation may be important because they do not receive adequate exposure to sunlight. This is especially the case if living in high latitudes where there is less opportunity for sunlight exposure. Major dietary sources of vitamin D are limited to animal foods. Vegans and those consuming very restrictive vegetarian diets are therefore at risk of deficiency. There have been reports of a high prevalence of rickets in children reared on macrobiotic diets (21). Alternative dietary sources include fortified soy milks and cheeses and vegan margarines. In some cases a vitamin D supplement may be required, particularly in children under 2 yr and lactating mothers with inadequate vitamin D intake.

3.8. n–3 Fatty Acids

Vegetarian diets can be lower in n–3 fatty acids, in particular the marine fatty acids eicosapentaenoic acid (EPA) and docosahexaenoic acid (DHA), and higher in n–6 fatty acids (linoleic acid). α-Linolenic acid, the n–3 fatty acid found in plant foods, can be converted to EPA and DHA, but the rate of conversion is very low, and can be further inhibited by a high intake of linoleic acid. These long-chain fatty acids are thought to be important for immune, cognitive, and cardiac function. Most studies show lower serum levels of EPA and DHA in vegans (18). Vegan sources of n–3 fatty acids include flaxseed and flaxseed oil, canola oil, olive oil, walnuts, and/or vegan DHA supplement in nongelatin capsules. Intake of n–3 fatty acids should be 1–2% of total energy intake (24).

4. SUMMARY

Many individuals and special interest groups claim that vegetarian diets can reduce the aging process, prolong life, and promote health and vitality. These claims are largely unsubstantiated in terms of reliable scientific evidence. Vegetarian and vegan diets may be associated with improved health outcomes especially for CHD. Vegetarian lifestyles often encompass attitudes and behaviors which can serve to improve overall health and well-being, including physical activity, not smoking, and limiting alcohol consumption.

It is widely recognized that over-reliance on one single food, or food group, will not provide the range of nutrients required for optimum health and well-being. This is the case for all diets – omnivorous, vegetarian, and vegan. All dietary practices should aim to meet current recommended nutrient intakes to prevent chronic diseases (24). A diet low in fat, sugar, and salt and rich in fruit, vegetables, and dietary fiber is encouraged. Variety in individual diets is also important. If a particular food or food group is not consumed routinely, alternative nutrient sources should be included.

Vegetarian and vegan diets can be balanced and healthy for all stages of life, provided appropriate preparation and planning is given (22). This is especially the case for groups at risk of nutrient deficiency including infants, small children, menstruating and lactating women, and athletes. Supplementation of vegan diets may be necessary if adequate intake of nutrients cannot be achieved.

The largest study done on the relationship between meat consumption and risk of death was carried out on half a million Americans who were aged 50 to 71 years at the start of the study. Over the next 10 years there were roughly 50,000 male deaths and 23,300 female deaths. One clear finding was that meat eaters typically have an unhealthy lifestyle: they smoke more, exercise less, are heavier, and eat a poorer diet. Conversely, the people who eat little meat tend to follow a much healthier lifestyle. When the researchers compared the extreme quintiles (i.e., the subjects who were in the highest and lowest fifths for consumption), thosewith a high intake of red and processed meat had about a 20–30% higher risk of death, after allowing for confounding variables. These extra deaths were split between cancer and cardiovascular disease.

SUGGESTED FURTHER READING

American Dietetic Association & Dietitians of Canada. Position of the American Dietetic Association and Dietitians of Canada: Vegetarian diets. J Am Diet Assoc 2003; 103: 748–765.

Mangels AR, Messina V. Considerations in planning vegan diets: Infants. J Am Diet Assoc 2001; 101:670–677.

Messina V, Mangels AR. Considerations in planning vegan diets: Children. J Am Diet Assoc 2001; 101:661–669.

Sinha R, Cross AJ, Graubard BI, Leitzmann MF, Schatzkin A. Meat intake and mortality: a prospective study of over half a million people. Arch Intern Med 2009; 169:562–571.

www.vrg.org The Vegetarian Resource Group provides information on vegetarianism, vegetarian books and recipes, and links to related sites.

www.soyfoods.com This U.S. Soy Foods Directory website is an essential resource for anyone interested in learning more about soy foods. The site includes a searchable database, recipes, and research information about the health benefits of soy foods.

REFERENCES

1. European Vegetarian Union. How many Veggies? Available at www.european-vegetarian.org/lang/en/info/howmany.php. Accessed January 20, 2008.
2. The Vegetarian Resource Group. How many Adults are vegetarian? www.vrg.org/journal/vj2003issue3/vj2003issue3poll.htm. Accessed January 20, 2008.
3. Chang-Claude J, Hermann S, Elber U, Steindorf K. Lifestyle determinants and mortality in German vegetarians and health conscious persons: results of a 21 year follow up. Cancer Epidemiol Biomarkers Prev 2005; 14: 963–968.
4. Fraser GE. Associations between diet and cancer, ischemic heart disease, and all cause mortality in non-Hispanic white California Seventh-day Adventists. Am J Clin Nutr 1999; 70(3 Suppl):532S–538S.
5. Key TJ, Fraser GE, Thorogood M, Appleby PN, et al. Mortality in vegetarians and non-vegetarians: detailed findings from a collaborative analysis of 5 prospective studies. Am J Clin Nutr 1999; 70(3 Suppl):516S–524S.
6. Key TJ, Appleby PN, Rosell MS. Health effects of vegetarian and vegan diets. Proc Nutr Soc 2006; 65:35–41.
7. Appleby PN, Davey GK, Key TJ. Hypertension and blood pressure among meat eaters, fish eaters, vegetarians & vegans in EPIC-Oxford. Public Health Nutr 2002; 5:645–654.
8. Sacks FM, Appel LJ, Moore TJ, et al. A dietary Approach to prevent hypertension: a review of the Dietary Approaches to Stop Hypertension (DASH) study. Clin Cardiol 1999; 22(7 Suppl):1106–1110.
9. Sabate J. The contribution of vegetarian diets to human health. Forum Nutr 2003; 56:218–220.

10. Rosell M, Appleby PN, Spencer EA, Key TJ. Weight gain over 5 yr in 21,966 meat eating, fish eating, vegetarian and vegan men and women in EPIC-Oxford. Int J Obes 2006; 30:1389–1396.
11. Willet WC. Diet, nutrition and avoidable cancer. Environ Health Perspect 1995; 103(8 suppl):165–170.
12. World Cancer Research Fund/American Institute Cancer Research Expert Report. Food, Nutrition, Physical Activity and the prevention of cancer: a Global Perspective. AICR, Washington, DC, 2007.
13. Norat T, Lukanova A, Ferrari P, Rivoli E. Meat consumption and colorectal cancer risk: dose-response meta-analysis of epidemiological studies. Int J Cancer 2002; 98: 241–256.
14. Gonzalez CA, Riboli E. Diet and cancer prevention: Where we are, where we are going. Nutr Cancer 2006; 56:225–231.
15. Jenkins DJ, Kendall CW, Marchie, A, et al. Type 2 diabetes and the vegetarian diet. Am J Clin Nutr 2003; 78(suppl):610S–616S.
16. Van Dam RM, Willet WC, Rimm EB, Stamfer MJ, Hu FB. Dietary fat and meat intake in relation to type 2 diabetes in men. Diabetes Care 2002; 25:417–424.
17. New SA. Intake of fruit and vegetables: implications for bone health. Proc Nutr Soc 2003; 62:889–899.
18. American Dietetic Association & Dietitians of Canada. Position of the American Dietetic Association and Dietitians of Canada: Vegetarian diets. J Am Diet Assoc 2003; 103: 748–765.
19. Mangels AR, Messina V. Considerations in planning vegan diets: Infants. J Am Diet Assoc 2001; 101:670–677.
20. Messina V, Mangels AR. Considerations in planning vegan diets: Children. J Am Diet Assoc 2001; 101:661–669.
21. Saunders TAB. Meat or wheat for the next millennium? A debate pro veg. The nutritional adequacy of plant-based diets. Proc Nutr Soc 1999; 58:265–269.
22. Hunt J. Bioavailability of iron, zinc and other trace minerals from vegetarian diets. Am J Clin Nutr 2003; 78(suppl):633S–639S.
23. Stabler SP, Allen RH. Vitamin B12 deficiency as a worldwide problem. Annu Rev Nutr 2004; 24:299–326.
24. World Health Organisation/Food Agriculture Organisation (WHO/FAO). Diet, Nutrition and the prevention of Chronic Diseases: Report of a joint WHO/FAO Expert Consultation. Technical Reports Series no 916. Geneva, WHO, 2003.

8 Dietary Recommendations for Non-alcoholic Beverages

Ted Wilson

Key Points

- Coffee, tea, and milk is either beneficial or at least health neutral for cardiovascular and cancer health, for this reason consumption should be promoted.
- Fruit and vegetable juices can be useful for improving nutritional health when the respective whole food is unavailable, but they can represent a source of excess caloric and sodium intake.
- Soft drinks represent a source excess caloric intake and their consumption should be limited.
- Energy drinks are popular with young people and no peer-reviewed papers have documented deleterious effects related to their consumption.
- Caffeine content in beverages varies widely, although adverse health effects from its consumption do not warrant general caution for non-pregnant persons.

  Key Words: Beverages; caffeine; tea; coffee; fruit juices; sports beverages; milk

1. WE ARE (MAINLY) WHAT WE DRINK

Beverages play a major role in determining nutritional health and water represents as much as 60% of the body weight in a lean person and as little as 45% in the obese. Nonalcoholic beverages include coffee, tea, milk, juices, soft drinks, energy drinks, sports drinks, drinks for weight management, and of course water. Alcoholic beverages also have major health implications and are discussed in the following chapter. The recommended intake, based on Dietary Recommended Intake (DRI), of water for non-exercising persons is 3.7 L/d for men and 2.7 L/d for women. This includes water obtained both from beverages and from food. Very few clinical recommendations exist to help physicians guide patients to achieving optimal beverage nutrition. This

From: *Nutrition and Health: Nutrition Guide for Physicians*
Edited by: T. Wilson et al. (eds.), DOI 10.1007/978-1-60327-431-9_8,
© Humana Press, a part of Springer Science+Business Media, LLC 2010

is surprising given that beverages provide about one fifth of our daily caloric intake, with the greatest caloric intake occurring in 19- to 39-yr-olds *(1)*. Beverages may also contain a wide range of amino acids, vitamins, minerals, and fats whose health effects are well understood, and polyphenolic compounds whose effects on health are poorly understood. Beverages are also the main source of caffeine. This chapter provides a short review of the beneficial and detrimental effects of major beverages, including coffee, tea, fruit juices, soft drinks, and energy drinks.

2. COFFEE CONSUMPTION POSES NO HEALTH RISK FOR MOST PERSONS

It is reasonable to believe that low-to-moderate coffee consumption (≤3 cups/d) should be safe for the typical consumer. Overall, epidemiological evidence shows that coffee intake poses little or no risk for most common neoplasms; indeed there may be an inverse relation between coffee consumption and risk of colorectal cancer *(2)*. Coffee consumption has also been associated with neutral or moderately beneficial effects on cardiovascular disease risk and overall mortality *(3)*. Additionally, recent evidence suggests that coffee consumption may be beneficial for preventing type 2 diabetes *(4)*. While caffeine provides its neurological effects, phenolic acids in coffee may also have significance relative to its other biological effects.

When estimating coffee consumption, it is important to consider the size of the container, the habit of refilling the cup, the variability of coffee drinking between different days (weekdays/weekends), and seasonal differences in intake.

Coffee caffeine concentration is dependent on the coffee type (American coffee, espresso, or mocha), and the amount and type of coffee bean used for brewing (Table 1). The decaffeination process is associated with a reduced phenolic content and the introduction of compounds, such as nitric acids and formaldehyde, which may have deleterious health effects. It is also noteworthy that decaffeination does not remove all of the caffeine; there are large variations in residual caffeine in "decaffeineated" coffee. A general guideline for coffee is at most 2–3 cups/d.

3. TEA CONSUMPTION IS PROTECTIVE AND SHOULD BE ENCOURAGED

After water, tea is the most popular beverage in the world, including Britain, China, Japan, and several other countries in Asia. Its popularity in

Table 1
Typical Caffeine Content of Commonly Consumed Drinks

Drink	Content (mg)	Drink (12 oz)	Caffeine Content (mg/serving)
Filter drip (6 oz)	130–189 (ave 150)	Jolt Cola	70
Espresso (1.3–2 oz)	100	Mountain Dew	55
Instant (6 oz)	50–130	Diet Mountain Dew	55
Decaffeinated (6 oz)	2–12	Surge	52
Green tea (6 oz)	10–15	Tab	47
Black tea (6 oz)	50	Diet Coke	45
Snapple iced tea (16 oz)	31	Dr Pepper	42
Lipton iced tea (16 oz)	18–40	Diet Dr Pepper	42
Nestea iced tea (16 oz)	16–26	Sunkist Orange Soda	42
Arizona iced tea (16 oz)	15–30	Pepsi-Cola	38
Hot chocolate (mix, 6 oz)	10	Diet Pepsi	36
Chocolate milk (6 oz)	4	Coca-Cola Classic	34
Milk chocolate (28 g)	6	Red Bull Energy Drink	32

Adapted from *(16)*

the United States is increasing, in part as a consequence of the favorable health benefits attributed to it. Leaves from the tea plant *Camellia sinensis* are the source of the primary tea types (green, black, and oolong). Industrial processing of green and black teas changes their respective polyphenolic profiles. Freshly brewed green tea contains (–)-epigallocatechin-3-gallate (EGCG) and other phenolics and black tea contains lower levels of these polyphenolic compounds. EGCG makes up more than 40% of the total polyphenolic mixture and appears to be the polyphenol most responsible for green tea's beneficial effects. Maximal plasma concentrations are achieved for EGCG 1.3–2.4 h after consumption. It is classified by the FDA as "generally recognized as safe" (GRAS) and is a popular food additive and nutraceutical supplement. Tea also contains caffeine (Table 1), though considerably less than coffee.

Green tea shows much potential as an anticancer agent; this is because many epidemiological studies have reported a protective association with the risk of cancer *(5)* and cardiovascular disease *(6)*. Black tea has also been demonstrated to be protective against cardiovascular disease by helping to improve endothelial cell function and vasodilation *(7)*. However, much of the generally optimistic epidemiological evidence concerning green tea is based heavily on studies in Japan and China where many people drink eight or more cups/d. Thus 1 or 2 cups/d may have a fairly small (though useful) effect. In Western populations the consumption of three or more cups/d of black tea has also been strongly associated with protection from CHD *(8)*. As general guide line consumption of up to 3–4 cups/d should be recommended *(5)*.

4. MILK IS GOOD FOR YOU

Milk has long been recognized as a way to improve calcium intake and bone health, especially when it is fortified with vitamin D, a topic discussed more thoroughly in Chapter 30. Milk is also an excellent source of potassium and magnesium. The popularity of clinical recommendations for milk has had its ups and downs and ups over the last 20 yr. Milk consumption by some persons who lack lactase in their intestine, results in lactose intolerance and a recommendation that it be avoided in the absence of lactase or the use of lactose-free dairy products. While persons of south-east Asian decent are most troubled by this condition, it can also be seen in many people of northern European descent.

Milk is an excellent source of protein, micronutrients, and fat. Surprisingly, the fat content of milk does not lead to deleterious changes in the lipoprotein profile nor does it lead to increased risk for heart disease. Indeed, the DASH study demonstrated that low-fat dairy consumption may reduce blood pressure *(9)*. Milk consumption may promote improved weight control, despite the added fat and calories. It has also been inversely correlated with the risk of developing insulin resistance. Milk consumption is arguably most important in younger persons who are developing bone mass. Unfortunately, in the last few decades milk consumption has gradually declined at the same time that soft drink consumption, and obesity, has steadily increased among this age group. Milk consumption should be promoted in persons who are not lactose intolerant. A general guideline for milk consumption should be 2–4 cups/d, with a suggestion of reduced or low-fat milk as a way to promote overall patient awareness of calorie intake saturated fat.

5. HEALTH BENEFITS OF FRUIT JUICES

The DASH study conclusively demonstrated that the inclusion of fruits and vegetables is associated with a reduction in blood pressure *(9)*. It is notable that persons in the lowest quartile of fruit and vegetable consumption are in the highest quartile for CVD and cancer. For these reasons the Five-A-Day program seeks to boost fruit and vegetable consumption. Because of their enjoyable taste, widespread accessibility, and ease of storage, juices are a popular way to increase fruit consumption. The American Dietetic Association recommends that juice consumption can be used to improve fruit and vegetable intake. However, patients should also be reminded that juice consumption is not a sole solution to improving dietary balance in light of several major points:

(a) Juices are a poor source of fiber, relative to their native whole form.
(b) They have a high content of simple sugars, and this can induce an excessive energy intake. Indeed, the energy content of apple juice and orange juice (OJ) (110 kcal/8 oz serving) is about 6% higher than that of cola drinks.
(c) The vitamin C content decreases as a function of time after production, and products should be consumed within a week of opening.
(d) The polyphenolic profile of juices is highly related to environmental conditions and the fruit source.
(e) Total consumption recommendations are difficult to make, but should probably not exceed two to three 8 oz cups/d.
(f) Consumers should be reminded that whole fruits provide a better nutritional value, although they may not be as available or cost-effective, although consumers generally prefer juice to whole fruit.

5.1. Health Benefits of Citrus Juice Consumption

OJ and grapefruit juice represent the two most commonly consumed citrus juices in the United States. OJ is the most nutrient-dense fruit juice commonly consumed in the United States. An 8-oz serving (1 cup) provides 120 kcal and 72 mg of vitamin C (120% of Daily Value). OJ is also a good source of potassium (450 mg or 13% of DV), folate (60 μg or 15% of DV), and thiamin (0.15 mg or 10% of DV). Grapefruit juice differs slightly from OJ in its nutrient profile. An 8-oz serving of grapefruit juice contains about 90 kcal and has the same amount of vitamin C as OJ. Grapefruit juice contains lower concentrations than OJ of potassium, the B-vitamins folate, thiamin, and niacin, and a different profile of phenolic acids, some of which may be responsible for an alteration of drug metabolism, a topic discussed at greater length in Chapter 35.

The rich content of various micronutrients found in citrus juices has several potential health benefits. Vitamin C is of course an important antioxidant and critical for production of collagen. Folate is a key nutrient responsible for prevention of neural tube defects. Potassium functions to maintain intracellular fluid balance and, as such, a high intake is associated with lower blood pressure and a reduced risk of stroke. Consumption of OJ may help lower the LDL/HDL ratio and components of citrus juice may also decrease LDL oxidation thus reducing the risk of CHD.

Epidemiological data, clinical investigations, and animal studies provide strong evidence that citrus juice consumption is beneficial with respect to CHD, cancer, and overall mortality. However, because the vitamin C in OJ readily oxidizes following exposure to air, citrus juices should be consumed within 1 wk of opening *(10)*.

5.2. Health Effects of Other Types of Fruit Juice

Cranberry juice has been used in folk medicine for millenia. Recent clinical studies have confirmed its usefulness for the prevention of urinary tract infections. The active antibacterial agents are proanthocyanidins specific to cranberries which prevent bacterial adhesion to the urinary tract. These anti-adhesive effects may also be associated with oral and gastric health benefits. Consumption of cranberry products is associated with beneficial antioxidant, vasodilatory, and antiplatelet aggregation properties that may make these products a viable substitute to red wine and Concord grape juice for protection from CHD *(11, 12)*. However, consumer and researcher understanding of how cranberries affect human health remains difficult to determine in part because of the large range of product sweeteners currently used and the differences in the amount of cranberry juice actually present in these beverages, which can range from 3 to 27% v/v.

Concord and purple grape juices contain an array of polyphenolic compounds that are similar to but not identical to those in red wine. The biological effects of grape juice have been demonstrated to include a small improvement in plasma lipid profile, vasodilation, and antiplatelet aggregatory activities. Pomegranate has been associated with improved vasodilation and a hypocholesterolemic effect, while apple juice has been less thoroughly linked to improved antioxidant capacity.

As with all things, moderation is best, clinicians may wish to remind their patients that many juices contain a high content of (natural) sugar. For instance, four cups of white grape juice would provide a caloric intake of around 600 kcal, equivalent to close to a third of the caloric needs for an elderly person wishing to lose or maintain weight.

5.3. And Don't Forget Vegetable Juices

Tomato juice has been popular for decades. Unfortunately, its health benefits are potentially reduced by the excessive content of added salt (as high as 560–660 mg sodium/cup). But in recent years numerous brands of vegetable juices have appeared on the market, V-8 being the classic example. Some varieties are low in salt, which is usually prominently stated on the label. These juices can have a low energy content (50 kcal/cup as compared to 110 kcal/cup in OJ and apple juice). It is also important to recognize that many vegetable drinks include pear, white grape, or other juices as a source of sweeteners. Sugar calories are indeed sugar calories, regardless of whether they come from high-fructose corn syrup, cane sugar juice, or pear juice.

There are several types of pseudo fruit juices that are, in reality, nutritionally the same as cola. These include fruit beverages, fruit nectar, fruit drink, and fruit punch. Consumers should not be fooled by pictures of fruit or vegetables on the main label; read the ingredients in the small print.

The cost of vegetable juice is similar to OJ thereby making these products a convenient and affordable way for people to inject more vegetables into their diets. The potential for many vegetable juices to be purchased and stored without refrigeration is an added consideration that makes them a good way to help people reach the five-a-day goal for fruit and vegetable consumption.

6. HEALTH EFFECTS OF SOFT DRINK CONSUMPTION

The impact of sugar from soft drinks and other sources is more thoroughly discussed in Chapter 3. His chapter also discusses this topic with respect to soft drink consumption patterns and manufacturing trends. A clear determination of the effects of soft drinks is compounded by many factors and they represent a significant source of caffeine (Table 1). Their consumption is positively correlated with body weight, and dental decay, and inversely correlated with dairy intake. The impact of soft drinks on total energy intake is widely variable between individuals. In light of this, soft drink contributions to total caloric intake and nutritional imbalance are greatest for teenagers. Soft drinks can contribute to a positive caloric balance and in adolescents intake can represent as much at 28% of total caloric intake.

In a perfect world we would have zero soft drink consumption and water would have many splendid tastes and qualities. Water consumption would also be supported by billion dollar advertising campaigns. In the light of reality it is perhaps sensible to suggest limiting soft drinks to no more than one to two cups/d, though none is clearly preferable. Given that the consumption of diet soft drinks is not typically associated with reductions in body weight, their consumption should be limited in a similar fashion.

7. WEIGHT LOSS AND WEIGHT MANAGEMENT BEVERAGES

For several reasons meal replacement beverages may have a place in the regular nutrition of many persons. A variety of meal replacement beverages (e.g., Slim-Fast, Met-Rx, and Atkins Nutritionals) provide consumers with a convenient way to consume a relatively balanced nutritional intake of about 200 kcal along with a typically large protein intake, as well as minerals and vitamins in a liquid format. The elderly often have a high risk for malnutrition, inadequate protein intake, and poor weight maintenance. For these persons liquid meal replacements may be useful and are commonly consumed because they are, above all, readily available and often quite palatable. One of their primary advantages is that most brands can be stored without refrigeration. Predictably, to improve palatability some beverages actually contain generous amounts of fat or sugars.

Surprisingly, older persons tend to consume more food during the meal following consumption of a liquid meal replacement, making these beverages useful for elderly persons attempting to gain weight, but detrimental for overweight persons attempting to lose weight *(13)*. Their effects in middle-aged persons are not as clear. While liquid meal replacements may be useful for some persons, the best nutritional advice for most people is to consume a balanced diet that emphasizes a variety of foods consumed in their solid form.

8. SPORTS BEVERAGES

A variety of beverages are consumed by athletes for a variety of reasons. Compromises in physical and mental performance can occur with loss in body water of as little as 2% of total body weight. They are also consumed to maintain electrolyte status as well as to improve physical performance and muscle mass. Sports beverages have been found to be generally effective for improving hydration and electrolyte status and physical performance. However, there are few peer-reviewed studies to support claims of improving muscle mass in body builders. Part of the difficulty in performing peer-reviewed studies is related to the ever-changing contents of sports beverages. However, a few consistent observations can be made about these beverages.

Athletes are prone to dehydration and sports beverages can and do improve hydration status. The key component to this, surprisingly, is taste: if people like the taste, then they are more likely to drink more of the beverage before or during exercise, thereby leading to greater improvements in their hydration status. In addition to taste, many beverages include sodium and similar concentrations of glucose. The presence of both sodium and glucose permits the intestine to co-transport the two substances into the blood. In addition, as sodium and glucose maintain spheres of hydration, this also enhances the rapid absorption of water from the intestine. However, beverages that contain an excessive amount of sugar (e.g., soft drinks) can actually promote a reduction in gastric emptying and an osmotic effect in the intestine that can lead to solvent drag of water into the intestine and dehydration.

Sports beverages can improve electrolyte status, although the effects are most significant for long-term exercise (e.g., a half marathon or mowing a lawn on a hot summer day for 2 h). However, if a person is adequately hydrated and has a proper electrolyte balance prior to beginning their exercise, electrolyte replenishment from a sports beverage is unlikely to facilitate a significant improvement in physical performance during longer-term periods of exercise.

Physicians will frequently suggest that persons achieve 30 min of moderate exercise, walking, etc., per day. It is worth reminding patients that drinking Gatorade (a 500 ml bottle provides $2\frac{1}{2}$ servings or 125 calories) could negate most of the caloric benefits from the exercise. Recommend paying close attention to the caloric content of the sports drink and remind them that unless it is an extremely hot day, dehydration is unlikely given this type of work load.

A trip to a health food store or examination of the advertisements in a body building magazine will demonstrate to the clinician that a variety of liquid supplements are marketed with the claimed ability to improve muscle mass, appearance, or performance. While many products include some sort of claim, often based on the findings from clinical studies, it is generally impossible to find the supporting studies published in credible peer-reviewed journals. This is a reality for most products; however, the popularity of these products is noteworthy and one needs to be mindful that many persons may use them, but not share this information with their clinician.

A typical product will come in a powdered form that provides a rich content of protein, vitamins, and minerals, but with a small content of carbohydrates and fats. Some products may also contain creatine phosphate, caffeine, or plant-derived extracts/compounds. The inclusion of these ingredients is poorly regulated by the FDA. The price of these products varies widely: from one to ten dollars per day, and given this high cost it is a tribute to the power of marketing that they are so popular. For these reasons, the author believes that clinicians should use their influence to counsel caution among users.

9. ENERGY DRINKS REMAIN CONTROVERSIAL BEVERAGES

The increasing popularity of what are popularly termed "energy drinks" is an American and global phenomenon. They are consumed for perceived enhancements in mental acuity, wakefulness, and physical performance. The safety of energy drinks remains controversial because of anecdotal and casual associations between their consumption and acute cardiac events. In light of these considerations the classic energy drink Red Bull® was banned in some European countries. Regardless of whether their consumption provides a measureable change in physiological/mental status, their popularity is very great with net sales of several billion dollars per year.

Energy drinks constitute a class of beverages whose ingredients are not uniform. While caffeine is a primary ingredient in most brands (Table 1), its content is quite variable (2.5–171 mg/oz). Energy drinks generally contain a variety of other compounds with potential for altering physiological/mental activity. These additional ingredients often include taurine (neurotransmitter function) and various B vitamins. In addition, most contain sugars, although some are nearly calorie free; caloric contents range from 10 to 150 kcal/8 oz serving.

While energy drinks are commonly believed to have significant physiological effects, documentation in this regard is relatively scant. Echocardiographic evidence suggests that Red Bull® consumption may improve stroke volume in persons with heart failure *(14)*. Consumption of energy drinks along with alcoholic beverages has been suggested to reduce the perception of alcohol-induced impairment of motor function. Surprisingly, in a study of 70 college-aged subjects who consumed a 240 mL serving of Red Bull or placebo, the author *(15)* did not observe any statistically significant changes in heart rate, ECG QRT-segments/intervals, or blood pressure during the 2 h following consumption. However, given the consistency of anecdotal reports linked to cardiac pathologies associated with energy drinks, especially when consumed with alcohol, caution seems warranted.

10. WHAT'S THE BUZZ REGARDING CAFFEINE?

Caffeine is a stimulant of the nervous system and can improve reaction times and wakefulness *(16)*. It is integral to the effects of many beverages and the content of caffeine varies widely in different beverages (Table 1). Caffeine has a profound stimulant effect in some persons, although individual sensitivities vary widely. It potentially induces its effects by acting upon adenosine receptors and/or by inhibiting phosphodiesterase to increase intracellular cAMP. Surprisingly few negative health effects have associated with caffeine consumption. However, as a cautious recommendation, the elderly and pregnant women may wish to limit their intake of caffeinated beverages. Given that caffeine has a half-life of 3–6 h, people may also consider it a causative agent for sleep disorders.

11. CONCLUSIONS

We are mainly what we drink. However, there are a variety of components in beverages, in addition to water, that may impact human health. In many cases, as with the micronutrients and phytochemicals in fruit and vegetable juices, these are likely to be beneficial. Coffee and tea generally have health-neutral to beneficial effects. Tea has been linked to reduced risk of CHD while coffee may be protective against type 2 diabetes. Milk has been determined to promote improved cardiovascular health and its fats may even improve weight control. But beverages can also be a major source of excessive caloric intake that may contribute to obesity and type 2 diabetes. Regarding sports drinks, energy drinks, and caffeine, caution should be an operative word; however, conclusive evidence to support health concerns regarding their consumption generally does not exist. No single beverage can replace water, that ubiquitous beverage, but even water has its faults when we consider the presence of potential pollutants.

SUGGESTED FURTHER READING

Wilson T, Temple NJ, eds. Beverages in Health and Nutrition. Humana Press, Totowa, NJ, 2004.

Binns CW, Lee AH, Fraser ML. Tea or coffee? A case study on evidence for dietary advice. Public Health Nutr 2008; 11:1132–1141.

Van Duyn MA, Pivonka E. Overview of the health benefits of fruit and vegetable consumption for the dietetics professional: selected literature. J Am Diet Assoc 2000; 100:1511–1521.

REFERENCES

1. Nielson SJ, Popkin BM. Changes in beverage intake between 1977 and 2001. Am J Prev Med 2004; 27:205–10.
2. Higdon JV, Frei B. Coffee and health: a review of recent human research. Crit Rev Food Sci Nutr 2006; 46:101–123.
3. Lopez-Garcia E, van Dam RM, Li TY, Rodriguez-Artalejo F, Hu FB. The relationship of coffee consumption with mortality. Ann Intern Med 2008; 148:904–914.
4. Campos H, Baylin A. Coffee consumption and risk of type 2 diabetes and heart disease. Nutr Rev 2007; 65:173–179.
5. Carlson JR, Bauer BA, Vincent A, Limburg PJ, Wilson T. Reading the tea leaves: anticarcinogenic properties of (-)-epigallocatechin-3-gallate. Mayo Clin Proc 2007; 82: 725–732.
6. Basu A, Lucas EA. Green tea CVD 2007.

7. Jochmann N, Lorenz M, Krosigk A, et al. The efficacy of black tea in ameliorating endothelial function is equivalent to that of green tea. Br J Nutr 2008; 99:863–868.
8. Gardner EJ, et al. Green tea CVD 2007
9. Appel LJ, Moore TJ, Obarzanek E, et al. A clinical trial of the effects of dietary patterns on blood pressure. N Engl J Med 1997; 336:1117–1124.
10. Johnston CS, Bowling DL. Stability of ascorbic acid in commercially available orange juices. J Am Diet Assoc 2002; 102:525–529.
11. Maher MA, Mataczynski H, Stephaniak HM, Wilson T. Cranberry juice induces nitric oxide dependent vasodilation and transiently reduces blood pressure in conscious and anaesthetized rats. J Medicinal Foods 2000; 3:141–147.
12. Wilson T, Porcari JP, Maher MA. Cranberry juice inhibits metal- and non-metal initiated oxidation of low density lipoprotein. J Nutra Funct Med Foods 1999; 2:5–14.
13. Stull AJ, Apolzan JW, Thalacker-Mercer AE, Iglay HB, Campbell WW. Liquid and solid meal replacement products differentially affect postprandial appetite and food intake in older adults. J Am Diet Assoc 2008; 108:1226–1230.
14. Baum M, Weiss M. The influence of a taurine containing drink on cardiac parameters before and after exercise measured by echocardiography. Amino Acids 2001; 20:75–82.
15. Ragsdale R, Gronli TD, Batool SN, et al. Effect of red bull energy drink on cardiovascular and renal function. Amino Acids 2009; doi: 10.1007/s00726-009-0330-z
16. Weinberg BA, Bealer BK. Caffeine and health. In: Wilson T, Temple NJ, eds. Beverages in Nutrition and Health. Humana Press, Totowa, NJ, 2004.

9 Should Moderate Alcohol Consumption Be Promoted?

Ted Wilson and Norman J. Temple

Key Points

- Alcoholic beverages contain a variety of phytochemicals, but there is little strong evidence regarding the effects of these substances on health.
- Alcohol creates many social problems, such as violence and accidents, as well as negative health effects, most notably those related to cancer and fetal alcohol syndrome.
- Moderate consumption of alcohol is generally defined as two drinks a day for a man or one for a woman. This is associated with significant protective effects against coronary heart disease and several other diseases and health problems.
- The relationship between alcohol consumption and overall mortality depends on age. Below age 40 alcohol is associated with an increased risk of death. For people older than about 50 or 60 alcohol consumption has a J-shaped relationship with risk of mortality; the lowest risk of death is seen in moderate drinkers.

Key Words: Alcohol drinking; alcohol-related disorders; coronary heart disease; mortality

1. INTRODUCTION

The widespread consumption of alcoholic beverages and their potentially conflicting health impacts makes a discussion of this topic vitally important for physicians. Alcohol consumption in large quantities is strongly linked to dramatic negative health consequences. But the long-term effects of moderate consumption – years rather than hours – are much less well understood. These contrasting actions of alcohol are briefly reviewed in this chapter and elsewhere in a more extensive review *(1)*.

From: *Nutrition and Health: Nutrition Guide for Physicians*
Edited by: T. Wilson et al. (eds.), DOI 10.1007/978-1-60327-431-9_9,
© Humana Press, a part of Springer Science+Business Media, LLC 2010

A drink technically contains 14 g of ethanol and is equivalent to 12 oz (356 ml) of regular beer, 4–5 oz (148 ml) of wine, or 1.5 oz (44 ml) of distilled spirits. Moderate consumption is generally defined as two drinks a day for a man or one for a woman. Many disease pathologies can be attributed to alcohol consumption including stroke, cancer, fetal alcohol syndrome, and a great number of cases of death from accidents or violence. The biological effects of a drink are mostly related to its ethanol content, both directly and as a result of ethanol metabolites, as well as to the other substances found in alcoholic beverages, including sugars and polyphenolic compounds. Ethanol is a nonnutrient and contributes 7 kcal/g to metabolic energy balance. It is either metabolized to ATP or utilized for fatty acid synthesis.

2. PHYTOCHEMICALS IN ALCHOLIC BEVERAGES

Alcoholic beverages also contain a variety of phytochemicals. These mostly come from the raw plant foods from which each beverage is fermented. Red wine contains phenolic compounds such as resveratrol, tannins, and catechins. These substances have been associated with antioxidant protection, vasodilatation, inhibition of platelet aggregation, and improved plasma cholesterol profile. Beer, particularly darker ones, tends to have a higher polyphenolic content and greater antioxidant capacity relative to light beers. Spirits and mixed drinks are another source of polyphenolic and other compounds; they provide much of the unique colors and flavors found in these beverages. As a result of the distillation process the content of phytochemicals in spirits is usually very low compared to wine and beer.

As is the case with fruit and vegetable juices, current knowledge regarding the thousands of phytochemicals in various plant foods is still surprisingly limited. While we can confidently state that a diet rich in foods that contain an abundance of phytochemicals is likely to be healthy and should be recommended, it is premature to make bold statements as to the disease-preventing action of specific substances.

3. HARMFUL EFFECTS OF ALCOHOL

Alcohol consumption may also alter the efficacy, metabolism, and effect of medications, a topic reviewed in Chapter 35. Circulating alcohol inhibits the secretion of anti-diuretic hormone by the neurohypothysis, causing a mild diuretic effect and an increased palatability for salty foods. The positive feedback loop between alcohol intake, diuresis, increased salt consumption, increased plasma osmolarity, and increased beer consumption in part explains why bars often provide, at no cost, salty peanuts, pretzels, and popcorn. For this same reason people, especially the elderly, may be at risk of excessive dehydration if they drink beer or other alcoholic beverages on hot afternoons following outside work or upon acute exposure to elevations above 10,000 ft.

It is well established that abuse of alcohol is associated with accidents, violence, and suicide. It is a factor in about a quarter of fatal car crashes in the United States. The most dramatic evidence of the dangers of binge drinking comes from Russia. Between 1984 and 1994 there was serious economic decline and great political turmoil in that country. One of the results of this was that during the late 1980s and the 1990s mortality rates jumped dramatically. This was reflected in a decline in life expectancy in men of 4 years. A major factor in this was apparently widespread alcohol abuse, particularly binge drinking, which led to large increases in deaths from accidents, homicide, and suicide, as well as heart disease and stroke.

Alcohol, though not technically a nutrient, is a source of calories. As alcohol has 7 kcal/g, one drink therefore delivers about 88 kcal of energy. Many alcoholic beverages have additional calories because of their content of carbohydrates. Typically, a glass of wine or a can of beer contains about 100–140 kcal. However, this can be quite variable; a sweet wine, for example, may have 240 kcal per glass while some brands of beer ("light beer") are low in sugar and therefore have few nonalcoholic calories.

Clearly, the calories delivered by alcoholic beverages are enough to tip the energy balance well into positive territory. It might be predicted, therefore, that alcohol consumption should be associated with excess weight gain. However, as so often happens in nutrition, predictions collapse in the face of reality (2). A solid body of evidence has appeared demonstrating that alcohol intake actually has an inverse association with weight. This may reflect reduced food intake in frequent consumers of alcohol. Another possible explanation is that the increase in basal metabolic rate caused by moderate alcohol consumption may offset the additional calories from alcohol-containing beverages.

For many persons, years of alcohol abuse eventually lead to chronic nutritional and health problems. Alcoholic beverages are relatively poor sources of nutrients, apart from some sugars and minerals, and in some cases, some amino acids. This is especially true for hard liquors. The body often compensates for high alcohol intake by decreasing the consumption of regular foods. As a result, there is a high probability of malnutrition in heavy drinkers, especially for folate and thiamin (Wernicke–Korsakoff syndrome). Alcohol-induced deficiencies of amino acids and excessive hepatic fatty acid synthesis can lead to the development of fatty liver, alcoholic hepatitis, and, eventually cirrhosis. In relation to other alcoholic beverages, the consumption of hard liquor is more strongly correlated with alcoholism, cirrhosis, stroke, and accidental death.

Alcohol use during pregnancy can induce fetal alcohol syndrome (FAS). This irreversible condition encompasses symptoms that include prenatal and postnatal growth retardation, mental retardation, and the hallmark clinical sign of abnormal facial features. FAS occurs at a level of alcohol intake which in a nonpregnant woman would not be considered alcohol abuse. A subclinical form of FAS is known as fetal alcohol effects (FAE). Children with FAE may be short or have only minor facial abnormalities, or develop learning disabilities, behavioral problems, or motor impairments. Women who have an occasional drink during pregnancy should not fear doing irreparable harm to their fetus, though it is now generally accepted that any woman who is or may become pregnant should abstain from alcohol.

Consumption of alcohol is associated with an increased risk of numerous types of cancer. This topic is also discussed in Chapter 33. The relationship between alcohol intake and risk is linear so that even moderate consumption levels poses some, albeit minor, risk of cancer. Alcohol acts as a cocarcinogen with cigarette smoke. The risk ratio (RR) with an alcohol intake of four drinks per day is estimated to be 1.9–3.1 for cancer of the mouth, throat, and esophagus, 1.6 for breast cancer, and about 1.1–1.4 for cancer of the stomach, colon-rectum, liver, and ovary. For all cancer combined a significant risk is seen starting at an alcohol intake of two drinks per day, with an RR of 1.2 at four drinks per day.

4. HEALTH BENEFITS ASSOCIATED WITH ALCOHOL CONSUMPTION

A substantial body of epidemiological evidence has accumulated over the past 20 years that shows a strong negative association between moderate alcohol consumption and risk of coronary heart disease (CHD). Our best evidence is that moderate consumption brings a reduction in risk of about 10–40%.

This epidemiological story has generated heated debate in the medical literature which reflects the pitfalls in interpreting the findings from epidemiological studies. One aspect of the debate relates to the challenge created by "sick quitters." This refers to persons with a diagnosis of a condition related to CHD, such as hypertension or diabetes, who quit drinking alcohol. This causes an artificial jump in the risk of CHD in nondrinkers and a lowering of the risk among drinkers.

A much more notorious problem concerns the so-called French Paradox (3). It was observed that France has a surprisingly low rate of CHD in comparison with some Northern European countries, such as the United Kingdom. This could not be easily explained by the "usual suspects" as France has high rates of both smoking and consumption of foods rich in saturated fat. It was reasoned that the explanation could be found in the popularity of red wine in that country. Endless repetition of this speculation, at least in some circles, gave red wine the status of a proven preventive of CHD.

However, a different story emerges when the epidemiological evidence is examined in its totality. In particular, the findings from cohort studies (as opposed to ecological studies based on comparisons of national averages) revealed the following. First, there is much erratic variation from one study to the next, and, second, there is no consistent pattern indicative of one type of alcoholic beverage being superior to any other with regard to the prevention of CHD. It is true that some studies have suggested a lower risk among wine drinkers than in those who consume other types of alcohol, such as beer. However, this finding can be explained by such factors as wine drinkers often having a relatively healthy lifestyle and a high socioeconomic status (a factor associated with a lower risk of CHD), as well as drinking pattern (a glass or two of wine with dinner several times a week is believed to be healthier than the same quantity of alcohol consumed in one or two "binges"). The conclusion from this is that all types of alcoholic beverage – wine, beer, spirits – are of similar potency for the prevention of CHD.

The major mechanism by which alcohol prevents CHD is believed to be by elevation of the blood level of HDL-cholesterol and by decreasing LDL cholesterol *(4)*. Alcohol may also exert an antithrombotic action, although this action has also been limited to a small increase in stroke.

The saga of CHD has overshadowed other findings concerning the health benefits of a moderate intake of alcohol. In each of these cases it is important to bear in mind the basic rule of epidemiology: it reveals association not causation. Therefore, we must be hesitant before jumping to the conclusion that a protective association proves that alcohol actually prevents particular diseases or health conditions.

For several aspects of poor health status there is a J-shaped relationship between alcohol consumption and risk *(4, 5)*. People who consume alcohol in moderation have a lower risk than that seen in either heavier drinkers or nondrinkers, while risk increases sharply in those with a high alcohol intake. Hypertension and the risk of stroke manifest this relationship. While a relatively high intake of alcohol (more than four drinks per day) is associated with an increased risk of both conditions, moderate consumers appear to be at relatively low risk. This association is seen most clearly in women and for ischemic stroke rather than hemorrhagic stroke.

That excessive alcohol intake leads to poor erectile function is well known. As Shakespeare put it: "It provokes the desire, but takes away from the performance" (Macbeth). But recent findings have pointed to a modest beneficial effect of moderate alcohol consumption. In the case of erectile dysfunction, therefore, a J-shaped curve appears to be true in more ways than one.

The same serendipitous discovery has also been made for the cognitive decline that occurs with aging. It is well known, of course, that heavy drinking has a damaging effect on brain function. But recent research has revealed that moderate drinkers actually have an enhanced cognitive ability or a slower rate of decline with aging (6, 7). And this may even extend to the risk of dementia, mostly Alzheimer's disease.

One of the most dramatic effects is seen with type 2 diabetes. Cohort studies report that moderate consumers of alcohol reduce their risk of the disease by between one third and one half. Several other conditions are also less common in those who drink moderately, including chronic obstructive pulmonary disease (COPD), gallstones, and hearing loss.

It needs to be emphasized again that there are several other confounding factors involved in the association between alcohol and health. These include genetics, nutrition (e.g., deficiencies of specific vitamins), and other aspects of lifestyle, such as smoking. The pattern of drinking is of particular importance. So far we have been talking about "moderation" with respect to alcohol intake. But there is a big difference between the man who has two glasses of wine or two cans of beer each evening and the man who has his weekly 14 drinks divided between a Friday night and a Saturday night. The latter pattern – binge drinking – is far less healthy than the former.

5. EFFECT OF ALCOHOL ON TOTAL MORTALITY

With the opposing health effects of alcohol, a critically important question is the effect of alcohol on total mortality. Here, age is an important variable. For younger people, alcohol can cause much harm while doing very little to improve the health. That is because the leading cause of death in Americans under age 40 is accidents, with homicide and suicide also being major causes, especially in men. They are all associated with alcohol. The sole positive attribute for people in this age group is providing enjoyment.

It is only among people older than about 50 or 60 where alcohol consumption in moderation causes a reduction in mortality. At that age the health benefits, especially the prevention of heart disease and stroke, dominate the picture. As a result it is among this age group that a J-shaped relationship is seen between alcohol intake and risk of mortality.

6. WHAT ADVICE SHOULD A PHYSICIAN GIVE?

Despite the potential health benefits of moderate drinking, medical experts should not recommend that non-drinkers commence light to moderate drinking. The reason for this is that around 5–10% of people in any society where alcohol is available become abusers of the beverage. However, if a person is a light drinker, there is also little reason to advise them to stop.

It is, of course, imperative that a person's past history be considered. For those with a history of alcoholism, the ability to "stop after just one drink" may not exist. Recommendations regarding alcohol consumption should remain in larger part a personal decision of the patient based upon clinical realities.

SUGGESTED FURTHER READING

Rimm E, Temple NJ. What are the health implications of alcohol consumption? Nutritional Health: Strategies for Disease Prevention, 2nd ed. Temple NJ, Wilson T, Jacobs DR, eds. Humana Press, Totowa, NJ, 2006, pp. 211–221.

Room R, Babor T, Rehm J. Alcohol and public health. Lancet 2005; 365:519–530.

National Institute on Alcohol Abuse and Alcoholism (NIAAA). http://www.niaaa.nih.gov/.

REFERENCES

1. Rimm E, Temple NJ. What are the health implications of alcohol consumption? Nutritional Health: Strategies for Disease Prevention, 2nd ed. Temple NJ, Wilson T, Jacobs DR, eds. Humana Press, Totowa, NJ, 2006, pp. 211–221.
2. Colditz GA, Giovannucci E, Rimm EB, et al. Alcohol intake in relation to diet and obesity in women and men. Am J Clin Nutr 1991; 54:49–55.
3. Renaud S, de Lorgeril M. Wine, alcohol, platelets, and the French paradox for coronary heart disease. Lancet 1992; 339:1523–1526.
4. Rimm EB, Williams P, Fosher K, Criqui M, Stampfer MJ. Moderate alcohol intake and lower risk of coronary heart disease: Meta-analysis of effects on lipids and haemostatic factors. BMJ 1999; 319:1523–1528.
5. Friedman LA, Kimball AW. Coronary heart disease mortality and alcohol consumption in Framingham. Am J Epidemiol 1986; 124:481–489.
6. Stampfer MJ, Kang JH, Chen J, Cherry R, Grodstein F. Effects of moderate alcohol consumption on cognitive function in women. N Engl J Med 2005; 352:245–253.
7. Espeland MA, Gu L, Masaki KH, et al. Association between reported alcohol intake and cognition: results from the Women's Health Initiative Memory Study. Am J Epidemiol 2005, 161.228–238.

10 Issues of Food Safety: Are "Organic" Apples Better?

Gianna Ferretti, Davide Neri, and Bruno Borsari

Key Points

- Organically grown foods have become increasingly popular with the consumer because of a desire to improve nutrition and prevent environmental contamination.
- Fruits and vegetables are cultivated according to different approaches: conventional (chemical-based agriculture), integrated farm management, organic agriculture.
- Experimental evidence suggests that higher levels of micronutrients and antioxidants are associated with organically grown fruit and vegetables.
- Cultivation systems affect the amount of chemical residues in produce and the risk of its possible biological contamination.
- Synthetic pesticide and additive residues can be avoided in properly managed organic systems.
- The differences between foods grown under different agricultural methods may not be enough to declare organic produce as superior quality food relative to their conventional or integrated counterparts.

Key Words: Organic food; pesticides; food safety

1. INTRODUCTION

The promotion of diets capable of insuring a balanced nutrient intake to enhance harmonious growth and health has become a priority in developed countries *(1)*. However, this may occur at the cost of increased levels of contaminants and agriculture no longer being sustainable. Since the 1970s US agricultural systems have been geared toward maximal "production," but in more recent times food "quality" has also become an important issue. Quality has translated to an increased public awareness of and demand for

From: *Nutrition and Health: Nutrition Guide for Physicians*
Edited by: T. Wilson et al. (eds.), DOI 10.1007/978-1-60327-431-9_10,
© Humana Press, a part of Springer Science+Business Media, LLC 2010

foods grown under organic conditions. Plants absorb minerals and trace elements from their environment, along with potentially harmful xenobiotics, and synthesize vitamins and other nutrients (fat, protein, fatty acids, amino acids, and sugars, as well as fiber). Animals eat plants thus incorporating nutrients into their own tissues as well as accumulating xenobiotics from pesticides and other toxins, when these are present in the environment.

In the meantime, organic agriculture has become one of the fastest growing markets in the American agricultural sector. Consumers' demand for organic foods has increased at an astonishing annual rate of about 20% per year and was estimated to be over $20 billion in 2003 *(2)*. Pricing for organic produce in 2004 was approximately 33% greater than conventionally grown produce *(3)*. However, an accurate determination of whether organically grown foods are of greater nutritional "quality" than conventional foods remains difficult to verify. Ascertaining that organically produced foods are better than conventional and that the benefits they possess are deserving of their added economic cost of production remains challenging to assess. In light of these discrepancies we support the idea that there are many reasons to believe that organically produced foods are worth this added production cost and wish to defend our position in this chapter.

1.1. Conventional and Organic Food Production Systems

Food production systems are designed according to an integration of resource use (environmental, genetic, technological, and human), services, and economic means. Conventional, large-scale food production relies heavily on pesticides, fertilizers, and fossil fuels, which pose substantial risks of contamination to plant and animal products. These constitute legitimate concerns to food systems safety and to the environment, with a reduction of biodiversity and an enhancement of soil degradation and erosion *(4)*. Two main alternative production systems are available at present *(5)*: integrated farm management (IFM) and organic agriculture (OA). IFM consists in employing multiple tactics (such as Integrated Pest Management, IPM), in a compatible manner to maintain pest populations at levels below those causing economic injury, while providing better protection to humans, domestic animals, plants, and the environment from the residues of agrichemical products. "Integrated" means that a broader, interdisciplinary approach is adopted in agriculture. This integration of techniques, however, should be compatible with the crop being produced and marketing systems in which farming takes place. OA instead has a more holistic approach. In practical terms, it is distinguishable from other farming methods by two main principles: first, synthetic soluble mineral inputs (fertilizers) are prohibited and, second, synthetic herbicides and pesticides are rejected in favor of natural pesticides and organic soil management practices. Food production systems based on these principles result in more costly products and less yields per acreage (5). However, this may provide superior nutritional attributes to the produce in comparison with conventionally grown foods (6). While it is the goal of organically produced foods to contain fewer added chemicals, some are permitted in production protocols, as outlined in Table 1, and this can be a surprising discovery to some consumers.

2. WHAT MAKES A FOOD SAFE?

Food safety hazards include contamination by biological, physical factors, or chemical substances which are summarized in Table 2. These may pose significant health risks to consumers. The contamination of food may occur through environmental toxins (heavy metals, PCBs, and dioxins) or through the intentional use of various chemicals, such as pesticides, animal drugs, and other agrichemicals. Food additives and contaminants resulting from food manufacturing and processing can adversely affect human health (7). It remains challenging to identify possible sources of food biological contamination that inevitably cause periodic accidents in any type of production system. Regretfully, this remains an endemic problem that since the dawn of human civilization has affected public and community health. Continuous efforts are made with the goal of reducing these and similar risks in any type of food production system. We remain convinced that the risk of food contamination increases where food is grown on the largest scale and for the most distant markets, whereas, conversely, potential risks for contamination by xenobiotics is minimized when food is grown under organic conditions.

3. NUTRITIONAL VALUE OF ORGANIC VERSUS CONVENTIONAL FRUIT AND VEGETABLES

Levels of macronutrients, micronutrients, and phytonutrients (e.g., flavonols and anthocyanidins) vary, within a relatively wide range, according to the plant species and plant organ (stem, leaf, fruit) being consumed. Phytonutrients have been suggested to have potential for health promotion (lycopene from tomatoes for improved vision) and disease prevention (soy isoflavones from beans for breast cancer risk reduction). External (genotype-independent) and internal (genotype-dependent) factors affect the levels of nutrients important for human health, and plant nutrient synthesis is also affected by the conditions of stress of the plant; however, molecular mechanisms are still not completely understood (8).

Table 1
Additives Legally Permitted for Use in the Preparation of Organic Foods Produce in Europe

Colorants	Foods
E153 – *Vegetable carbon*[a] E160b – Annatto, Bixin, Norbixin	Concentrated fruit juices, jams, jellies, and liquorice Concentrated fruit juices, jams, jellies
Alkali, Anticaking Agent, Dough Conditioner, Drying Agent, Firming Agent E170 – Calcium carbonates	Some bakery products, frozen desserts, and flour
Preservatives E220 – Sulfur dioxide or E223 (Sodium metabisulphite) or E224 (Potassium metabisulphite)	Wine, dried fruit
Acidity Regulators, Anticaking Agents, Anti-Foaming Agents, Bulking Agents, Carriers and Carrier Solvents, Emulsifying Salts, Firming Agents, Flavor Enhancers, Flour Treatment Agents, Foaming Agents, Humectants E270 – Lactic acid, E290 – Carbon dioxide E500 – Sodium carbonates, E509 – Calcium chloride	Bread, cakes, snacks
Antioxidant E306 – Tocopherol-rich extract	Fruit juice, cakes, snacks
Emulsifiers, Stabilizers, Thickeners, and Gelling Agents E322 – Lecithin E400 – Alginic acid, E406 – Agar E407 – Carrageenan, E410 – Locust bean gum E410 – Sodium alginate and E402 (Potassium alginate), E412 – Guar gum	Bakery products, cheese, frozen desserts, fruit butters, jellies, and preserves

E414 – Arabic gum
E415 – Xanthan gum
E440(i) – Pectin
E464 – Hydroxypropylmethylcellulose

Cheese, including
processed cheese, ice
cream, jelly and
preserves, and
dressings
Canned fruit, fruit
butters, jellies

Packaging Gases
E938 – Argon; E939 – Helium
E941 – Nitrogen, E948 – Oxygen

[a]Banned as a food additive in the United States

Table 2
Food Safety: Factors Involved in Food Production and Storage

Physical hazards: foreign objects (e.g., wood, plastic, glass) from the
environment or equipment
Biological hazards: micro-organisms such as bacteria, viruses, parasites,
and moulds (source of aflatoxins)
Chemical risks in food: acrylamide, PCBs and dioxins; persistent organic
pollutants (POPs); organic compounds that are resistant to
environmental degradation through chemical, biological, and photolytic
processes
Allergenes: milk, eggs, fish, crustacean shellfish, tree nuts, peanuts,
soybeans
Antimicrobials: cephalosporin antibiotic resistance
Food additives and contaminants: melamine

3.1. Comparison of Organically Grown and Conventionally Grown Products

Organically grown products tend to have a higher content of dry matter
and secondary plant metabolites than conventionally grown products (9).
Winter and Davis (10) reviewed the literature concerning the comparison of
the nutritional quality of organic and conventional foods. Their findings are
summarized here for several common fruits and vegetables.

3.1.1. GRAPES AND WINE

The content of resveratrol, a phenolic grape (*Vitis vinifera*) phytoalexin, in
organic wine was 26% higher in organic than in conventional wines in paired
comparisons of the same grape variety (11). However, polyphenoloxidase
enzyme levels in organic and conventional grapes did not differ; although

diphenolase activity was two times higher in organic grapes than conventional grapes *(10)*.

3.1.2. ORANGES

Higher levels of total phenolics, total anthocyanins, and ascorbic acid are typically observed in organic oranges and juices relative to their nonorganic counterparts. Organic orange extracts improve free radical and oxidative damage to rat cardiomyocytes and differentiated Caco-2 cells when compared with conventional extracts from conventionally grown sources *(12)*.

3.1.3. APPLES

Apples are one of the main sources of flavonoids in the Western diets, providing approximately 22% of the total phenols consumed per capita in the United States *(13)*. The nutrient content of organic and conventional apples has been widely investigated. Genotype-related differences may contribute to the higher contents of antioxidants such as polyphenols and flavonols in organic apples *(10)*. In a recent study, higher levels of antioxidants in local varieties of apples (Mela Rosa) compared with Golden Delicious apples were verified, with higher levels observed even after storage both in organic and conventional agriculture *(14)*. In other experimental trials, the quality attributes of apples coming from different regions, and different production systems, did not differ significantly, at harvest, or after storage *(15)*.

3.1.4. PEACH AND PEARS

The concentration of polyphenols and the activity of polyphenoloxidase (PPO), together with the content in ascorbic acid, citric acid, and alpha- and gamma-tocopherol, are higher in organic peach (*Prunus persica* L., cv. Regina bianca) and pear (*Pyrus communis* L., cv. Williams) *(10)*.

3.1.5. TOMATOES

The comparison of the antioxidants content between organically and conventionally grown tomatoes revealed equal or higher vitamin C, carotenoids, and polyphenols (except for chlorogenic acid) than conventional tomatoes. The concentration of vitamin C and polyphenols remained higher in purees after processing from organic tomatoes. However, in vivo studies indicate that plasma levels of the two major antioxidants, vitamin C and lycopene, are not significantly modified after 3 weeks of tomato puree consumption *(10)*.

Although organic fruits and vegetables have higher contents of antioxidants and micronutrients when compared to equivalent conventional produce, it remains difficult to insure their superior nutritional quality and healthy attributes.

3.2. Other Causes of Differences Between Organic and Conventional Foods

Differences among food production systems also emerge from the farming protocols and delivery systems. These may be more or less sensitive to a sustainable approach to food production and environmental stewardship. It is also worth noting that "stewardship" and "value system" concerns may impact human nutrition and health by affecting consumers' selection and consumption of foods. Anemia resulting from iron deficiency among "true" vegan vegetarians is one such example where philosophical decisions about "what to eat or not to eat" may affect people's health. Concerns in this regard are important to nutritionists and have led to recent discussions about the need for improvements in the USDA inspection process of evaluating meats and produce and their quality.

3.2.1. PESTICIDES

Nearly all pesticides are prohibited in organic farming and residues are rarely found. However, the use of biological measures to control pests can be utilized; for example, applying BT-producing bacteria to plant leaves in order to control insect–crop infestations. By contrast, in conventional foods, there is growing concern about the "cocktail effect" that multiple pesticide residues have on human health. Although these residues may be below thresholds that guarantee food safety, they pose great concern to an increasing number of consumers.

3.2.2. FOOD POISONING

The risk of biological contamination, both in the field and post-harvest, may affect food quality and safety. However, there is no evidence linking organically produced foods to an increased risk of food poisoning. A recent survey gave organic food a clean bill of health and confirmed expectations that organic methods, such as careful composting of manure, minimize risks of food contamination (16). Spadaro and his coworkers (17) found no significant difference between conventional and organic apple juices for patulin and other fungal contaminants. Nonetheless, as we have already pointed out, mycotoxins and bacteria in food and feed pose a constant threat to the transport and storage of food, and, inevitably, to the health of consumers (18).

3.2.3. GMOs

Genetically modified organisms (GMOs) and their derivatives are prohibited in organic food production. There is currently insufficient published evidence to reach any definitive conclusion regarding the safety of genetically modified foods for human consumption. This big question remains unanswered although the industry assures absolute safety. However, the reluctance of the USDA to label GMO foods is not helping a growing segment of society to accept these foods willingly, and this skepticism for GMOs has sparked even more interest in organically produced food.

3.2.4. ANTIBIOTICS

The routine, growth-promoting or prophylactic use of antibiotics is prohibited in organic standards for animal husbandry *(16)*. There is growing concern over the risk to human health and concerns that micro-organisms may develop antibiotic resistance because of the misuse and overuse of antibiotics in livestock rearing *(7)*. A recent report suggests that bacterial isolates from foods produced from organically raised animals were less resistant to antimicrobial treatment when compared to conventionally raised animal foods *(10)*. Concerns of microbial pathogenesis have not been fully addressed by the USDA, although these concerns are an additional source of consumer interest in organically produced foods.

3.2.5. FOOD ADDITIVES

More than 500 additives are permitted for use in nonorganically processed foods, compared with about 30 permitted in organic food processing (Table 1). Even though organic standards limit the use of additives linked to allergic reactions, headaches, asthma, growth retardation, hyperactivity in children, heart disease, and osteoporosis *(16)*, some of them could trigger allergic reactions in consumers who are already predisposed to these and similar conditions.

3.2.6. FOOD PALATABILITY

Given that the incidence of cardiovascular disease and cancer is negatively correlated with increasing daily fruit and vegetable intakes, by simply increasing food palatability one may increase fruit and vegetable intake and reduce the incidence of these chronic diseases. The few consumer taste tests data suggest that organic apples "taste" better than their conventionally produced counterparts, and improved taste is of course one way to improve consumption. A small body of observational and clinical evidence supports the hypothesis that consumption of organically produced food is beneficial to human health *(9)*. Although, the higher prices could limit a further expansion of the actual organic food niche, we envision that in a not far future, high quality, environmentally sound food will become a standard for consumers. In the meantime we support large-scale consumption of IFM food as a temporary solution to an achievement of quality food for all, as a higher emphasis on organic farming spurred by a more equitable allocation of resources in its favor will reduce production costs while making organic foods more affordable to a progressively largest segment of consumers. The higher price of organic foods should not deter consumers from choosing these as by making this decision consumers promote a form of agriculture that is more environmentally sound, while compensating the grower with a more realistic amount of money that more accurately reflects the true cost of food production.

4. CONCLUSION

Recent accidents in the US food system have resulted in the withdrawal from the market of contaminated tomato, spinach, corn, and other commodities. These incidents indicate that large-scale, highly centralized food systems remain fragile and that their ability to ensure food safety remains questionable.

Consumers wishing to improve their intake of minerals, vitamins, and phytonutrients while reducing their exposure to potentially harmful pesticide residues, nitrates, GMOs, and artificial additives used in food processing should, wherever possible, choose organically produced fruits and vegetables. The compositional data of organic and conventional vegetables could be used in public health campaigns to increase the consumption of products able to provide improved health protection and the prevention of chronic diseases. However, the crucial question of whether organic is "worth the extra cost" will probably remain one that needs to be determined by consumers only.

Further research is urgently needed to clarify the exact relationship between agricultural management and the nutritional quality of crops. However, decisions on appropriate sites, cultivars, and harvest criteria can differ between the organic and nonorganic sectors of agriculture. A better understanding of the cultivation systems available to consumers has become crucial to an improved understanding of public health enhancement.

REFERENCES

1. World Health Organization. Diet, Nutrition and the Prevention of Chronic Diseases. World Health Organization, Geneva, 2003.

2. Kortbech-Olesen R. Market. In: Yussefi M, Willer H, eds. The World of Organic Agriculture. IFOAM, Tholey-Theley, Germany, 2003, pp. 21–26.

3. Oberholtzer L, Greene C, Lopez E. Organic Poultry and Eggs Capture High Price Premiums and Growing Share of Specialty Markets. US Department of Agriculture, L, LDP-M-150-01December 2006.

4. Gliessman SR. Agroecology. The Ecology of Sustainable Food Systems. CRC Press, Boca Raton, Fl, 2007, p. 384.

5. Trewavas A. A Critical Assessment of Organic Farming-and-Food Assertions with Particular Respect to the UK and the Potential Environmental Benefits of No-Till Agriculture. Crop Protection 2004, 23, pp. 757–781.

6. Morgan K, Murdoch J. Organic vs. conventional agriculture: knowledge, power and innovation in the food chain. Geoforum 2000; 31:159–173.

7. Fox MW. Eating with Conscience. The Bioethics of Food. New Sage Press, Troutdale, OR, 1997, p. 192.

8. Wu X. Lipophilic and hydrophilic antioxidant capacities of common foods in the United States. J Agricol Food Chem 2004; 52:4026–4037.

9. Di Renzo L, Di Pierro D, Bigioni M, et al. Is antioxidant plasma status in humans a consequence of the antioxidant food content influence? Eur Rev Med Pharmacol Sc 2007; 11:185–192.

10. Winter C, Davis S. Organic foods. J Food Sci 2006; 71:117–124.

11. Dani C, Oliboni LS, Vanderlinde R, Bonatto D, Salvador M, Henriques JA. Phenolic content and antioxidant activities of white and purple juices manufactured with organically-or conventionally-produced grapes. Food Chem Toxicol 2007; 45:2574–2580.

12. Tarozzi A, Hrelia S, Angeloni C, et al. Antioxidant effectiveness of organically and non-organically grown red oranges in cell culture systems. Eur J Nutr 2006; 45:152–158.

13. Lotito SB, Frei B. Consumption of flavonoid-rich foods and increased plasma antioxidant capacity in humans: Cause, consequence, or epiphenomenon? Free Radic Biol Med 2006; 41:1727–1746.

14. Ferretti G, Marchionni C, Bacchetti T. Valutazione della qualita' nutrizionale dei frutti di mele del germoplasma marchigiano. In: Virgili S, Neri D, eds. Mela rosa e mele antiche. Valorizzazione di ecotipi locali di melo per un'agricoltura sostenibile. ASSAM, Ancona, Italy, 2002, pp. 53–65.

15. Ròth E, Berna A, Beullens K, et al. Postharvest quality of integrated and organically produced apple fruit. Postharvest Biol Techn 2007; 45:11–19.

16. Soil Association. Organic Farming, Food Quality and Human Health: A Review of the Evidence. www.soilassociation.org. (ISBN 0 905200 80 2). Bristol, UK, 2007, p. 87.

17. Spadaro D, Ciavorella A, Frati S, Garibaldi A, Gullino ML. Incidence and level of patulin contamination in pure and mixed apple juices marketed in Italy. Food Control 2007; 18:1098–1102.

18. McHughen A. Toppling the organic house of cards (Book review). Nature Biotechn 2007; 25:522–523.

11 What Is a Healthy Diet? From Nutritional Science to Food Guides

Norman J. Temple

Key Points

- This chapter summarizes the key features of a healthy diet.
- Various food guides are described and critically evaluated. These include MyPyramid, Harvard's Healthy Eating Pyramid, DASH Eating Plan, Canada's Food Guide, and Traffic Lights Food Guide.

Key Words: Food-based dietary guidelines; food guides; Mypyramid

1. DEFINING A HEALTHY DIET

Since the 1970s our knowledge of the relationship between diet, health, and the risk of disease, especially chronic diseases of lifestyle, has increased tremendously. However, the application of this knowledge to clinical practice and to public health has not been as thorough. This has taught us the essentials of what people need to eat for optimal health. This information is described throughout this book. Based on this information we can summarize the essential features of a healthy diet, meaning one that assists in achieving optimal health and minimizes risk of chronic disease.

1.1. Controlling Fat Intake and BMI

There is perhaps no better starting point than weight control. Control the weight. The ideal BMI is generally agreed to be in the range 18.5–25. Alas, an epidemic of obesity has swept the western world for the past quarter

From: *Nutrition and Health: Nutrition Guide for Physicians*
Edited by: T. Wilson et al. (eds.), DOI 10.1007/978-1-60327-431-9_11,
© Humana Press, a part of Springer Science+Business Media, LLC 2010

century, leading to a secondary epidemic of diabetes and other conditions. All physicians therefore need to make weight control a priority issue. This was well put by Orson Welles: "My doctor told me to stop having intimate dinners for four. Unless there are three other people."

Integral to this is the encouragement for all patients to engage in regular physical activity. For health, an appropriate goal is 30 min of exercise, of at least moderate intensity, such as brisk walking, on most days of the week. Increasing the intensity to vigorous (such as jogging or fast walking) or duration (to 1 h) is better. A popular gadget these days is a pedometer with a target of 10,000 steps per day. Where weight loss is a goal of exercise, then the laws of physics are crystal clear: more exercise is better.

Recommendations for fat intake have been in flux in recent years: from "less than 30%" of energy intake to a more liberal 20–35%. An important reason for this increase in the upper limit is because the emphasis on a low-fat diet had an unexpected negative consequence: many low-fat foods, such yoghurt and cookies, have had their fat partially replaced with highly refined carbohydrates negating the intended nutritional advantage. However, a diet low in fat – around 25% of energy – but also low in refined carbohydrates, is probably ideal. A key reason for this is the strong link between a high intake of fat and excessive weight gain.

1.2. All Fats Are Not Alike

The type of fat is of great importance. The cause-and-effect relationship between saturated fat, blood cholesterol, and heart disease has been well known for decades. More recent evidence suggests a role for saturated fats in other conditions, such as diabetes. For this reason, the diet should be limited in its content of meat (especially red meat with a high fat content), milk with 2% or more fat, and hard margarine. Tropical oils (palm and coconut) are also rich in saturated fats and should be avoided for that reason.

Closely related to saturated fats are the *trans* fats, which have also been linked to the risk of heart disease. These fats are formed in oils during the hydrogenation process. *Trans* fats are commonly found in hard margarine and in many baked goods such as donuts, croissants, chips, and cookies. As far as possible these fats, including margarine containing hydrogenated fats, should be avoided. Changes in labeling laws have greatly improved public awareness in the United States and there have been decreases in their use for processed foods.

The body requires essential polyunsaturated fats for normal functioning. Vegetable oils, such as corn oil, sunflower oil, and most brands of soft margarine, are rich sources. However, these fats mostly provide $n–6$ fats, such as linoleic acid. What is often lacking is $n–3$ fats. Sources include flaxseed oil (a rich source), followed by soybean oil and then canola oil. Fatty fish, such as sardines, mackerel, salmon, trout, and herring, are also a rich source of n–3 fats. However, whereas the n–3 fats in plant oils are mainly linolenic acid, fish oils are particularly rich in the long-chain types (DHA and EPA) that appear to be most protective against heart disease.

Among meat and fish products, cold-water fatty fish is most preferred, followed by low-fat fish, poultry, lean red meat, regular cuts of red meat, and, lastly, processed meat. Beans and lentils make an excellent alternative to meat and can be well recommended.

1.3. Carbohydrates; Good and Bad

If fats are reduced, then carbohydrates must increase. And the healthiest way to increase carbohydrate consumption is with whole grain cereals. Much evidence has accumulated of the protective association of whole grains with heart disease, type 2 diabetes, and cancer.

Most people need to reduce their intake of refined sugars: less is definitely better. In this context "sugar" means both sucrose and high-fructose corn syrup that is ubiquitous in soft drinks. A reasonable upper limit is 10% of energy. Sugar is linked to obesity and dental caries. Nutritionally speaking, refined cereals, such as white bread and white rice, lie midway between whole grains and sugar.

1.4. Whole Fruits and Vegetables Are Better

A generous intake of fruit and vegetables is strongly recommended. There are several good reasons for this. In particular, these foods provide significant protection against cancer and several other diseases. The protective substances include dietary fiber, various nutrients (potassium, folate, vitamin C, and many others). But as with the health benefits of whole grains it is most unclear how much of this can be attributed to fiber and specific micronutrients and how much to phytochemicals. However, the evidence is sufficiently strong that phytochemicals are important for health and it is recommended that everyone consume a variety of fruit and vegetables (dark green vegetables, orange fruit, and vegetables, etc.). Potatoes are the least favored of the vegetables, mainly because of their minimal content of phytochemicals. Dietary supplements are not a substitute for the consumption of fruit and vegetables; a major reason is that supplements lack phytochemicals.

An important benefit of fruit and vegetables is that they have a low energy density (kcal per 100 g). As a result they satisfy the appetite after only a relatively small quantity of kcals has been consumed. No one ever got fat by eating too many apples or carrots or drinking too much tomato soup!

Whole fruit is superior to fruit juice because of its fiber content (and like-wise for vegetables and vegetable juice). But juices are a convenient way to boost the intake of fruit and vegetables. We live in a world where sugar-rich soft drinks are consumed in vast quantities, especially by young people. Almost anything that displaces them is a big improvement. For that reason juices can play a valuable role in the diet.

It is important to avoid being confused by pseudo-juice products. Drinks labeled as "fruit nectar," "fruit beverage," or "fruit punch" contain little or no actual fruit juice. Despite the pictures of fruit that often appear prominently on the labels, these products are little more than fruit-flavored sugar water.

1.5. Coffee, Tea, and Alcohol

What about tea and coffee? Considering the vast quantities that are con-sumed, they are amazingly free of evidence of harmfulness. Of the two, tea is by far the healthier. Most of its phytochemicals survives the boiling process. In the case of black tea there is evidence that it may offer some modest pro-tection against heart disease. Coffee seems rather neutral, healthwise, except for its interference with sleep.

Alcohol in excess creates many problems, especially violence and acci-dents. It is also a significant factor in cancer. However, in moderation alcohol can be beneficial for the health. It reduces the risk of heart disease and also appears to help prevent hypertension and several other chronic conditions. The balance between risks and benefits of moderate consumption of alcohol are strongly age related: alcohol has a net benefit with people over age 50 or 60, whereas with people below age 40 the harm caused by alcohol domi-nates the picture. Arguably, the most prudent policy is one that explains that alcohol in moderation – up to two drinks a day for men and one drink a day for women – will likely have several health benefits for people in middle age and older, while also stressing the hazards of abuse. Quite apart from the total alcohol intake, an important factor is drinking pattern. Occasional heavy drinking can lead to a much increased risk of death.

1.6. The Problem with Salt

Increasing the salt content of a food is a common way to improve the palatability and the sales of a processed food product. This may benefit some sectors of the food industry. However, there is a rock solid body of evidence that lowering the salt content of the diet must be a priority issue. The average American consumes around 9 g of salt a day. Current recommendations call for this to be reduced to below 6 g (or 2300 mg sodium). However, an intake of half of this level is highly desirable. This could have a major public health benefit as it would significantly lower the prevalence of both hypertension and of mildly elevated levels of blood pressure. This would, in turn, prevent a great many cases of heart disease and stroke.

1.7. Supplements: There Is No Shortcut to a Balanced Diet

An important question concerns the use of supplements. Many people are of the opinion that a multivitamin is also advisable for the general population. While this is of dubious value for those who eat a nutritious diet, it makes sense for the large sections of the population whose diet is habitually poor. A multivitamin – meaning pills containing a broad spectrum of vitamins and minerals – is also advisable for women who could become pregnant and those who are pregnant or breastfeeding. This is especially the case in order to ensure sufficient intake of folic acid and of iron. Another valuable supplement is fish oil, especially for people who seldom eat fatty fish. An appropriate dose is a teaspoon a day of cod liver oil (pills cost several times more for the same amount). There is now strong evidence for the benefit of vitamin D, especially for those aged over 50. In addition to its well-known function in maintaining bone health it also appears to have a potent cancer-preventing action, and some evidence also suggests that it may prevent a few other diseases. The problem of insufficient vitamin D gets steadily worse the further north one lives; for example, everyone living in the northern states will be unable to synthesize the vitamin in their bodies for around 5 months during the winter. For those living north of the sunshine states a recommended intake of vitamin D from supplements is 1000 IU (25 mcg) per day. This refers to the total supplementary intake from all sources including multivitamin pills and fish oil.

1.8. How Safe Is Our Food?

"Doctor. Should I buy organic food?" Organic foods are grown without synthetic pesticides. It is almost certainly preferable to reduce one's intake of pesticides. But the quantities consumed from conventionally grown food are extremely small. Organic foods are usually much more expensive than regular supermarket food, typically by 50% or more. This extra cost is probably an unjustified expense for most of the population.

No account of a healthy diet is complete without also considering how to design it in a manner that is environmentally friendly. Here are some good rules to follow. The single biggest dietary change that we should aim for is the reduction in consumption of meat. This is because meat production requires huge amounts of land, energy, and water. In this regard four-legged meat is twice as bad as chicken. By contrast, beans and lentils are much more environmentally friendly, quite apart from their nutritional advantages. In order to reduce transportation people should, where feasible, buy food grown as near as possible to where they live. Another important factor is that people should buy food with minimal packaging and this should be recycled. If food is packaged, then a large size is preferable. An especially environmentally unfriendly product is bottled water, particularly brands transported from distant locations.

2. FOOD GUIDES

There are several food guides available. These provide advice for the general public on how to select a diet that enhances health and helps to prevent disease. The challenge in constructing a food guide is to translate nutrition knowledge into a format that is easy for people to understand and to apply to their everyday lives.

While the details vary from country to country, there is broad agreement as to the key message. Here are the recurring themes in different food guides:

- eat plenty of whole grains, fruit, and vegetables
- consume an appropriate amount of meat (but not too much), meat alternatives (such as beans and lentils), and milk (or milk products)
- limit the intake of alcohol, sugar, and of foods rich in fat, in general, and saturated fat, in particular.

If there is one place where "the devil is in the detail," it is in food guides. Beyond the key themes above, there are a multitude of differences over such things as where to place potatoes (with or separate from other vegetables), where to put legumes (with vegetables or as an alternative to meat), and whether to keep fruit and vegetables together in the same group. Quite apart from these issues there are big differences around the world in the visual design of food guides. The intention in all cases is to convey to the general population what proportion of the diet should come from each food group. Some countries have used a dinner plate design while the United States has opted for a pyramid.

Deciding on the "right" answer to each of these questions and then designing the "best" diet goes far beyond questions of the nutrient content of various foods and describing a healthy diet; we must also consider the vital matter of how best to educate people as to the fundamentals of a healthy diet and how to persuade them to actually eat that diet. Fail to do that and everything is a waste of time! For that reason a vital consideration in designing food guides is to make them user friendly. In the next section attention is turned to food guides that are available.

2.1. MyPyramid

Until 2005 the guide disseminated to the general public in the United States was the Food Guide Pyramid. It was a simple matter to look at this one-page document and figure out how many servings should be eaten from each food group. But this all changed with the launch of MyPyramid (www.mypyramid.gov). Unlike all other food guides around the world this one requires the use of the internet. The user enters his or her profile (age, sex, and physical activity) and then receives a personalized set of diet recommendations. The obvious challenge with this food guide is the matter of user accessibility. It seems highly probable that there are millions of people who are willing to read a simple, printed food guide, much as one reads a TV guide, but simply cannot be bothered to use a website for this purpose.

In most countries, Canada for example, the folks who write the food guide belong to the health department of the government, but in the United States they work for the Department of Agriculture. That department therefore has a serious conflict of interest: it must help make farming and food production profitable (which often means boosting the sale of less than healthy foods) while at the same time advising people how to eat for health. As a result there is a strong suspicion that both the old and new pyramids are compromises between these two opposing forces. Marion Nestle of New York University described MyPyramid as "a disaster" (1). This is how nutrition experts from Harvard School of Public Health described MyPyramid and the Food Guide Pyramid (2): "The problem was that these efforts, while generally good intentioned, have been quite flawed at actually showing people what makes up a healthy diet. Why? Their recommendations have often been based on out-of-date science and influenced by people with business interests in their messages."

So what should a physician do to help his or her patients? MyPyramid, despite its faults, is still an option. For patients who are happy to use the internet it provides much information. The diet can be easily modified based on height, weight, and whether a person wishes to lose weight. It is also available in Spanish, and that certainly helps.

2.2. Harvard's Healthy Eating Pyramid

In view of the criticisms leveled against MyPyramid (and its predecessor), it should come as little surprise that alternative food guides have been developed. There are two American ones that deserve serious consideration. One is the Healthy Eating Pyramid (HEP) produced by the Department of Nutrition of the Harvard School of Public Health (2).

The general design of HEP is similar to the Food Guide Pyramid but with one notable exception: it does not specify the number of servings from each food group. Instead, it tells users that "The Healthy Eating Pyramid doesn't worry about specific servings or grams of food, so neither should you. It's a simple, general guide to how you should eat when you eat."

A detailed comparison between HEP and MyPyramid shows that HEP recommends more fruit (but about the same amount of vegetables) and places more emphasis on whole grains, fish, poultry, nuts, seeds, beans, and vegetable oils *(3)*. At the same time it recommends that the following foods be used "sparingly": red meat, butter, refined grains, and potatoes. It also recommends much less milk and other dairy foods; it suggests that these foods can be replaced by vitamin D and calcium supplements. HEP recommends only half as many "discretionary calories" (foods rich in solid fat and sugar, and alcohol). The diet is actually quite similar to the Mediterranean diet. In comparison with MyPyramid the most notable differences in the composition of HEP is that it provides more fiber (43 vs. 31 g), more polyunsaturated fat (11.9 vs. 8.9% of energy), but less saturated fat (6 vs. 8% of energy) and less salt. These figures are estimates based on diets supplying about 2000 kcal *(3)*.

2.3. DASH Eating Plan

This grew out of the DASH trial (Dietary Approaches to Stop Hypertension). That intervention tested a diet that emphasizes fruit, vegetables, and low-fat dairy products, while also providing a reduced intake of fat and saturated fat. The DASH diet succeeded in significantly lowering elevated blood pressure levels *(4)*. The National Heart, Lung, and Blood Institute (NHLBI) then turned the DASH diet into a diet for the general population. This is known as the DASH Easting Plan (dashdiet.org) *(5)*.

Compared with MyPyramid, the DASH Eating Plan recommends a greater emphasis on lean meat, poultry, and fish (rather than red meat) and also on nuts, seeds, and beans. This food guide recommends a large cut in oils (2–3 vs. 6 teaspoons) and in discretionary calories (32 vs. 267 kcal). The diet supplies more fiber (39 vs. 31 g), but much less fat, saturated fat, and polyunsaturated fat (19 vs. 29%; 5 vs. 8%; and 6.0 vs. 8.9% of energy, respectively). As before these figures are estimates based on diets supplying about 2000 kcal *(3)*.

The most striking differences between the three food guides are as follows. Compared with MyPyramid, both HEP and the DASH Easting Plan provide about one-third more fiber and about one-third less saturated fat. Whereas HEP provides a generous amount of polyunsaturated fat (both *n*–6 and *n*–3 fats), the DASH Eating Plan is essentially a low-fat diet with a much reduced intake of all classes of unsaturated fat (but with significantly more protein and carbohydrate). On balance, HEP and the DASH Easting Plan are both excellent diet guides. This author's personal preference would be either HEP but with a bit less unsaturated fat or else the DASH Easting Plan but with rather more polyunsaturated fat (both n–6 and n–3 fats).

2.4. Canada's Food Guide

A full revised version of this food guide was published in 2007 (http://www.hc-sc.gc.ca/foodguide) (6). It is similar to the old Food Guide Pyramid with respect to the number of servings from each food group. And like that food guide it is easy to understand, though the presentation is quite different. There are several notable features. The recommended number of servings of fruit and vegetables (which are lumped together in one food group) has now overtaken grains. Supplements are specifically recommended for particular groups: 400 IU of vitamin D per day for men and women over age 50 (remember this is for people living in Canada) and a multivitamin containing folic acid for women who could become pregnant and those who are pregnant or breastfeeding. Anyone wishing to use this food guide should request a printed copy as this makes using it much easier than reading it via the internet.

2.5. Traffic Lights Food Guide

A radically different approach to food guides is to use a traffic lights design. This food guide is simplicity itself. Within each food group, foods have been categorized as follows: green (eat freely, based on recommended amounts), amber (eat in limited amounts), or red (these are treats; eat little or none). This food guide design is a logical development of traffic lights food labels which are becoming increasingly used in the UK and other countries (7).

The author has designed a version of this food guide (see Table 1). Food guides typically categorize foods into two broad classes: those that are recommended and those that should be eaten only in limited quantities. But nutrition science informs us that many foods belong somewhere in between. For that reason one important advantage of the traffic lights design is that foods are divided into three classes.

Little research has been done to determine whether a traffic lights design will lead to people eating a healthier diet. Until that research is done, it is a matter of speculation as to whether this design is superior to the type of food guides discussed earlier.

Table 1

Traffic Lights Food Guide. Eat a Mixture of Foods from the Different Food Groups but Carefully Follow the Rules Given Below

Food Group	Green (Eat Freely Based on Recommended Amounts)	Amber (Eat in Limited Amounts)	Red (Eat Little or None)
Fruit/vegetables	Nearly all fruits and vegetables	Potatoes, fruit juice	French fries
Grain products	Whole grains, such as whole wheat bread, oats, dark rye bread, and popcorn	Refined cereals, such as white rice, white bread, and corn flakes	Cookies, muffins, popcorn with salt/butter
Milk products	Skim and 1% milk, fortified soy milk	2% Milk, low-fat cheese	Whole milk, regular cheese, cream cheese, ice cream
Meat, fish, beans, nuts	Fish, beans, lentils, nuts	Lean beef, chicken	Bacon, most regular cuts of red meat, eggs
Oils, fats	Most vegetable oils, soft margarine (from canola oil or soy oil)	Olive oil	Hard margarine, butter

Golden Rules for a Healthy Diet

1. Eat only enough to satisfy your appetite. If you are gaining excess weight or you wish to lose weight, then eat less.
2. Eat 5–10 servings a day of grain products. Of this, at least three servings (preferably more) should be whole grains. One serving is a slice of bread, a cup of breakfast cereal, or half a bagel.
3. Eat 5–10 servings a day of whole fruit and vegetables. One serving is an apple, a banana, a cup of salad, or half a cup of other vegetables. In addition, up to one cup of juice (2 servings) may be consumed. Aim for a mixture of different types of fruit and vegetables. Fresh or frozen is better than canned.

4. Consume two or three servings a day of milk products (more for adolescents and women who are pregnant or breastfeeding). One serving is a cup of milk or yogurt, or an ounce and a half (45 g) of cheese.
5. Consume 1–3 servings a day of meat, fish, beans, peas, lentils, and nuts. A serving is 3 ounces (90 g) of fish or meat, or half a cup of cooked beans.
6. Aim for about three teaspoons a day of margarine, oils, and salad dressing, or double that if you eat little or no other sources of polyunsaturated fats, such as nuts or fish.
7. Minimize your consumption of sugar. This includes sugar in coffee and soft drinks, and drinks labeled as fruit beverage. Also, minimize your consumption of foods rich in both fat and sugar, such as cakes and donuts.
8. Cut down on the amount of salt in your diet. Remember: most salt in the diet comes from processed foods, such as most types of bread, margarine, and canned foods.
9. It is OK to consume alcohol provided that this is done responsibly. Never drink and drive, never drink if pregnant, and do not get drunk. An acceptable intake is one drink a day for women and two drinks a day for men.

SUGGESTED FURTHER READING

Dietary Guidelines. This document is published by the Department of Health and Human Services (HHS) and the Department of Agriculture (USDA). It gives a summary of dietary advice. The latest edition was published in 2005 and has a length of about 70 pages. Available from http://www.health.gov/dietaryguidelines.

Temple NJ, Wilson T, Jacobs DR, Jr (eds). Nutritional Health: Strategies for Disease Prevention, 2nd ed. Humana Press, NJ, 2006.

Duyff R. American Dietetic Association. American Dietetic Association Complete Food and Nutrition Guide. Wiley, Hoboken, NJ, 2006.

REFERENCES

1. Nestle M. Eating made simple. Sci Am 2007 (Sept): 60–63.
2. http://www.thenutritionsource.org, Last accessed June 2, 2008.
3. Reedy J, Krebs-Smith SM. A comparison of food-based recommendations and nutrient values of three food guides: USDA's MyPyramid, NHLBI's Dietary Approaches to Stop Hypertension Eating Plan, and Harvard's Healthy Eating Pyramid. J Am Diet Assoc 2008; 108:522–528.
4. Sacks FM, Svetkey LP, Vollmer WM, et al. Effects on blood pressure of reduced dietary sodium and the Dietary Approaches to Stop Hypertension (DASH) diet. DASH-Sodium Collaborative Research Group. N Engl J Med 2001; 344:3–10.
5. dashdiet.org, Last accessed June 2, 2008.
6. http://www.hc-sc.gc.ca/foodguide, Last accessed June 2, 2008.
7. http://www.eatwell.gov.uk/foodlabels/trafficlights, Last accessed August 23, 2008.

12 Achieving Dietary Change: The Role of the Physician

Joanne M. Spahn

Key Points

- The worldwide obesity epidemic has increased the impetus for development of clinic-based strategies targeting delivery of nutrition advice and counseling in the primary-care setting.
- Nutrition counseling is most effective when targeted to patients at the highest risk, supported by counseling and referral of appropriate clients to nutrition intervention programs.
- Client-centered counseling strategies engage the patient in development and implementation of an action plan designed to enhance self-management practices.
- The 5A-counseling model is a recognized evidence-based method for conducting minimal contact behavior change interventions.
- Application of a combination of motivational interviewing and cognitive-behavioral strategies is effective in precipitating nutrition-related behavior change.

Key Words: Client-centered counseling; clinical care guidelines; behavior change; motivational interviewing; evidence-based counseling methods; stages of change; cognitive-behavioral theory; physician interventions

1. INTRODUCTION

Healthy People 2010 established a national goal to increase the proportion of physician office visits that include nutrition counseling or education for patients with a diagnosis of cardiovascular disease, diabetes, or hyperlipidemia, from 42 to 75% (1). Early intervention by medical providers has the potential to have enormous impact on disease prevention, mitigation of disease progression, improving the quality of life of patients, and decreasing health-care expenditures. Inclusion of nutritional status as a routine

From: *Nutrition and Health: Nutrition Guide for Physicians*
Edited by: T. Wilson et al. (eds.), DOI 10.1007/978-1-60327-431-9_12,
© Humana Press, a part of Springer Science+Business Media, LLC 2010

component of care heightens patients' awareness of the critical link between diet and health and enhances the credibility of the health-care professional in addressing nutrition-related issues. This chapter provides guidance on techniques and tools for optimizing the delivery of nutrition counseling in a busy primary-care practice setting.

2. EFFICACY OF NUTRITION COUNSELING BY PHYSICIANS

Numerous recent studies describe brief and effective clinic-based strategies for delivering nutrition advice and counseling in the primary-care setting, targeted to patients with diabetes, hyperlipidemia, hypertension, or who need weight control or general diet improvement (2–4). These interventions involved a client-centered approach, supported by a variety of office-based systems (office prompts, algorithms, and diet assessment tools), and resulted in significant nutrition-related behavior changes. Physician advice is a catalyst for diet-related behavior change (5, 6). Patient retention of nutrition advice is significantly better (95% vs. 27%, $P < 0.01$, related to specific foods; 90% vs. 20%, related to food preparation methods) when received by providers trained in nutrition counseling (7). Advice provided by trained providers was more extensive, specific, and culturally relevant, and communication skills were used to enhance rapport and ensure that patients understood the advice. Ockene and colleagues reported that a brief patient-centered counseling approach (average of 8.2 min for the initial counseling intervention), with and without office system support, is the key to achieving significant change at 1-year in percentage of energy intake from saturated fat, weight, and blood lipid levels (2). Referrals to a registered dietitian or community-based nutrition intervention program are excellent strategies to increase the intensity of interventions but cannot substitute for ongoing involvement of the patient's primary physician.

Physicians are ideally positioned to influence patients to seriously consider dietary change to improve health, especially when they make referrals to dietitians. A listing of dietitians available in all geographic areas can be found on the American Dietetic Association web site (www.eatright.org). Group interventions, such as behavioral therapy or self-management education programs, are efficacious and cost-effective strategies for supporting diet and physical activity lifestyle change (8–11).

3. MEDICAL OFFICE SYSTEM SUPPORT

Given the time constraints in primary-care practice, nutrition counseling is best targeted to patients at the highest risk, needs to be brief, integrated within an organized office system, and include referral of

Table 1
Web-Based Nutrition Education Resources

Source of Information	Internet Site
American Dietetic Association	http://www.eatright.org/
Fit Day (Internet Weight Loss and Diet Journal)	http://www.fitday.com/
My Pyramid Tracker	http://www.mypyramidtracker.gov/
NHLBI Health Information for the Patient, Public, and Professional	http://www.nhlbi.nih.gov
NIH Office of Dietary Supplements, Dietary Supplement Fact Sheets	http://dietary-supplements.info.nih.gov (then click on "Health Information")
Nutrition Academy Award Products	http://www.nhlbi.nih.gov/funding/training/ naa/products.htm
The Weight-control Information Network (WIN)	http://win.niddk.nih.gov/

appropriate patients to a nutrition professional. Clinical care guidelines for overweight, hypertension, diabetes, and heart disease are available at www.guidelines.gov website. The Nutrition Academy Award Program web site, referenced in Table 1, provides assessment criteria to identify patients who would benefit most from nutrition intervention. Other chapters in this book also cover these topics. Use of an office system facilitates an evidence-based approach, ensuring efficient and consistent data collection, assessment and documentation of counseling, simplified tracking of care through the use of flowcharts, chart reminders, reminder postcards for patients, and coordinated educational materials and strategies *(12)*.

The principles for organizing an office system to support delivery of nutrition care advice and counseling include *(13)*:

1. Policy development;
2. Determining baseline rates for target populations (e.g., patients with diabetes, hyperlipidemia, hypertension, obesity);
3. Defining staff roles and identifying a process champion;
4. Identifying and adapting screening, assessment, and intervention tools;
5. Setting a start date; planning periodic communication to assess implementation and chart reviews.

Routine documentation of a core set of nutrition-related data such as height, weight (a BMI chart posted by the scale aids support staff in documenting BMI), waist circumference, and activity level sets the stage for the provider to address diet related to clinical care. Patients may complete assessment forms while waiting to see the provider. The WAVE (Weight, Activity, Variety and Excess) and REAP (Rapid Eating and Activity Assessment for Patients) are two such tools designed to target healthy eating and cholesterol reduction *(14–16)*. Each assessment tool provides a brief diet assessment and facilitates meaningful counseling in 1–9 min. The Nutrition Academy Award Program web site is an easy way to access these tools. Table 1 identifies sources of high-quality education literature, interactive media, and self-monitoring tools (provided in a variety of languages and suitable for low-literacy clients), which target a wide variety of nutrition-related issues.

4. CLIENT-CENTERED THERAPY

Client-centered counseling is designed to place much of the responsibility for the intervention process on the client. By adopting a facilitation role, the counselor fosters a greater openness and trust. Use of informal clarifying questions increases the client's insight and self-understanding. Establishing client rapport is a prerequisite for free expression of thoughts and feelings that, particularly in the unmotivated client, may not be "politically correct." The goal is to move from the traditional hierarchical relationship to one of partnership.

This approach toward counseling is particularly useful in diet counseling as it is the client who ultimately determines what change he or she is willing and able to make. The physician brings a depth of medical knowledge, which can help to frame the problem, and motivate and guide the client to set realistic goals. The client knows best what lifestyle changes can be made and can identify barriers and solutions relevant to their situation. The client-centered approach takes the pressure off the provider to have all the answers and represents a shift in the typical relationship between physician and client, which may be a bit unfamiliar to both parties. The ultimate goal of counseling is to actively engage the patient in self-management practices necessary to change and maintain a healthy diet. The traditional doctor–patient approach (e.g., "I want you to walk 45 min everyday, and lose 10 pounds") is likely to antagonize many patients. They may well give the impression to the doctor that they agree with the plan, but will then go and find a doctor who will give them a pill to fix the problem.

5. THE 5 A'S COUNSELING MODEL

The 5 A's is an evidence-based method for conducting minimal contact interventions targeting behavior change *(17)*. Adoption of this approach for physician-provided nutrition counseling allows others to collaborate in developing tools and materials to support the process. The five A's include

- *Assess*: ask about/assess diet, diet history, and readiness to change.
- *Advise*: give clear, specific, and personalized lifestyle change advice, including tailored information about personal health risks/benefits.
- *Agree*: collaborate with patient to identify nutrition-related goals and strategies the patient is willing to implement.
- *Assist*: use behavior change strategies to assist the patient in achieving agreed-upon goals by acquiring knowledge, confidence, and social/environmental support for behavior change.
- *Arrange*: schedule follow-up contacts (in person or by phone) to provide ongoing support. Referral to more intensive counseling may be appropriate for high-risk patients.

The NAA *Medical Nutrition Handbook* provides excellent counseling guides to support both 5- and 15-min brief nutrition interventions using the 5 A algorithm *(18*; available at website).

6. MODELS FOR INDUCING CHANGE

6.1. Transtheoretical Model and Stages of Change

This model attempts to describe a sequence of cognitive and behavioral stages people use over time to achieve intentional behavior change. The core concept, known as Stages of Change, reflects an individual's attitudes, intentions, and behavior related to change of a specific behavior. Stages of change are identified as precontemplation, contemplation, preparation, action, and maintenance. Table 2 outlines treatment strategies endorsed by the transtheoretical model *(19)*. Strategies targeted to the early stages of change target motivation, and those used in the later stages are more consistent with strategies used in behavioral therapy.

6.2. Motivational Interviewing

Motivational interviewing, which integrates well within the transtheoretical model, facilitates the client in exploring and resolving their own uncertainty and building confidence and enhancing commitment to change. The four guiding principles of the technique include expression of empathy, development of discrepancy, roll with resistance, and support self-efficacy (client confidence in their ability to accomplish a specific task). The

Table 2
Stages of Change and Stage Appropriate Treatment Strategies

Stage of Change	Treatment Strategies
Precontemplation	Personalize assessment information, educate about risk, acknowledge patient's emotions related to condition
Contemplation	Increase patient's confidence (self-efficacy), discuss ambivalence and barriers to change, reinforce past accomplishments, encourage a support network, emphasize expected benefits
Preparation	Facilitate client setting of small, specific, realistic goals to build confidence; reinforce small accomplishments
Action	Provide tailored self-help materials; refer to a behavioral program or self-management program
Maintenance	Help patient anticipate and prepare for high-risk situations, link patient with community support groups, encourage continued self-monitoring and goal setting, if patient ready to continue

tone of the counseling session is totally nonjudgmental and the counselor uses open-ended questions and reflective listening to frame discrepancies between client goals and actions. Conflict and confrontation are avoided by rolling with resistance – verbalizing the understanding that the client is in the best position to determine when change can occur. The process stresses the use of reflective listening skills, rather than the drive to provide information; it supports enhancement of self-efficacy and optimism for change (20). This is a major paradigm change from the counseling that is frequently employed by physicians and which is oriented around problem solving. Further descriptions of this technique can be found at http://www.motivationalinterview.org/.

6.3. Cognitive-Behavioral Theory

Cognitive-behavioral theory is based on the assumption that all behavior is learned and is directly related to internal factors (e.g., thoughts and thinking patterns) and external factors (e.g., environmental stimuli and feedback) that are related to the problem behavior. Patients are taught to utilize a variety of behavioral and cognitive strategies to recognize behaviors that lead to inappropriate eating and replace them with more rational thoughts and actions. The behavioral strategies most suited to minimal contact

Table 3
Behavioral Strategies Useful to Support Dietary Change

Strategy	Application
Self-monitoring	Cornerstone of therapy, used in goal setting/progress assessment
	Provide rationale and instruction for self-monitoring
	Assist patient in reviewing log and identifying patterns
	Assist with goal setting and problem solving
	Celebrate successes
Goal setting	Collaborative activity
	Identify goal that client is willing to expend effort to achieve
	Discuss pros and cons of goal
	Document and track progress toward long- and short-term goal
	May need to provide information/skill development
	Encourage strategies to build confidence
	Celebrate successes
Problem solving	Define the problem
	Brainstorm solutions
	Weigh pros and cons of potential solutions
	Patient selects/implements strategy
	Evaluate outcomes/adjust strategy

interventions are outlined in Table 3 and include self-monitoring, goal setting, and problem solving.

6.4. Incorporation of Behavioral Theory Tenets to the 5A Model

The 5A model provides specific guidance on how to integrate motivational interviewing, the transtheoretical model, and cognitive-behavioral therapy principles into a minimal contact dietary intervention. A quick assessment allows for tailoring of counseling goals. For those patients not ready to make dietary changes, the goal of the intervention is to enhance readiness/motivation. The intervention addresses the client's ambivalence about change; motivational interviewing is an appropriate strategy. Clients ready to change will be more open to utilize behavior therapy strategies such as self-monitoring, goal setting, and problem solving. The 5A model outlined in Table 4 guides the content of the brief nutrition encounter.

Table 4
Incorporation of Behavioral Theory Tenets to the 5A Model

Assess
Diet
Diet readiness
Diet history
	Diet: Recommend use of a brief nutrition assessment tool such as the WAVE or REAP (good waiting-room activity). To address the topic you might say:
	    "What you eat is very important for your health and for the management of your [blood cholesterol, blood pressure, etc.].
	    May I discuss your diet with you today?"
	This invitation gives the client some control over the encounter. If the answer is "no," end the discussion. If the patient is uncertain or says "yes," avoid giving advice, but continue the assessment.
	
	Disease-specific assessment criteria should be addressed.
	
	Diet readiness to change: You may ask the client to rate on a scale of 1–10 (10 being fully ready to take action) how ready they feel to take action to improve their diet right now. The focus of the intervention will vary based upon the readiness score:
	    o If score is low *(1–4)*, inform, raise awareness, explore beliefs/attitudes, and encourage change
	    o If score is moderate *(5–7)*, explore patient's ambivalence and, if willing, negotiate a small, specific behavior change goal.
	    o If score is high *(8–10)*, focus on goal setting/problem solving

Advise	You might say: "Based upon your health risk [specify] and current diet assessment, I recommend we focus on _____ [excess saturated fat intake, excess carbohydrate intake, low fruit/vegetable intake]."
	
	Aim for a strong, succinct, clear, personalized message about what you think the patient should do, delivered with concern and conviction, and related to the benefits to be derived from this change
	For patients not ready to change, but open to a discussion about diet change, rather than giving specific advise, you could briefly explore the patient's ambivalence to change by asking:
	    "Why did you rate yourself a—on the scale from 1–10?"
	    "What would need to happen for you to be more ready to change?"

"What would be some advantages to making a diet change?"

"What are the disadvantages to making a diet change?"

"Have you attempted to change your diet? What worked or didn't?"

"Would family/friends help you to change your diet?"

You might end the intervention here by saying: "I respect your decision to not make a change right now. You are the best judge of what is right for you, but when you are ready, I will be willing to assist you."

Agree   For patients ready to make diet change, you might ask:

"What do you think needs to change in your diet?"

"What are your ideas for making that change?"

- Negotiate behavior change goals
- Encourage self-monitoring
- Briefly discuss barriers and guide use of problem solving

Assist   Provide handouts web resources based upon patient goals/interests

Provide lists and recommendations for community resources

Arrange   Follow up by phone, e-mail, or an office visit in 2–4 wk, if specific behavior change goals are set

If patient is at high risk or has a chronic disease diagnosis, consider a referral to a registered dietitian for more intensive counseling

7. SUMMARY

Over the past dozen years a growing body of literature has emerged that describes brief and effective clinic-based strategies for delivering nutrition advice and counseling in the primary-care setting. The effectiveness of physician interventions with and without office system support significantly enhances patient outcomes. The 5A model for minimal contact interventions targeting behavior change is one such starting point. Numerous organizations have developed nutrition-specific tools and counseling guides to support this intervention model. Physician knowledge of behavior change models relevant to individual-level interventions facilitates tailoring of nutrition counseling to meet patient needs. Tailoring of nutrition education materials and referral to nutrition experts, behavior therapy, self-management education programs, or community programs, can enhance counseling intensity and support patients' development of self-management practices necessary to achieve and maintain healthy diets.

SUGGESTED FURTHER READING

Kreuter MW, Chheda SG, Bull FC. How does physician advice influence patient behavior? Evidence for a priming effect. Arch Fam Med 2000; 9:426–433.

Kristal AR, Glanz E, Curry S, Patterson RE. How can stages of change be best used in dietary interventions? J Am Diet Assoc 1999; 99:683.

Miller WR, Rollnick S. Motivational Interviewing: Preparing People for Change, 2nd ed. Gilford Press, New York, 2002. www.motivationalinterview.org

www.nhlbi.nih.gov/funding/training/naa/products.htm. The Nutrition Academy Award (NAA) Program website contains many tools designed to support incorporation of brief nutrition interventions into routine office practice.

http://naa.medicine.wisc.edu. The *Medical Nutrition Handbook* provides excellent counseling guides to support both 5-minutes and 15-minutes brief nutrition interventions using the 5 A algorithm.

http://win.niddk.nih.gov/index.htm. The Weight-control Information Network (WIN).

REFERENCES

1. US Department of Health and Human Services. Healthy People 2010: Understanding and Improving Health, 2nd ed. US Government Printing Office, Washington, DC, 2000.
2. Ockene IS, Hebert JR, Ockene JK, et al. Effect of physician-delivered nutrition counseling training and an office-support program on saturated fat intake, weight, and serum lipid measurements in a hyperlipidemic population: Worcester Area Trial for Counseling in Hyperlipidemia (WATCH). Arch Intern Med 1999; 159:725–731.
3. Clark M, Hampson SE, Avery L, Simpson R. Effects of a tailored lifestyle self-management intervention in patients with type 2 diabetes. Br J Health Psychol 2004; 9:365–379.
4. Ashley JM, St Jeor ST, Schrage JP, et al. Weight control in the physician's office. Arch Intern Med 2001; 9:1599–1604.
5. Kreuter MW, Chheda SG, Bull FC. How does physician advice influence patient behavior? Evidence for a priming effect. Arch Fam Med 2000; 9:426–433.
6. Kant AK, Miner P. Physician advice about being overweight: association with self-reported weight loss, dietary, and physical activity behaviors of US adolescents in the National Health and Nutrition Examination Survey, 1999–2002. Pediatrics 2007; 119:142–147.
7. Pelto GH, Santos I, Gonçalves H, Victora C, Martines J, Habicht JP. Nutrition counseling training changes physician behavior and improves caregiver knowledge acquisition. J Nutr 2004; 134:357–362.
8. Deakin T, McShane CE, Cade JE, Williams RD. Group based training for self-management strategies in people with type 2 diabetes mellitus. Cochrane Database Syst Rev 2005; 18(2):CD003417.

9. Norris SL, Engelgau MM, Narayan KM. Effectiveness of self-management training in type 2 diabetes: a systematic review of randomized controlled trials. Diabetes Care 2001; 24:561–587.
10. Norris SL, Lau J, Smith SJ, Schmid CH, Engelgau MM. Self-management education for adults with type 2 diabetes: a meta-analysis of the effect on glycemic control. Diabetes Care 2002; 25:1159–1171.
11. Rickheim PL, Weaver TW, Flader JL, Kendall DM. Assessment of group versus individual diabetes education: a randomized study. Diabetes Care 2002; 25:269–274.
12. Agency of Healthcare Research and Quality (AHRQ). Putting Prevention into Practice. A Step-by-Step Guide to Delivering Clinical Preventive Services: A Systems Approach. AHRQ Pub. No. APPIP01-0001. AHRQ, Rockville, MD, 2001. Available from: http://www.ahrq.gov/ppip/manual
13. Eaton CB, McBride PE, Gans KA, Underbakke GL. Teaching nutrition skills to primary care practitioners. J Nutr 2003; 133:563S–566S.
14. Barner C, Wylie-Rosett J, Gans K. WAVE: A pocket guide for a brief nutrition dialogue in primary care. Diabetes Educ 2001; 27:352–358, 361–362.
15. Gans KM, Ross E, Barner CW, Wylie-Rosett J, McMurray J, Eaton C. Quick assessment tools designed to facilitate patient centered counseling REAP and WAVE: new tools to rapidly assess/discuss nutrition with patients. J Nutr 2003; 133:556S–562S.
16. Gans KM, Risica PM, Wylie-Rosett J, et al. Development and evaluation of the nutrition component of the Rapid Eating and Activity Assessment for Patients (REAP): a new tool for primary care providers. J Nutr Educ Behav 2006; 38:286–292.
17. Five major steps to intervention (the "5 A's"). US Public Health Service, Agency for Healthcare Research and Quality, Rockville, MD. Available from: http://www.ahrq.gov/clinic/tobacco/5steps.htm Accessed on November 19, 2008.
18. Nutrition Academic Award Program. University of Wisconsin Medical School Division of Cardiology Department to Medicine. Medical Nutrition Handbook. Available from: http://www2.medicine.wisc.edu/home/naa/naamain. Accessed on November 19, 2008.
19. Kristal AR, Glanz E, Curry S, Patterson RE. How can stages of change be best used in dietary interventions? J Am Diet Assoc 1999; 99:683.
20. Miller WR, Rollnick S. Motivational Interviewing: Preparing People for Change, 2nd ed. Gilford Press, New York, 2002.

13 Dietary Supplements: Navigating a Minefield

Norman J. Temple
and Asima R. Anwar

Key Points

- Use of dietary supplements has increased rapidly in recent years and around half of people in North America regularly use supplements.
- A wide variety of supplements are sold. In some cases there is strong evidence supporting their efficacy but in many other cases there is little or no supporting evidence.
- Supplements are marketed by a variety of different methods, including health food stores, multilevel marketing, bulk mail, spam e-mails, Internet websites, and infomercials on TV.
- A large part of marketing practices involves giving unreliable or dishonest information that is not supported by scientific studies.
- There is very little regulation of the marketing of supplements in the United States. However, Canada is now in the process of enforcing reasonably strict regulations.
- Suggestions are given on counseling patients so that they can better evaluate claims made by the sellers of supplements.

Key Words: Dietary supplements; vitamin supplements; herbs; health claims; regulations; physician advice

1. INTRODUCTION

Dietary supplements refer to any substance taken in addition to regular food. Supplements include vitamins, minerals, amino acids, herbs, enzymes, and various substances extracted from plants and animals. They are sold as liquids, tablets, capsules, and powders. By definition these products are not conventional foods but are designed to supplement the diet.

From: *Nutrition and Health: Nutrition Guide for Physicians*
Edited by: T. Wilson et al. (eds.), DOI 10.1007/978-1-60327-431-9_13,
© Humana Press, a part of Springer Science+Business Media, LLC 2010

There has been a rapid increase in recent years in the sales of dietary supplements. Much of this can be traced to the passing of the Dietary Supplement and Health Education Act (DSHEA) in 1994, a law that gave the supplement industry much wider freedom to use dishonest marketing. The sales of dietary supplements in the United States doubled after, to almost $18 billion in 2000 *(1)* and has been steadily increasing since. Surveys reveal that around half of adults in the United States take supplements regularly *(2, 3)*. Canadian surveys are broadly similar *(4)*. The profiles of people most likely to use dietary supplements are female, older, white, nonsmokers, regular exercisers, and better educated *(3)*.

Physicians and other health professionals need to be aware of issues related to supplements. Patients may seek advice from their physician concerning supplements. Ideally, physicians should be able to give reliable information. Unfortunately, most physicians receive very little training in this area. This does not mean that physicians should have a detailed knowledge of all supplements, but rather that they know where to obtain information combined with having a good basic knowledge.

2. COMMON SUPPLEMENTS

A wide variety of supplements are sold. The quality of the evidence supporting their efficacy covers a wide spectrum: some are based on solid science and are recommended in other chapters, whereas at the other end the sales spiel more closely resembles astrology than it does astronomy.

2.1. Supplements with Strong Supporting Evidence

Supplements where the case for benefit is strongest are fish oil, calcium, vitamin D, and multivitamins. Vitamin D is discussed in Section 1.7 of Chapter 11. Multivitamins – meaning pills containing a broad spectrum of vitamins and minerals – can be especially valuable for many women during their reproductive years in order to achieve an adequate intake of iron and folic acid.

Minerals for which there is reasonably good evidence in support of supplementation are

• Calcium. This mineral has a preventive action against osteoporosis as discussed in the Chapter 30. The group for whom there is the strongest case for supplementation is women over the age of 50 as they are at most risk of skeletal calcium loss while also having an inadequate dietary intake of calcium. An appropriate supplement provides 500 mg calcium per day, preferably a cheap brand from a drug store. Many brands also contain vitamin D.

- Selenium. As discussed in Vitamins and Minerals: A Functional Approach by Boyle Struble, there is evidence for its efficacy as a cancer chemopreventive. However, this is still to be confirmed in further randomized clinical trials clinical trials (RCTs). It seems prudent to take a supplement supplying 50 micrograms (μg) per day. Many brands of multivitamin pills contain it, though at a lower dose.

It is in the area of herbs where the supporting evidence is highly contentious. Only two herbs are backed by fairly solid supporting evidence of effectiveness:

- Ginkgo biloba. Clinical trials suggest that this herb slows the progression of early stage dementia, especially Alzheimer's disease. It is also effective for cerebral insufficiency (5).
- St John's Wort. Emerging evidence suggests that it may be effective in the treatment of mild to moderate depression. It has also been reported to have fewer side effects than drugs (5).

2.2. Antioxidants

Many supplements are sold with a claim of being "rich in antioxidants," the obvious implication being that such products will improve health or prevent disease. This can sound very impressive. In support of this it has been firmly established that antioxidants are important for the body's defenses. However, nutritional studies do not categorically support a blanket claim that all antioxidants generally promote health. In fact, the reverse may also be true.

Several large RCTs have been conducted in which β-carotene or vitamins C or E have been given to patients. These are the three major antioxidant vitamins. The dose has typically been several times higher than the RDA. A recent major meta-analysis concluded that supplementing with these vitamins leads to an increase of about 5–6% in all-cause mortality (6, 7).

As was discussed in Chapter 25, the consensus among nutrition scientists is that while foods naturally rich in antioxidants, such as fruit and vegetables, are excellent for health. The reasons for this are complex and not universally understood. Therefore, when sellers of supplements state in their advertisements that a product is "rich in antioxidants," that is weak evidence that it will improve health or prevent disease.

2.3. Detoxification

For the sellers of supplements, detoxification is much like the word antioxidants: it provides a simple concept that most people can easily grasp and that can be used to provide an apparently scientific reason why a particular product will do wonders for the health. Detoxification is, of course, a well-established biochemical process. However, herbal treatments, in particular, are routinely sold with the promise that they will stimulate the liver – and perhaps some other organs as well – so that detoxification is accelerated and the body is cleansed. This will then lead to all sorts of benefits, such as more energy. However, supporting empirical evidence is lacking.

2.4. Boosting the Immune System

Many supplements come with the claim that they somehow stimulate the immune system. Much like detoxification this is usually associated with herbs. For some herbs there is supporting evidence, Echinacea for example. But in most cases the claims come minus credibility.

2.5. Herbs and Herbal Cocktails

Unlike conventional drugs, herbal supplements generally lack standardization of active ingredients. There can be much variation between different brands of what is supposedly the same herb due to such factors as the actual species of plant used, the part of the plant used, and the extraction method.

Many supplements consist of a mixture of herbs. Often the label will give the ingredient list as a dozen or so herbs, each with a Latin name. As very little research has been conducted on mixtures of herbs, there is no good reason to be confident that such supplements will achieve any clinically valuable benefits. Moreover, such herbal cocktails pose a risk of inducing harmful side effects that will be very difficult to relate to any specific herb or herb combination. Polypharmacy is always hazardous, whether it is based on conventional drugs or herbal cocktails.

2.6. Exotic Fruit Juices

In recent years several exotic fruit juices have appeared on the market. The main ones are acai, goji, mangosteen, and noni. They are sold by multilevel marketing and through health food stores. They invariably come with promises of wonderful benefits, but at an exorbitant price. A health food store in Edmonton, Canada, known to one of us (NT) charges about $50–60 per liter for these juices. By contrast, the local supermarket sells vegetable juices for less than $3 per liter.

2.7. Weight loss Products

With the huge obesity epidemic that has swept North America, it is scarcely surprising that supplement manufacturers have jumped on the bandwagon. New products appear with bewildering regularity. Typically, such products come with thin promises based on even thinner evidence. But what they do produce, very often, is a photo of a young woman with a BMI of about 20.

2.8. A Repeating Story

What we see, time and time again, is weak evidence dressed up as solid science. The marketers of supplements like to use scientific evidence the way a drunk uses a lamp post: more for support than illumination. Sometimes the marketers go to the extreme and claim that their product cures almost anything and everything, even cancer.

The following are the major types of claim made in support of the efficacy of supplements: (i) mere speculation (e.g., that detoxification will improve health or that an exotic fruit juice is rich in antioxidants and will therefore improve health); (ii) a change in functioning of the body (e.g., a change in one parameter of the immune system, and based on that it is claimed that the body will be less likely to develop infections); (iii) weak clinical evidence (e.g., a particular herb has been used by many herbalists for decades and they claim it is effective); and (iv) anecdotal evidence, often from an unqualified person with a serious conflict of interest ("Many of my customers have tried [the product] and it works very well."). A slight variation of anecdotal evidence is the use of testimonials ("Jim from Miami says: 'Thanks to Speedy Fat Burn I have lost 25 pounds in one month.' "). But what is lacking, in the great majority of cases, in the claims of those marketing supplements is consistent evidence from well-conducted RCTs, with clinical endpoints, showing real health benefits, and published in peer-reviewed journals.

Dietary supplements are a multibillion dollar industry, but integral to its success has been the widespread use of blatantly misleading marketing. This strategy has been so successful because most of the population has a weak grasp of science, especially biomedical science (8).

2.9. Potential Hazards from Supplements

One of the most common mantras of those in the supplement industry is that supplements are safe. Now it is certainly true that undesired side effects induced by supplements are rather uncommon. However, they do occur, especially with herbs. For example, in a recent study a chemical analysis was conducted on traditional Ayurvedic medicines that were being sold in the United States via the Internet. The findings revealed that 21% of these herbal preparations exceeded one or more standards for acceptable daily intake of lead, mercury, or arsenic (9). Quite apart from toxic contaminants, many herbs interact with various drugs. Another problem that is probably quite common, though hard numbers on this seem to be lacking, is that many people with a health problem that could be helped by a conventional medical treatment turn instead to useless supplements.

3. HOW DIETARY SUPPLEMENTS ARE MARKETED

Dietary supplements are marketed in diverse ways *(3)*. They can be purchased in three main ways: in pharmacies, supermarkets, and health food stores; directly from people engaged in multilevel marketing; and by mail order. Their sales are promoted using all forms of marketing methods, including advertisement in newspapers (sometimes as multi-page supplements), bulk mail ("junk mail"), spam e-mails, and Internet websites, as well as by infomercials on TV.

3.1. Direct Contact with Consumers

Health food stores (HFS) are a popular source of dietary supplements. HFS staff seldom have any proper scientific knowledge regarding the topics on which they freely dispense advice. But what they do have is a strong economic incentive to sell products. As a result, a request for advice will typically be responded to by a recommendation to take a particular supplement: advice that usually suffers from a serious lack of credible supporting evidence. In addition, studies in Hawaii, Canada, and the UK have shown that when the same question is asked in different HFS, there is a huge variation in the advice that is given *(3)*.

It is usually a different story in pharmacies. As pharmacists are trained health professionals and must abide by a code of ethics, customers requesting advice are far less likely to be recommended to buy useless supplements.

3.2. Multilevel Marketing

Dietary supplements are also sold by direct marketing – a strategy in which company salespeople recruit other salespeople. The foot soldiers and everyone up the chain get a commission for their sales. Its focus is profit, not consumer health.

The people who control this form of marketing often engage in unscrupulous activities. On one occasion flyers were distributed in Edmonton promoting a particular product where the person behind it was described as "the world's leading viroimmunologist." In another case, the mastermind was referred to as "Widely regarded as the world's #1 nutritionist" and the product as "The biggest discovery in nutrition in the last 40 years!"

3.3. Sources of the Supplemental Message

The supplement message is delivered by a variety of means including infomercials, bulk mail, and the Internet. Infomercials are TV programs produced and paid for by commercial companies. They resemble regular TV programs but are, in reality, a form of advertising. They typically last for 30 min and air during the night. Bulk mail ("junk mail") is a common form of advertising, especially for supplements that promise weightloss. Spam e-mails are a cheap and easy way for manufacturers to promote their dietary supplements to tens of thousands, if not millions, of people. As a result large numbers of products are being touted, most of them of highly dubious value. In recent years vast numbers of spam e-mails have been sent out promoting sex-related nutritional supplements. Spam e-mails typically work by directing the person to a website. There are many websites selling all types of supplements; they are, in effect, virtual health food stores. They often flout US law *(10)*.

3.4. The Object of the Exercise

The purpose of all this huge marketing enterprise is, of course, to maximize sales. As mentioned earlier, there are some supplements for which solid evidence exists justifying their value. Examples include vitamin D, calcium, and fish oil. Each of these cost around $3 or $4 per month. But go into a health food store, tell the salesperson that you do not have enough energy, you have an ache in your knee, and your mother died of cancer and you will likely be told to take a handful of supplements, each costing between $20 and $60 per month. This might easily add up to $100–200 per month. And it is quite likely that the recommended supplements would have little or no beneficial effect on health.

4. REGULATIONS ON THE MARKETING OF SUPPLEMENTS

4.1. United States

In 1994 Congress passed a new law regulating the marketing of dietary supplements: the Dietary Supplement and Health Education Act (DSHEA). This law freed dietary supplement manufacturers from many FDA regulations *(11)*. Whereas under the former law manufacturers were required to prove that a dietary supplement is safe, now, under DSHEA, the FDA must prove regulations that a supplement is unsafe. This shift in regulatory policy places burdens on a federal agency with important public health responsibilities but limited resources.

Manufacturers are now free to make health-related claims (structure/function claims) but are not permitted to state explicitly that the product will cure or prevent a disease. They must also state that the FDA has not evaluated the agent. What this means is that a manufacturer may now claim that a supplement "boosts the immune system," "makes the body burn fat while you sleep," or "fights cholesterol," provided they stop short of saying that the supplement prevents infectious disease, cures obesity, or prevents heart disease. Needless to say, most consumers will be confused by the distinction between the two sets of claims.

DSHEA was engineered by the supplement industry for its own benefit *(11)*. It allows sellers of supplements to make unscientific claims, unsupported by any good evidence, and claim that these are established facts. The law is, in effect, a Bill of Rights for modern day snake oil salesmen.

The Journal of the American Medical Association *(12)* published an editorial deploring this state of affairs: "The public should wonder why dietary supplements have effectively been given a free rise. New legislation is needed for defining and regulating dietary supplements." A similar article was published in the New England Journal of Medicine *(13)* with a focus on herbal supplements.

4.2. Canada

The situation in Canada was for years every bit as dishonest as that in the United States. But over the last several years Canada has carried out a radical reform of the system *(3)*. A new organization has been set up, the Natural Health Products Directorate, that will regulate dietary supplements. The mission of this organization is to ensure that Canadians have access to natural health products (NHPs) that are safe, effective, and of high quality. The new regulations cover not only conventional supplements but also include homeopathic remedies, traditional medicines (e.g., Chinese), and probiotics. A key feature of the new regulations is that the requirements for safety and good manufacturing practices fall on the companies that manufacture, package, label, import, or distribute NHPs. By 2010, when the new system is scheduled to be fully implemented, all manufacturers, importers, packagers, and labelers of NHPs must have site licenses, and any new NHP must have a product license. The regulations require a pre-market review of products to assure that label information is truthful and health claims are supported by appropriate types of scientific evidence.

5. HELPING PATIENTS MAKE INFORMED CHOICES ABOUT DIETARY SUPPLEMENTS

As mentioned earlier the use of supplements by patients can pose hazards, including both toxicity and interference with the action of prescription drugs. These problems arise most often with herbs. Patients often do not tell their physician about their use of supplements. Physicians need to have more awareness of these problems. In addition, as the general population is exposed to enormous amounts of marketing activity for supplements, much of which is misleading, physicians therefore have a responsibility to assist their patients in evaluating health claims. Indeed, physicians are well positioned to help counter the bogus marketing of supplements. They meet with patients regularly, and they are widely seen as a credible and impartial source of information.

Physicians can offer the following simple rules to help their patients evaluate product authenticity. First, suspicious claims for supplements often have the following features:

- The use of testimonials
- A claim that the product is a "scientific breakthrough"
- Touting the product as an effective treatment for a broad range of ailments. If things are too good to be true, they probably are.

Additional guidelines that physicians can usefully convey to patients are as follows:

- Ignore all advice given by persons who have a financial interest in selling supplements, especially when they appear to have no relevant qualifications. This includes staff in health food stores and people engaged in multilevel marketing; and statements on flyers that arrive in the mail, on infomercials, and on websites of supplement manufacturers.
- If in doubt about a supplement, obtain advice from a legitimate health professional, such as a physician, dietitian, or pharmacist.
- Always use common sense. A healthy dose of skepticism is a consumer's best protection against fraudulent and misleading marketing.
- For further information check at credible sources of information. Several health-related organizations supply information on supplements at their websites. These include the following:
  Mayo Clinic http://www.mayoclinic.com
  National Center for Complementary and Alternative Medicine (NCCAM) http://nccam.nih.gov/
  Medline Plus http://medlineplus.gov/
  MEDLINE http://www.ncbi.nlm.nih.gov/PubMed/
  The National Cancer Institute's website gives reliable information about various supplements claimed to be effective in the prevention or treatment of cancer
  http://www.cancer.gov/cancertopics/treatment/cam

SUGGESTED FURTHER READING

Temple NJ, Morris DH. Marketing dietary supplements for health and profit, 2nd ed. In: Temple NJ, Wilson T, Jacobs DR, eds. Nutritional Health: Strategies for Disease Prevention. Humana Press, Totowa, NJ, 2006, pp. 299–312.

National Council Against Health Fraud (NCAHF)
http://www.ncahf.org
Quackwatch http://www.quackwatch.org

REFERENCES

1. Nutrition Business Journal's annual industry overview VII. Nutrition Business Journal. May/June 2002.
2. Radimer K, Bindewald B, Hughes J, Ervin B, Swanson C, Picciano MF. Dietary supplement use by US adults: data from the National Health and Nutrition Examination Survey, 1999–2000. Am J Epidemiol 2004; 160:339–349.
3. Temple NJ, Morris DH Marketing dietary supplements for health and profit, 2nd ed. In: Temple NJ, Wilson T, Jacobs DR, eds. Nutritional Health: Strategies for Disease Prevention. Humana Press, Totowa, NJ, 2006, pp. 299–312.
4. Troppmann L, Johns T, Gray-Donald K. Natural health product use in Canada. Can J Public Health 2002; 93:426–430.
5. http://www.mayoclinic.com. Last accessed August 28, 2008.
6. Bjelakovic G, Nikolova D, Gluud LL, Simonetti RG, Gluud C. Antioxidant supplements for prevention of mortality in healthy participants and patients with various diseases. Cochrane Database Syst Rev 2008: CD007176.
7. Bjelakovic G, Nikolova D, Gluud LL, Simonetti RG, Gluud C. Mortality in randomized trials of antioxidant supplements for primary and secondary prevention: systematic review and meta-analysis. JAMA 2007; 297:842–857.
8. Blendon RJ, DesRoches CM, Benson JM, Brodie M, Altman DE. Americans' views on the use and of dietary supplements. Arch Intern Med 2001; 161:805–810.
9. Saper RB, Phillips RS, Sehgal A, et al. Lead, mercury, and arsenic in US- and Indian-manufactured Ayurvedic medicines sold via the Internet. JAMA 2008; 300:915–923.
10. Morris CA, Avorn J. Internet marketing of herbal products. JAMA 2003; 290: 1505–1509.
11. Nestle M. The Politics of Food. How the Food industry Influences Nutrition and Health. University of California Press, Berkeley, 2002.
12. Fontanarosa PB, Rennie D, DeAngelis CD. The need for regulation of dietary supplements – lessons from ephedra. JAMA 2003; 289:1568–1570.
13. Marcus DM, Grollman AP. Botanical medicines – the need for new regulations. N Engl J Med 2002; 347:2073–2076.

14 Taste Sensation: Influences on Human Ingestive Behavior

Bridget A. Cassady and Richard D. Mattes

Key Points

- Taste sensations serve multiple feeding-related functions.
- There are inherent likes and dislikes for taste qualities, but all are modifiable through dietary experience.
- Mere exposure to the taste of food elicits numerous physiological responses that may prime the body to efficiently absorb and utilize ingested nutrients.
- Gustatory disorders can increase an individual's risk to environmental toxin exposure, diminish quality of life, and negatively influence diet and nutritional status, but most affected patients adapt and experience no taste-related chronic health disorder.

Key Words: Taste; gustation; sweetness; perception; sensory; genetics

1. INTRODUCTION

All of life is a dispute over taste and tasting. Friedrich Nietzsche

The adverse effects of overconsumption and poor diet quality on public health are a growing concern. In attempts to improve nutritionally modifiable health disorders, attention has focused on determining factors that influence individual decisions about where, when, what, and how much to eat. While hunger is a key motivator in the initiation of feeding, sensory properties of food are thought to be the primary determinants of food choices in environments where food supplies are abundant and readily accessible. Though the chemical senses (i.e., gustation, olfaction, and chemesthesis [chemical irritation]) are often considered minor senses, they have played a fundamental

From: *Nutrition and Health: Nutrition Guide for Physicians*
Edited by: T. Wilson et al. (eds.), DOI 10.1007/978-1-60327-431-9_14,
© Humana Press, a part of Springer Science+Business Media, LLC 2010

role in survival. Taste, in particular, has been associated with food selection, avoidance of toxins, and promotion of nutrient ingestion.

The colloquial use of the term "taste" generally refers to the flavor of food, but flavor is actually a product of input from all of the anatomically and functionally distinct sensory systems. From a biological perspective, taste refers only to sensations stemming from stimulated taste receptor cells in the oral cavity *(1)*. This chapter briefly reviews the mechanisms and functions of the taste system and highlights current knowledge of inherent and acquired preferences for specific qualities and nutrients in humans, as well as the dietary implications of taste abnormalities.

2. ANATOMY AND PHYSIOLOGY OF THE TASTE SYSTEM

Taste cells are specialized epithelial cells that differentiate from surrounding epithelium. Approximately 50–150 taste cells cluster into onion-like configurations to form taste buds. Taste buds are dispersed in various regions on the tongue and also on the hard and soft palate, pharynx, larynx, esophagus, and epiglottis. Furthermore, taste cells similar to those present in the oral cavity have recently been identified in the lumen of the gut *(2)*. Mammals are believed to taste many compounds, but unlike smell, the repertoire of human taste sensations is limited and currently categorized into only five distinguishable qualities: sweet, salty, sour, bitter, and umami (the taste of monosodium glutamate [MSG], from the Japanese word for "deliciousness"). Although less well established, there is also accumulating evidence supporting a taste component for fat.

3. INNATE VS. ACQUIRED TASTES FOR SPECIFIC MACRONUTRIENTS AND SALT

Taste, more than the other chemical senses, is reported to convey information about the nutrient composition of a food. Sweetness denotes the presence of carbohydrate; umami is indicative of protein sources; electrolytes are detected, in part, by saltiness; acids are sour; and bitterness is a signal for toxins. Fat is unusual in that the predominant form of dietary fat, triglyceride, is tasteless, but adds to a foods flavor via its contribution to texture and as a carrier of sensory stimuli. In contrast, free fatty acids are likely effective taste stimuli, but are strongly disliked. Understanding the extent to which taste signals for nutrients are inherent and/or learned and adaptable is essential to establishing the significance of taste in nutrition.

3.1. Carbohydrate

There is strong evidence that humans have an innate liking for sweet taste. Fetal drinking is stimulated by the addition of sodium saccharine into amniotic fluid *(3)*. Preterm infants with little or no extrauterine taste experience display strong sucking responses upon stimulation with glucose and sucrose *(4)*. Full-term newborns display greater ingestion with sweeter stimuli and oral exposure to sweet taste consistently elicits facial expressions and responses (i.e., smiling, licking, relaxation) that are indicative of liking. These responses are proposed to predict early weight gain *(5)*, and thus obesity throughout the life cycle. However, this remains to be documented. One mitigating factor is the fact that preferences for sweet foods are modifiable through dietary experience and typically diminish after adolescence *(6)*. Preference differences for sweet taste have also been observed between races, sexes, and geographical locations and are mainly attributed to personal experiences and cultural beliefs. Recent evidence indicates there is a significant gene linkage to sugar intake *(7)*, but translation of this to behavior is currently premature.

Sweet taste has been linked to appetite regulation in humans. Short-term studies reveal that sweetness stimulates motivation to eat when a nonnutritive sweetener (e.g., saccharin, aspartame) is provided in the absence of energy (e.g., chewing gum and beverages). This augmentation of hunger is not observed when nonnutritive sweeteners are ingested with energy sources or when nutritive sweeteners are consumed *(8)*. Nonetheless, in environments where highly palatable food and energy-containing beverages are readily accessible and affordable, nutritive sweeteners have been hypothesized to promote excess intake of energy and, as a consequence, increased adiposity. Soft drink consumption, in particular, has been implicated because consumption has markedly increased in the past few decades and is presently the single largest contributor of energy (primarily as carbohydrate) in the diet. However, the involvement of sweetness, sweeteners (both nutritive and nonnutritive), and sweet-tasting energy-yielding beverages to the overweight and obesity epidemic is controversial, a topic also discussed in this chapter.

3.2. Protein

Humans are purportedly able to detect amino acids via sensory cues during the perinatal period. The prototypical example is the sensation accompanying exposure to monosodium glutamate (MSG), as well as the combination of glutamate and 5′-nucleotides such as inosine monophosphate (IMP-5). The savory taste of MSG is termed "umami" and is a common flavor enhancer in food. Glutamate, an amino acid, is found in many vegetables and in the majority of protein-containing foods, whereas IMP-5 is present in meats and several varieties of fish. In infants, oral stimulation with sodium and potassium salts of glutamate elicits facial responses similar to those following oral exposure to sweet taste, and thus are also interpreted as inherently pleasant *(9)*. Taste thresholds for MSG and IMP-5 have recently been shown to positively predict liking and preference for high-protein foods *(10)*.

The observation that elimination of only one essential amino acid rapidly results in a modification of feeding behavior that tends to correct the deficiency suggests there is a protein appetite *(11)*. This is further supported by evidence that protein-energy malnourished (PEM) infants display greater preferences for soup supplemented with casein hydrolysate (a protein source) as opposed to unsupplemented soup *(12)*. Healthy infants do not share these preferences, as the taste of casein hydrolysate is generally regarded as aversive and rejected. No differences are noted for responses to salty, sour, or bitter stimuli between PEM and healthy infants, indicating a specific protein-taste effect. Marginally protein-adequate elderly individuals also exhibit high hedonic (i.e., liking or palatability) ratings following exposure to soups supplemented with casein hydrolysate in comparison to unsupplemented versions *(13)*. While physiological state may alter amino acid taste responses, cultural influences also heavily influence taste preferences. The degree to which selected cultures prefer the taste of MSG and IMP-5 is attributed to the high frequency of consumption of these compounds *(14)*.

3.3. Fat

Dietary fat contributes approximately 30–45% of total dietary energy in Western societies, a topic also discussed in Chapter 1. While considerable efforts have been made to moderate dietary fat consumption, data from four National Health and Nutrition Examination Surveys (NHANES) show only small decreases in the percentage of energy from fat in the United States. Lack of dietary change may be due, in part, to the sensory appeal of fat-containing foods. Fats are thought to be detected mainly by their textural properties, but accumulating evidence indicates that there may be gustatory elements as well. Humans are able to detect free fatty acids in the oral cavity when nongustatory cues (i.e., olfactory, visual, tactile) are controlled. Such oral exposure to dietary fat results in postprandial increases of plasma triglycerides that are more robust than responses from texturally matched nonfat stimuli. There are mixed data regarding a genetic basis for fat sensitivity. However, no systematic study of a genetic basis for fat taste has been undertaken.

The preferred concentration of fat in foods is also modifiable. Reductions in oral exposure to dietary fat produce an elevated preference for foods with lower fat levels. This is in contrast to preferences of individuals with continuously higher levels of oral fat exposure *(15)*. Such adaptations in taste preferences are estimated to take approximately 8–12 weeks to evolve. Their role in improving long-term compliance to therapeutic diets has yet to be determined.

3.4. Sodium Chloride

Excess sodium intake has been linked to elevated blood pressure and increased risk of cardiovascular disease and stroke. The mean daily sodium intake of many Western nations exceeds 10 g/day, far surpassing physiological need. Approximately 40% of calories are derived from salt-rich foods *(16)*. Only 5–10% of dietary sodium intake is obtained in the form of table salt. The majority is derived from salt in processed foods. Given its ubiquity, voluntary reductions in sodium intake involve substantial effort. Mounting evidence suggests that the taste of salt is inherently appealing to humans, but this does not manifest until approximately 6 months of age.

Culture and dietary experiences play key roles in determining and altering preferred levels of salt in foods. Chronic (i.e., 8–12 weeks) reduction of sodium consumption results in preference shifts toward lower salt levels in food. These reductions in sodium are dependent on oral exposure frequency more so than total dietary sodium intake, as changes in palatability ratings are not noted in individuals reducing intake but maintaining sensory exposure. Thus, one can modify their preference for salt, but any new preference will only hold as long as the level of exposure remains in that range.

4. GENETIC VARIATIONS IN TASTE

Approximately 85% of Asians, 80% of African Americans, and 70% of Caucasians in the United States are sensitive to the bitter taste of 6-*n*-propylthiouracil (PROP) and phenylthiocarbamide (PTC) at very low concentrations, classifying them as "tasters." Taste sensitivity to these compounds is purportedly associated with an individual's general taste sensitivity, food preferences, diet selection, and risk for several diet-related chronic diseases. Such associations are based on the assumption that PROP tasters, due to greater papillae density and taste bud number *(17)*, are more sensitive to the bitter notes in foods compared to non-tasters. However, with few exceptions, the published literature offers little support for a significant influence of PROP/PTC taster status on diet selection.

5. PHYSIOLOGICAL RESPONSES TO TASTE PERCEPTION

In addition to guiding food choice, the thought of food or exposure to its taste, sight, sound, odor, or texture elicits multiple physiological responses referred to as preabsorptive or cephalic phase responses (Fig. 1). These responses are mediated by vagal activation. Though small in magnitude and short-lived (i.e., direct effects generally occur in seconds to minutes and persist only for minutes), cephalic phase responses are anticipatory and mimic those that occur during ingestion, digestion, absorption, and metabolism of foods. Gustatory stimulation, especially when coupled with oral mechanical activity (i.e., chewing and swallowing), is the most potent cephalic phase trigger. The perceived palatability of a stimulus has been directly correlated with response magnitude and aversive stimulation may attenuate responses *(18)*. Evidence of dietary implications of cephalic phase responses is only now emerging. For example, a cephalic phase mediated increase in efficiency of digestive responses has been proposed to allow for greater food intake, decreased intermeal interval, and enhanced ability to maintain energy balance *(19)*.

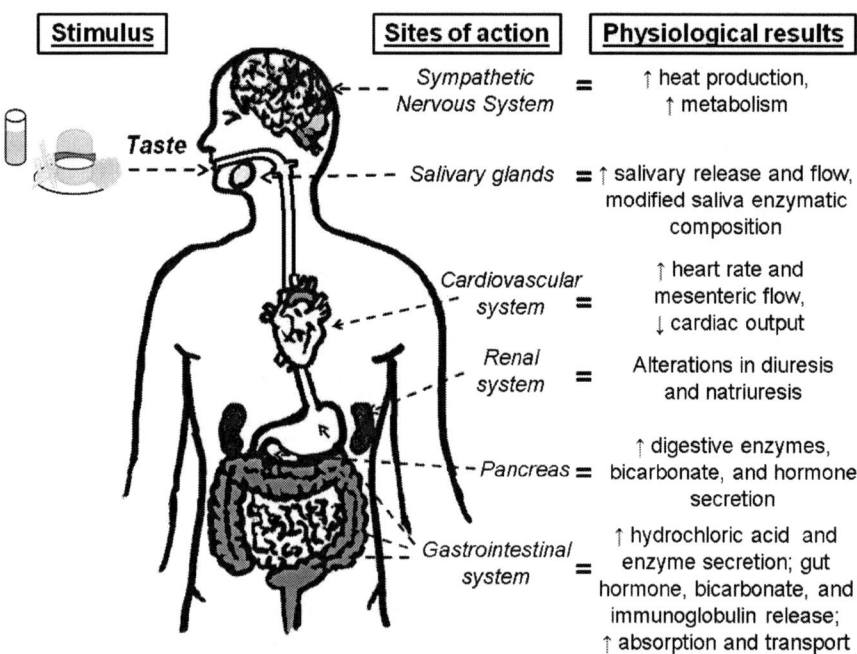

Fig. 1. Cephalic phase responses stimulation from taste components in foods. Reprinted with modification from Mattes RD. Physiologic responses to sensory stimulation by food: nutritional implications. J Am Diet Assoc 1997;97:406–413 with permission from Elsevier.

6. TASTE SENSATION ABNORMALITIES AND EFFECTS ON NUTRITIONAL STATUS

Taste loss, ageusia, is extremely rare; present in less than 1% of patients evaluated in taste and smell clinics. Hypogeusia, the most common complaint, refers to the partial loss of taste sensation to some or all taste qualities. The principal etiologies of hypogeusia are oral infections, oral appliances, medications, or severe trauma *(20)*. Taste distortions, known as dysgeusias, are characterized by the presence of phantom or inappropriate sensations. With rapid turnover rates of approximately 7–10 days, taste cells are highly vulnerable to metabolic toxins.

A high percentage of patients with taste and/or smell abnormalities report altered eating patterns, increased seasoning use, and diminished quality of life. However, nutrient and energy intake are generally within normal ranges. Clinically significant increases or decreases of body weight (>10% of pre-disorder weight) occur in a minority of patients *(21)*. When they occur, increases in weight may be the result of greater food consumption in efforts to achieve preferred intensity levels of sensory stimulation or an attempt to mask a persistent unpleasant sensation, whereas decreases may be the consequence of a lack of interest in food or a belief that food exposure provokes unpleasant sensations.

7. NUTRITIONAL IMPLICATIONS OF TASTE IN SELECTED POPULATIONS

7.1. Age

Aging is often associated with diminished appetite, lower food intakes, and weight loss. These declines have been attributed to deficits in gustatory function. While chemosensory dysfunction is more prevalent in the elderly, the contribution of this change to alterations of ingestive behavior has not been established. Taste is generally less affected than olfaction and diminished function is not biologically inevitable. Indeed, changes of taste are most likely attributable to effects of chronic diseases and medication use *(22)*. Where changes do occur, they are not uniform (i.e., affecting all qualities equally) and this precludes simple global therapeutic recommendations such as flavor fortification.

7.2. Obesity

Studies of threshold sensitivity and intensity sensation to graded stimulus concentrations have not revealed significant differences between lean and obese individuals. Some data suggest that obese individuals have greater preferences for sweet, high-fat foods compared to lean controls *(23)*, but this is not a robust finding. There is no specific recommendation to moderate energy intake in the obese based on their sensory function.

7.3. Hypertension

Evidence linking sodium intake to blood pressure has prompted study of the association between indices of salt taste and hypertension. Arguments have been made that lower sensitivity or intensity perception leads to greater intake to achieve a desired sensation or that greater sensory perception leads to greater intake as it facilitates detection and ingestion of a desired quality. Thus, an association can be viewed as compatible with any teleological argument. However, the data are not compelling for any relationship between salt taste and intake or blood pressure. Detection thresholds, intensity judgments, and hedonic ratings are generally similar in hypertensive and normotensive individuals. This also holds in salt-sensitive individuals, whose blood pressure is responsive to dietary sodium intake *(24)*. Some of the reported differences in salt taste among hypertensives may be attributable to effects of medications *(22)*. Accordingly, there is no basis to presume that differences in sodium intake between hypertensive and normontensive individuals are attributable to a differential response to the taste of or preference for salt.

7.4. Diabetes

Diabetic patients may experience alterations in sensory function, most notably for sweetness. Glucose taste thresholds may be higher in glucose intolerant patients. Taste alterations appear to become increasingly severe with the advancement of diabetes-related neuropathies. However, diabetic patients and healthy controls have similar hedonic responses to sweet stimuli and exhibit no sensory-related changes of dietary habits. A possible exception is women with gestational diabetes who reportedly have heightened preferences for and intake of sweet-tasting foods *(25)*.

8. SUMMARY

Taste clearly provides cues about food quality. There are innately more and less preferred sensations, but all are modifiable through dietary experience. Thus, innate responses hold limited predictive power for food choice. Primary abnormalities of taste may take various forms, but most individuals make suitable adjustments and maintain body weight and nutritional status. Changes of taste have been reported in various pathologies, but they are not uniform, of high prevalence, or strongly predictive of food choice. Given these observations, the question may be asked why taste is almost universally reported to be the most important factor in food choice. The answer largely lies in the inappropriate colloquial use of the term "taste," when actually referring to flavor and the observation that we like what we eat more than we eat what we like. That is, familiarity with the sensory properties of foods, determined largely by culture and personal lifestyle, strongly influences hedonic responses and ingestive behavior. These factors coupled with genetic variation, lead to unique expectations about the sensory properties of foods. Thus, assuming a static measure of taste function will predict ingestive behavior is comparable to expecting indices of vision to predict preferences and purchasing decisions for paintings.

SUGGESTED FURTHER READING

Monell Chemical Senses Center's website: http://www.monell.org.
Doty RL, ed. Handbook of Olfaction and Gustation, 2nd ed. Marcel Dekker, New York, 2003.
Prescott J, Tepper BJ, eds. Genetic variation in taste sensitivity. Marcel Dekker, New York, 2004.
Zafra MA, Molina F, Puerto A. The neural/cephalic phase reflexes in the physiology of nutrition. Neurosci Biobehav Rev 2006;30:1032–1044.
Rankin KM, Mattes RD. Toxic agents, chemosensory function, and diet. In: Massaro EJ, ed. Handbook of Human Toxicology. CRC Press, Boca Raton, FL, 1997, pp. 347–367.

REFERENCES

1. Kare MR, Mattes RD. A selective overview of the chemical senses. Nutr Rev 1990;48:39–48.
2. Egan JM, Margolskee RF. Taste cells of the gut and gastrointestinal chemosensation. Mol Interv 2008;8:78–81.
3. DeSnoo, K. Das trinkende Kind im Uterus. Monatsschr Geburtshilfe Gynaekol 1937;105:88–97.
4. Tatzer E, Schubert MT, Timischl W, Simbruner G. Discrimination of taste and preference for sweet in premature babies. Early Hum Dev 1985;12:23–30.
5. Stunkard AJ, Berkowitz RI, Stallings VA, Schoeller DA. Energy intake, not energy output, is a determinant of body size in infants. Am J Clin Nutr 1999;69:524–530.
6. Mojet J, Christ-Hazelhof E, Heidema J. Taste perception with age: generic or specific losses in threshold sensitivity to the five basic tastes? Chem Senses 2001;26:845–860.
7. Rankinen R, Bouchard C. Genetics of food intake and eating behavior phenotypes in humans. Annu Rev Nutr 2006;26:413–434.
8. Mattes RD, Popkin BM. Nonnutritive sweetener consumption in humans: effects on appetite and food intake and their putative mechanisms. Am J Clin Nutr 2009; 89: 1–14.
9. Steiner JE. Human facial expressions in response to taste and smell stimulation. Adv Child Dev Behav 1979;13:257–295.
10. Prescott J, Laing D, Bell G, et al. Hedonic responses to taste solutions: a cross-cultural study of Japanese and Australians. Chem Senses 1992;17:801–809.
11. Leung PM, Rogers QR. Effect of amino acid imbalance and deficiency on dietary choice patterns of rats. Physiol Behav 1986;37:747–758.
12. Vasquez M, Pearson PB, Beauchamp GK. Flavor preferences in malnourished Mexican infants. Physiol Behav 1982;28:513–519.

13. Murphy C, Withee J. Age and biochemical status predict preference for casein hydrolysate. J Gerontol 1987;42:73–77.
14. Luscombe-Marsh ND, Smeets AJ, Westerterp-Plantenga MS. Taste sensitivity for monosodium glutamate and an increased liking of dietary protein. Br J Nutr 2008;99:904–908.
15. Mattes RD. Fat preference and the adherence to a reduced-fat diet. Am J Clin Nutr 1993;57:373–381.
16. Mattes RD, Donnelly D. Relative contributions of dietary sodium sources. J Am Coll Nutr 1991;10:383–393.
17. Beauchamp GK, Cowart BJ, Moran M. Developmental changes in salt acceptability in human infants. Dev Psychobiol 1986;19:17–25.
18. Tepper BJ, Nurse RJ. Fat perception is related to PROP taster status. Physiol Behav 1997;61:949–954.
19. Wicks D, Weirght J, Rayment P, Spiller R. Impact of bitter taste on gastric motility. Eur J Gastroenterol Hepatol 2005;17:961–965.
20. Power ML, Schulkin J. Anticipatory physiological regulation in feeding biology: cephalic phase responses. Appetite 2008;50:194–206.
21. Mattes RD, Cowart BJ. Dietary assessment of patients with chemosensory disorders. J Am Diet Assoc 1994;94:50–56.
22. Doty R, Shah M, Bromley S. Drug-induced taste disorders. Drug Saf 2008;31:199–215.
23. Drewnowski A, Brunzell JD, Sande K, Iverius PH, Greenwood MR. Sweet tooth reconsidered: taste responsiveness in human obesity. Physiol Behav 1985;35:617–622.
24. Mattes RD, Westby E, De Cabo R, Falkner B. Dietary compliance among salt-sensitive and salt-insensitive normotensive adults. Am J Med Sci 1999;317:287–294.
25. Tepper BJ, Seldner AC. Sweet taste and intake of sweet foods in normal pregnancy and pregnancy complicated by gestational diabetes mellitus. Am J Clin Nutr 1999;70: 277–284.

15 Pregnancy: Preparation for the Next Generation

Jennifer J. Francis

Key Points

- Ideally, good nutrition practices begin in the preconception period.
- Weight gain during pregnancy should be based on prepregnancy body mass index (BMI).
- Most nutrient requirements during pregnancy can be met through a carefully selected diet. However, all women of childbearing age should take a folic acid supplement, and some high-risk women can benefit from iron and/or calcium supplements.
- Nutrition remains an important concern during the postpartum period, especially for women who choose to breastfeed their infants.
- Referrals should be made for women in high-risk pregnancies, low-income women with high risk for poor nutrition, and women with concerns about breastfeeding.

Key Words: Pregnancy; nutrient requirements; weight gain; high-risk pregnancies; food safety; breastfeeding

1. INTRODUCTION

Nutrition is a modifiable factor that has a tremendous impact on healthy pregnancy outcomes. Some effects of good nutrition during pregnancy can be appreciated immediately, such as reduced risk of maternal anemia and improved maternal glucose control. Others are evident upon the birth of the infant, such as healthy birth weight and absence of congenital defects. Still other benefits of a healthy diet during pregnancy may not be apparent for years to come.

From: *Nutrition and Health: Nutrition Guide for Physicians*
Edited by: T. Wilson et al. (eds.), DOI 10.1007/978-1-60327-431-9_15,
© Humana Press, a part of Springer Science+Business Media, LLC 2010

More and more evidence is coming to light supporting the fetal-origins hypothesis, which theorizes that in utero conditions have profound and long-lasting effects on fetal DNA and the subsequent health of offspring *(1)*.

Ideally, good nutrition practices should be encouraged beginning at the preconception period and continue on through pregnancy, lactation, and the postpartum period.

2. NUTRITION IN THE PRECONCEPTION PERIOD

Recent data indicate that nearly 35% of live births were the result of unintended pregnancies *(2)*. In this light, it is clear that issues pertaining to childbirth readiness should be discussed with all women of childbearing age at primary-care visits.

Achieving and/or maintaining a healthy body weight is a goal that should be considered well in advance of pregnancy. This is because weight loss can interfere with efforts at conception and is not recommended during pregnancy.

Since eating habits can be difficult to change, it is essential to establish positive behaviors before conception. Habits that promote optimal nutrition include

- eating three meals and – two to three snacks per day,
- choosing minimally processed foods rather than foods with added salt, sugar, and fat,
- following the recommendations of the USDA MyPyramid Food Guide,
- limiting caffeine to less than 300 mg/day,
- avoiding alcohol.

In addition, the physician should screen for conditions, habits, and practices that might interfere with good nutrition, including lactose intolerance, iron deficiency anemia, vegan diets, pica, use of megadose vitamin and mineral supplements, use of herbal supplements, and extreme weight loss/fad diets.

Women with pre-existing disease conditions with a nutrition component should be referred to a registered dietitian (RD) for medical nutrition therapy. These include diabetes, hypertension, HIV/AIDS, and phenylketonuria; gestational diabetes is a condition that sometimes develops as a result of pregnancy and is discussed later in this chapter.

Folic acid has been proven to reduce the risk of neural tube defects when taken in the periconception period. Since the neural tube is formed and closes within the first month of pregnancy, and many women are not aware that they are pregnant until after this critical period, folic acid supplementation is most effective at preventing defects when taken preconceptionally. The current recommendation is that all women of childbearing age take a supplement every day containing 400 µg folic acid *(3)* in addition to consuming foods that are good sources of folic acid, including leafy green vegetables, citrus fruits, and fortified cereals. Women in the lowest socioeconomic brackets deserve special consideration as they tend to have the highest risk for neural tube defects *(4)* and may be least likely to use supplements *(5)*.

3. NUTRITION DURING PREGNANCY

The goal of nutrition during pregnancy is twofold; to reduce adverse outcomes in the mother and in the fetus. Maternal outcomes that can be affected by nutrition status include risk for maternal anemia, gestational diabetes, preeclampsia, postpartum infections, and complications of labor and delivery. For the infant, low birth weight (<2,500 g), small for gestational age, prematurity, fetal death, infant death, macrosomia, and some congenital defects are all poor birth outcomes that can be affected by nutrition status.

3.1. Weight Gain in Pregnancy

Weight gain guidelines for pregnant women are dictated primarily by the woman's prepregnancy body mass index (BMI). Weight gain guidelines are outlined in Table 1 *(6)*. Pregnant adolescents, black women, and women whose weight falls at the lower end of their BMI category should strive for gains toward the upper end of the recommendation. Short women and women whose weight falls at the upper end of their BMI category should aim to limit their weight gain toward the lower end of the recommendation.

Table 1
Recommended Weight Gain in Pregnancy

Body Mass Index (BMI)	Suggested Weight Gain (lbs)
<19.8 (underweight)	28–40
19.8–26.0 (healthy weight)	25–35
26.0–29.0 (overweight)	15–25
>29 (obese)	At least 15

Source: Institute of Medicine. Nutrition During Pregnancy. I. Weight gain. II. Nutrient Supplements. National Academies Press, Washington DC, 1990. These recommendations are currently being reviewed; updates are anticipated for 2009.

In addition to total weight gain, the pattern of weight gain is also important. For women who begin pregnancy in the healthy weight range, a gain of 3–5 pounds in the first trimester should be followed by steady gains of approximately one pound per week thereafter. Underweight women should gain slightly more during these periods, and overweight women should gain slightly less. Any sudden and drastic gain in weight should be investigated carefully, as sudden changes in weight indicate fluid retention and possible hypertension.

3.2. Energy and Macronutrient Needs During Pregnancy

Calorie needs during pregnancy are not increased in the first trimester, but are increased by 340 kcal/day in the second trimester and by 450 kcal/day in the third trimester. Individuals who engage in little physical activity may need less, and the converse is true for individuals who are very active. The best way to assess whether caloric intake is sufficient is by monitoring weight gain.

Protein needs are increased by approximately 25 g/day, for a total of 71 g/day. Selecting the recommended number of servings from the MyPyramid Food Guide will adequately provide for protein needs. Protein supplements, such as high-protein drinks, are not recommended.

An adequate supply of carbohydrates is necessary to provide energy to the fetal brain and to spare protein for tissue growth. Approximately 175 g/day of carbohydrate are required during pregnancy. Again, this amount is adequately provided by a healthy diet, and most women have no difficulty achieving this. Some women who have adopted very low-carbohydrate diets should be counseled on the importance of including complex carbohydrates in their meals and snacks.

Essential fatty acids are required for proper development of the fetal central nervous system. Including vegetable oils, seeds, nuts, and fish in the diet provides both n–3 and n–6 fatty acids. Several research studies have shown a clear positive association between fish intake during pregnancy and indicators of neurodevelopment of the child, including cognition and visual acuity (7,8). Although fish are the richest source of n–3 fatty acids, intake should be limited due to concerns about mercury, as discussed below.

Fluid needs during pregnancy are generally accommodated for in response to increased levels of thirst. Water, diluted fruit juices and unsweetened beverages are the best choices for hydration.

3.3. Vitamin and Mineral Needs During Pregnancy

The requirements for many vitamins and minerals are increased during pregnancy. A carefully chosen diet of nutrient-dense foods is sufficient to cover most vitamin and mineral needs. However, there are some nutrients that remain a concern during pregnancy. See Table 2 for recommended intakes for selected nutrients (9).

Table 2
Recommended Dietary Allowance (RDA) and Adequate Intake (AI) for Selected Nutrients in Pregnancy

Life Stage	RDA Folate (µg/day)	RDA Vitamin D (µg/day)	RDA Vitamin A (µg/day)	RDA Vitamin B12 (µg/day)	RDA Iron (mg/day)	AI Calcium (mg/day)	AI Vitamin D (µg/day)
Pregnancy, 14–18 yr	600	5	750	2.6	27	1,300	5
Pregnancy, 19–30 yr	600	5	770	2.6	27	1,000	5
Pregnancy, 31–50 yr	600	5	770	2.6	27	1,000	5
Lactation, 14–18 yr	500	5	1,200	2.8	10	1,300	5
Lactation, 19–30 yr	500	5	1,300	2.8	9	1,000	5
Lactation, 31–50 yr	500	5	1,300	2.8	9	1,000	5

Institute of Medicine. Dietary Reference Intakes: The Essential Guide to Nutrient Requirements. National Academies Press, Washington DC, 2006.

Folic acid is essential in the earliest days of pregnancy for proper closure of the neural tube, and for this reason, folic acid supplements are recommended for all women who could become pregnant. In addition, adequate folic acid may have a protective effect against the risk of a host of other adverse outcomes via its role in converting homocysteine to methionine. Elevated levels of homocysteine throughout pregnancy have been linked to the risk for rupture of the placenta, still birth, preterm delivery, preeclampsia, congenital defects, and low birth weight. In this light, it seems wise to continue folic acid supplementation even after the critical period for preventing neural tube defects. In addition to folic acid supplements, women should be encouraged to choose a diet with rich sources of folate.

For women who have previously been pregnant with a child affected by neural tube defects, up to 4 mg/day of folic acid are recommended *(10)*. Although this amount exceeds the Upper Limit (UL) for folic acid, this level has not been shown to be harmful.

Vitamin D plays an essential role in fetal growth and deposition of calcium in the fetal skeleton and teeth. Primary sources of vitamin D include exposure to the sun and vitamin D fortified milk. Women who have dark skin, use sunscreen, avoid sun exposure, live in northern climates, or avoid milk may have low blood levels of vitamin D. In such cases, moderate amounts of sun exposure and increased intakes of fortified dairy products are the preferred methods for increasing vitamin D status. However, in cases of extreme deficiency where the above recommendations are not possible or practical, supplementation may be necessary to prevent osteomalacia in the mother, or rickets in her offspring.

Excess intake of vitamin A is a concern during pregnancy, as it is a known teratogen and may cause birth defects. In addition to avoiding supplements with more than 5,000 IU of retinol or retinoic acid, women should be warned against the use of oral acne medications, such as Accutane, which is derived from vitamin A. Beta carotene, the precursor form of vitamin A found in plant foods, is nontoxic.

Although the requirement for vitamin B_{12} is increased during pregnancy, needs are easily met by a mixed diet that includes foods of animal origin. Vegan diets may be deficient in vitamin B_{12} and, therefore, women who consume no animal products must use a supplement or choose foods that are fortified with vitamin B_{12} to meet their needs.

Calcium metabolism changes dramatically during pregnancy. While absorption, bone turnover, and excretion increase, the fetus and placenta accumulate calcium. By these mechanisms, calcium balance is adequately maintained without increasing dietary intake over prepregnancy requirements. However, women with calcium intakes less than the Adequate Intake (AI) may suffer from decreased maternal and fetal bone density, decreased postpartum bone remineralization, and breastmilk with decreased concentrations of calcium.

Women with chronically low intakes of calcium should be encouraged to increase their intake of dairy foods and/or other foods that are good sources of calcium including fortified cereals, juices, soymilk, dark green leafy vegetables, and legumes. The calcium in dairy foods is the most bioavailable. For those who are unable to sufficiently increase their dietary intake, a daily supplement containing 1.5–2 g of calcium may be helpful.

Iron requirements are increased to support increases in maternal and fetal hemoglobin production. Although the maternal body compensates with increased absorption, fetal needs appear to take precedence over maternal needs, leading to iron deficiency and/or iron deficiency anemia. Iron deficiency anemia during pregnancy is linked to increased risk for preterm birth, low birth weight, fatigue, and reduced resistance to infection in the mother, and lower intelligence quotients and abnormal behavior scores in children born to anemic mothers.

Because plasma volume increases at a more rapid pace than red blood cell production, hemodilution is a normal effect of pregnancy. Therefore, the cutoff values used for screening for anemia are different for pregnancy. Hemoglobin values less than 11 g/dL in the first trimester and less than 10.5 g/dL in the second and third trimesters indicate anemia.

Iron requirements are increased by a greater percentage during pregnancy than are calorie needs. These increased needs during pregnancy are hard to meet through diet alone. For this reason, many practitioners routinely prescribe supplements with 30 mg of iron for all pregnant women beginning at the second trimester. Others prefer to screen for anemia before recommending a supplement. Women diagnosed with anemia may be prescribed larger dose supplements, with 60–180 mg iron. However, high doses of iron are associated with adverse gastrointestinal effects, including nausea, cramps, and constipation. A balance between increased dietary intake from food and a tolerable level of supplemental iron must be sought.

In the past, it was believed that low sodium diets would help prevent water retention, edema, and hypertension. It is now known that sodium plays an important role in fluid balance during pregnancy, and women should not be advised to restrict their sodium intake.

3.4. Substances to Limit or Avoid in Pregnancy

The surgeon general recommends that women who are pregnant or who could become pregnant abstain from drinking alcohol to prevent the array of birth defects associated with fetal alcohol spectrum (11). Women should be counseled to quit smoking before becoming pregnant, but quitting at any time during pregnancy will confer benefits as second-hand smoke can also harm the infant after birth. Caffeine consumption should be limited to less than 300 mg/day or about three cups of coffee. Artificial sweeteners such as aspartame, sucralose, and saccharine are safe to use in moderation. The safety of many herbal supplements and remedies has not been tested, and practitioners should question their patients about their use of these products.

3.5. Food Safety During Pregnancy

There are a few basic steps that can greatly reduce the risk of foodborne illness during pregnancy: washing hands often before and during food preparation and before eating; keeping raw foods separate from cooked and ready-to-eat foods; cooking foods to proper temperatures; and promptly refrigerating leftover foods and cold foods brought home from the grocery store. Women should be cautioned against eating raw or undercooked meat and eggs, including raw cookie dough, Caesar dressing, soft cooked eggs, and rare hamburgers.

The bacteria *Listeria monocytogenes* can cause miscarriage, premature labor, and infant death. It is unique because it can grow at refrigerated temperatures. For this reason, pregnant women should avoid eating unpasteurized dairy products, including unpasteurized cheeses, deli meats, deli salads, smoked seafood, and pâtés. Processed and cured meats like hot dogs must be heated until steaming.

The bacteria *Toxoplasma gondii* is commonly known to infect cat litter, but can also be present in raw and undercooked meats and on the surface of fruits and vegetables. Avoiding touching cat litter, thoroughly cooking meats, and rinsing fruits and vegetables before eating can reduce the risk of exposure.

The mercury content of fish is also a concern for pregnant women *(7)*. Pregnant women should avoid eating shark, swordfish, king mackerel and tilefish, albacore (white tuna), walleye, and bass. Other fish should be limited to less than 12 oz/wk, and light tuna should be limited to less than 6 oz/wk *(12)*.

3.6. Translating Nutrition Guidelines into Practical Advice About Food

Women do not eat grams of macronutrients or milligrams of minerals, they eat portions of food. It is therefore reassuring to know that most nutrient needs will be met by a carefully selected, nutrient-dense diet. If women are familiar with a few basic concepts, they can make their food choices wisely. Food guidelines for pregnant and lactating women can be found at http://www.mypyramid.gov.

4. SPECIAL CONCERNS DURING PREGNANCY

4.1. Common Complaints

The hormonal changes that occur during pregnancy can cause a host of uncomfortable symptoms for women, including morning sickness, heartburn, constipation, and food cravings. Women should be discouraged from taking herbal or "folk" remedies for these ailments as the safety of many of these treatments has not been tested.

Despite its name, morning sickness can strike at any time of the day. Many women suffer from nausea and vomiting only in the early part of pregnancy, but for others, the symptoms can last for the entire three trimesters. The following suggestions may alleviate the discomfort of morning sickness: having something dry to eat like toast or crackers before getting out of bed in the morning, consuming small frequent meals rather than three large meals, consuming liquids separately from meals and snacks. Food odors that cause queasiness are often less offensive if foods are eaten cold, and often fresh air can also help.

Heartburn can occur as the growing fetus pushes up on the mother's internal organs, creating pressure on the lower esophageal sphincter. Helpful suggestions are to avoid spicy or greasy foods, consume liquids separate from meals, eat small frequent meals, and avoid lying down or exercising immediately after meals. Antacid tablets may help as well.

The hormones of pregnancy can alter the muscle tone of the gastrointestinal tract and cause constipation, which may lead to hemorrhoids if there is much straining with bowel movements. Women should take care to get adequate fiber and water during pregnancy, preferably from whole grain foods, fresh fruits and vegetables, and legumes. Bulk-forming laxatives may also provide some relief.

While most cravings women experience during pregnancy are not harmful, neither do they have any basis in physiological need. However, some women develop cravings for non-food items, a condition known as pica. Clay, dirt, laundry starch, and freezer frost are some of the substances most often craved by women with pica. These items can cause toxicities, parasitic infection, or intestinal blockage. Women with diabetes can experience blood sugar abnormalities if large amounts of starch are eaten. If non-food items replace nutritious foods in the diet, nutrient deficiencies can occur. Women with pica are also often found to be anemic. Whether pica is the cause of the anemia or if the reverse is true remains to be seen.

4.2. High-Risk Pregnancies

Gestational diabetes mellitus (GDM) is a condition of poor glucose tolerance diagnosed during pregnancy. Although blood glucose control usually returns to normal postpartum, women diagnosed with GDM are at higher risk for type 2 diabetes later in life. Other consequences of GDM include increased risk for preeclampsia and complications during labor and delivery. Infants born to mothers with GDM are at higher risk for some birth defects, macrosomia and related outcomes such as shoulder dystocia. Women at high risk for GDM include those with a family history of diabetes, overweight, age over 35, a previous pregnancy affected by GDM, or from high-risk ethnic groups, such as Hispanic, black, Native American, south or eastern Asian, and Pacific Islanders. People from these groups should be screened with a 50 g 1 hour oral glucose challenge as early as possible in pregnancy. Other women are usually screened between 24 and 28 wk gestation. A team approach is required, including the patient, the physician, a registered dietitian, and a diabetes educator. Medical nutrition therapy for GDM includes meeting calorie needs as appropriate for recommended weight gain, carbohydrate control (40–45% of total calories coming from carbohydrates spread out evenly through the day), avoidance of concentrated sweets, high fiber intake, avoidance of excess weight gain, and moderate exercise. Regular blood glucose monitoring by the patient is recommended. If diet and exercise fail to bring blood glucose levels under control, insulin may be necessary.

Gestational hypertension is high blood pressure first diagnosed in pregnancy, usually around 20 wk gestation. This may progress to preeclampsia, a condition of hypertension and proteinuria. Women with preeclampsia are at high risk for preterm delivery and progression to eclampsia, a life-threatening condition characterized by convulsions, coma, and death. The exact cause of preeclampsia is unknown, though it seems to be related to abnormal implantation followed by oxidative stresses that reduce blood flow to the placenta. In this light, prevention measures are limited, but women at their ideal body weight with diets that include healthy amounts of antioxidants and minerals are best prepared for pregnancy. Calcium supplementation may help high-risk women, though this has not been proven *(13)*. Low-sodium diets are not beneficial for preventing or treating preeclampsia. Once preeclampsia is diagnosed, dietary measures are largely ineffective at controlling blood pressure, and treatment usually relies on pharmaceutical methods.

A multifetal pregnancy requires weight gains higher than for a singleton pregnancy, with early weight gain being of particular importance. While the Institute of Medicine guidelines recommend gains of 35–45 pounds for twin pregnancy *(6)*, other research shows that weight gains in excess of this, and dependent on prepregnancy BMI (underweight, 50–62 pounds; healthy weight, 40–54 pounds; overweight, 38–47 pounds; obese, 29–38 pounds) are more appropriate *(14)*. More research is needed to determine the exact nutrient requirements consistent with healthy outcomes.

5. NUTRITION FOR LACTATION

Breastmilk is the gold standard for human nutrition *(15)*. The decision to breastfeed is often influenced by external factors, such as the support, or lack thereof, by family, friends, and health professionals, by work, school, or family responsibilities, and by the woman's knowledge of the benefits of breastfeeding.

Women should be provided with information regarding the benefits of breastfeeding early in pregnancy, and often throughout the pregnancy. Benefits for the mother include increased levels of oxytocin, leading to increased uterine contractions, reduced postpartum bleeding, faster return of the uterus to prepregnancy size, and delayed return of menstruation. Women who breastfeed their infants also have improved bone density, reduced risk of breast and ovarian cancer, and reduced risk of rheumatoid arthritis.

Many women are concerned that they may not be able to breastfeed but they should be assured that the vast majority of women are physically able to produce enough milk for their babies, and that breast milk is produced on demand, i.e., the more often they feed their infants, the more breast milk they will produce. Breastfeeding is medically contraindicated in only a few conditions: active tuberculosis, illegal drug use, HIV or AIDS (in developed nations), and galactosemia in the infant.

Nutrition needs during lactation can be provided by a carefully selected diet. Energy needs are increased by 500 kcal/day over prepregnancy needs, but some of these calories may be provided by maternal fat stores. Moderate calorie restriction and moderate exercise are acceptable ways to reduce postpartum weight without affecting the quality of breast milk. Protein and fatty acid requirements are not elevated during lactation, but carbohydrate needs are increased to provide glucose for the lactose content of breast milk. Vitamin and mineral status in the lactating mother generally does not affect the quality of breast milk, unless deficiencies are prolonged and severe. Increased needs of some vitamins and minerals during lactation are to support the mother's nutrition status. DRIs for selected nutrients are presented in Table 2.

6. NUTRITION FOR THE POSTPARTUM PERIOD

Practitioners can use postpartum visits as an opportunity to encourage women to develop strategies to return to or achieve a healthy BMI. These visits are also the ideal time to discuss preparations for future pregnancies, much as described above for preconception.

7. REFERALS FOR SERVICES

There are some circumstances in which referrals for additional services should be made. Pregnant women with poor weight gain, hyperemesis gravidarum, chronically poor diets, phenylketonuria, chronic diseases such as hypertension and diabetes, or a history of substance abuse may be referred to a registered dietitian for medical nutrition therapy *(12)*. Lactating women who are experiencing difficulty with the breastfeeding process should be referred to a certified lactation consultant. The Supplemental Food Program for Women, Infants and Children (WIC) serves low-income pregnant, breastfeeding, and postpartum women, as well as children up to 5 years of age who are at high risk for medical or nutritional problems. Through WIC, women can receive health referral services, supplemental food vouchers, and nutrition assessment, education, and counseling.

8. SUMMARY

For most women, good nutrition during pregnancy, including increased energy needs, can be achieved through a carefully selected nutrient-rich diet. Good nutrition practices should begin in the preconception period. Women are best prepared for pregnancy when they are at or near their ideal body weight, eat a nutrient-dense diet, take a folic acid supplement, and abstain from tobacco and alcohol. Weight gain during pregnancy should be based on prepregnancy BMI. Some women may benefit from iron or calcium supplements. Pregnant women should take extra precautions to avoid any foodborne illness. Common complaints of pregnancy may often be relieved through dietary measures; herbal supplements have not been shown to be safe. High-risk pregnancy conditions, such as gestational diabetes, preeclampsia, and multifetal pregnancy, are best treated using a team approach. Nutrition continues to be important in the postpartum period, particularly for mothers who choose to breastfeed their infants. Women with chronic disease, who are low income and at high risk for poor nutrition, or who have concerns about breastfeeding should be given referrals for specialized services. Appropriate weight gain, adequate nutrient intakes, and avoidance of harmful substances, such as alcohol and tobacco, are the key components of optimal prenatal nutrition. Women in high-risk pregnancies should be referred to a dietitian for medical nutrition therapy.

SUGGESTED FURTHER READING

USDA Daily Food Guide http://www.mypyramid.gov
Maternal and Child Health Bureau http://www.mchb.hrsa.gov
March of Dimes http://www.marchofdimes.com

La Leche League http://www.llli.org

Institute of Medicine. Nutrition During Pregnancy. I. Weight gain. II. Nutrient supplements. National Academies Press, Washington DC, 1990.

Kaiser L, Allen LH. Position of the American Dietetic Association: nutrition and lifestyle for a healthy pregnancy outcome. J Am Diet Assoc 2008; 108:553–561.

REFERENCES

1. Thompson JN. Fetal nutrition and adult hypertension, diabetes, obesity and coronary artery disease. Neonatal Netw 2007; 26:235–240.
2. Fertility, Family Planning, and Reproductive Health of U.S. Women: Data from the 2002 National Survey of Family Growth. Available at: http://www.cdc.gov/nchs/data/series/sr_23/sr23_025.pdf. Last accessed January 31, 2008.
3. Lu MC. Recommendations for preconception care. Am Fam Physician 2007, 76. 397–400.
4. Wasserman CR, Shaw GM, Selvin S, et al. Socioeconomic status, neighborhood conditions and neural tube defects. Am J Public Health 1998; 88:1674–1680.
5. Cena ER, Joy AB, Heneman K, et al. Folate intake and food related behaviors in nonpregnant, low-income women of childbearing age. J Am Diet Assoc 2008; 108:1364–1368.
6. Institute of Medicine. Nutrition During Pregnancy. I. Weight gain. II. Nutrient supplements. National Academies Press, Washington DC, 1990.
7. Oken E, Radesky JS, Wright RO, et al. Maternal fish intake during pregnancy, blood mercury levels, and child cognition at age 3 years in a US cohort. Am J Epidemiol 2008; 167:1171–1181.
8. Hibbeln JR, Davis JM, Steer C, et al. Maternal seafood consumption in pregnancy and neurodevelopmental outcomes in childhood (ALSPAC study): an observational cohort study. Lancet 2007; 369:578–585.
9. Institute of Medicine. Dietary Reference Intakes: The Essential Guide to Nutrient Requirements. National Academies Press, Washington DC, 2006.
10. Korenbrot CC, Steinberg A, Bender C, et al. Preconception care: a systemic review. Matern Child Health J 2002; 6:75–88.
11. Surgeon General's Advisory on Alcohol Use in Pregnancy. Available at: http://www.surgeongeneral.gov/pressreleases/sg02222005.html. Last accessed January 17, 2008.
12. What You Need to Know about Mercury in Fish and Shellfish. Available at www.epa.gov/waterscience/fish/advice/. Last accessed September 12, 2008.
13. Trumbo PR, Ellwood KC. Supplemental calcium and risk reduction of hypertension, pregnancy-induced hypertension, and preeclampsia: an evidence-based review by the US Food and Drug Administration. Nutr Rev 2007; 65:78–87.
14. Kaiser L, Allen LH. Position of the American Dietetic Association: nutrition and lifestyle for a healthy pregnancy outcome. J Am Diet Assoc 2008; 108:553–561.
15. Gartner LM, Eidelman AI. Breastfeeding and the use of human milk section on breastfeeding. Pediatrics 2005; 115:496–506.

16 Infants: Transition from Breast to Bottle to Solids

Jacki M. Rorabaugh and James K. Friel

Key Points

- Exclusive breastfeeding is recommended for the first 6 months of life.
- Formula feeding is only recommended to mothers who cannot or choose not to breastfeed.
- Breast milk has a degree of bioactivity, antioxidant ability, immunological defenses, minerals, and fatty acids not yet found in formula. These lacking elements may help explain the health benefits associated with breast milk. Formula manufacturers are trying to introduce these missing elements into formula.
- Complementary feeding should begin at 6 months of age with breast milk continuing until at least 1 year of age.
- Complementary feeding should help promote a positive association with hunger, food, appetite, and the person feeding. Infants should also learn gross motor skills and form relationships.

Key Words: Infants; breast milk; breastfeeding; formula; growth

1. WHAT IS THE BEST MILK FOR AN INFANT?

Breastfeeding is recommended for the first year of life *(1, 2)*. Exclusive breastfeeding is recommended for the first 6 months of life. Formula feeding is recommended only for those who choose not to or cannot breastfeed. The consumption of whole or reduced-fat cow's milk is not recommended during the first year of life *(3)*. About two out of three mothers in the United States initiate breastfeeding and one out of five continue to 6 months.

From: *Nutrition and Health: Nutrition Guide for Physicians*
Edited by: T. Wilson et al. (eds.), DOI 10.1007/978-1-60327-431-9_16,
© Humana Press, a part of Springer Science+Business Media, LLC 2010

Breastfeeding is rarely contraindicated. Infants who have galactosemia or whose mother uses illegal drugs, has untreated active tuberculosis, or has been infected with HIV should not breastfeed. However, neither smoking nor environmental contaminants, moderate alcohol consumption, and the use of most prescription and over-the-counter drugs should preclude breastfeeding.

With all the best intentions and technological expertise, "humanized" infant formulas do not compare to mother's own milk. It is therefore logical and appropriate for health professionals to encourage the consumption of human milk whenever possible. However, once the information is presented, there is no justification for attempting to coerce women into making a feeding choice (4). Sometimes a formula-fed child and rarely a breastfed infant develop sensitivity to cow's milk, either cow's milk allergy (CMA) or lactose intolerance. Secondary lactase deficiency does occur in infancy, most often following a gastrointestinal disorder.

While human milk is "uniquely superior" for infant feeding and is species specific, the most acceptable alternative is commercial formulas. Manufacturers do their utmost to mimic human milk. A "formula" is just that: an equation that is proprietary, consisting of a composite mix of nutrients, emulsifiers, and stabilizers. Formulas in North America that are marketed for term infants are either (a) cow milk-based (casein or whey predominant), (b) soy protein-based, or (c) protein hydrolysate-based. The use of soy-based formulas, speciality formulas, or formulas for the feeding of the premature infant is beyond the scope of this review.

The success of formula manufacturers is due to (a) aggressive marketing, (b) lack of support for breastfeeding from family, friends, and the medical profession, (c) cultural and public perception, (d) convenience, and (e) some government programs giving infant formula away for free. With the increase in working mothers, formula feeding becomes a practical and attractive alternative. Guidelines for formula composition have evolved over the years to provide not only what must be in a formula but minimum and maximum levels as well. Standards may vary between countries.

2. NUTRIENT CONTENT OF BREAST MILK AND INFANT FORMULA

The composition of a formula depends on many factors and differs between manufacturers. For example, cholesterol exists in human milk but is not added to formula because the public perceives it as "bad." Human milk has a caloric density of 670 kcal/L. Most term formulas are designed to have the same caloric density. Low-iron formulas are marketed even though health professionals do not recommend their use as a standard feed. They remain on the market because the public and some health professionals perceive them as beneficial in dealing with problems such as colic and constipation.

The nutrient composition of milk changes over time. The composition of human milk also changes during feeding so that most of the fat in human milk occurs in the latter part of feeding, probably saturating the infant and providing a signal for terminating feeding. It appears that the infant who is breastfed has more control over the amount consumed at a feeding than does the formula-fed infant (4). Frequent feedings with small amounts at each feeding, as is seen in infants who are breastfed ad libitum, may lead to favorable changes in metabolism (5). These differences may affect feeding habits later in life.

Protein content of human milk is high during early lactation (colostrum) and then gradually declines to a low level of 0.8–1% in mature milk. The high protein concentration of colostrum is largely due to very high concentrations of secretory IgA and lactoferrin. These proteins provide protection against bacteria giving benefits in early life beyond the role of building blocks for tissue synthesis. Indeed, human milk is truly the first and foremost "functional food."

Milk proteins are separated into various classes, mainly caseins (10–50% of total) and whey (50–90% of total) proteins (6). Milk fat globule membrane proteins and protein derived from cells present in milk comprise 1–3%. For some years manufacturers prepared their formula with either a whey or a casein base. For the term infant, there appears to be no advantage nutritionally of whey-predominant over casein-predominant formulas. Interestingly, digested fragments of human casein, but not bovine, may exert physiological effects such as enhancing calcium uptake by cells and playing a role in infant sleeping patterns (6). Little is known about the role of hormones that are present in human milk; they may play a role in the developing infant.

Human milk contains significant amounts of polyunsaturated fats. These include 10–12% linoleic acid (18:2, n–6), 1–2% linolenic acid (18:3, n–3), and a small but significant amount of long-chain (n–6) and (n–3) fatty acids (7). While the level of total polyunsaturated fats in human milk varies with the intake of the mother, it is generally 13–20%. Long-chain fatty acids present in human milk, but not currently in formula, may confer some developmental advantage. Formula contains more of the shorter chain fatty acids.

The primary carbohydrate source in formula and human milk is lactose with very small amounts of other sugars. No minimum or maximum level of carbohydrate is set for North America. Corn syrup solids and/or maltodextrin may be used in certain formulas (4).

Minerals can be divided broadly into macro, micro, and ultra-trace elements. Mineral concentrations differ in human milk over the first 3 months of lactation (8). The levels of Zn, Cu, Rb, and Mo decrease over time, suggesting homeostatic regulation and possible essentiality for human infants *(8)*. In general, the mineral content of human milk is not influenced by maternal diet, parity, maternal age, time of milk collection, different breasts, or socioeconomic status *(9)*.

The ultra-trace elements (<1 μg/g dry diet) exist naturally in human milk but depend on protein sources in formulas where they occur as contaminants. Although many of these elements have no specified human requirement, we believe that recommendations for ultra-trace elements need to be established.

Human milk has all the essential vitamins required by the infant but is low in vitamins D and K. Vitamin K is given to all infants at birth and vitamin D (also considered to be a hormone) is usually recommended as a supplement for breastfed infants. Minimum and maximum levels of vitamins are regulated for formulas so that they are complete. Formula labels state the amount of all nutrients, including vitamins that must be present when the shelf life expires. Because of this, "overage" is necessary as some vitamins will break down over time. Thus, as much as 60% over label claim might be present for different nutrients, primarily vitamins *(10)*.

The use of supplements for human milk-fed infants is controversial. Some see supplements as undermining the integrity of human milk and implying that milk is not adequate. Nonetheless, human milk is neither a perfect nor a complete food *(11)*. There are good data to support the administration of vitamin K soon after birth to prevent hemorrhagic disease of the newborn and vitamin D supplements during early infancy to prevent rickets *(2, 11)*.

Current practice is for iron supplements to be deferred until 4–6 months of age. Some authorities *(11)* recommend iron supplements of 7 mg/day, beginning in the first few weeks of life. A significant increase in iron status has been documented in infants receiving a modest iron supplement (7.5 mg/day) *(12)*. Fluoride supplements once recommended for all infants are no longer recommended during the first year of life *(11)*.

Formulas that conform to specification of Canadian/American guidelines do not require supplementation with any minerals or vitamins as they are complete. A controversial nutrient is iron. The amount of iron fortification required is not yet certain; however, formulas providing low intakes of iron (<4 mg/L) may lead to anemia. It was believed that consuming iron-fortified formulas would result in intolerance and gastrointestinal distress, but these theories have been discredited *(13)*. See Fomon *(4)* for a review of regulations for the nutrient content of infant formulas.

In general, the content of protein, lipid, carbohydrate, energy, minerals, and most water-soluble vitamins in human milk is not affected by poor maternal nutrition *(14)*. Fat-soluble vitamins and fatty acids are affected by maternal diet *(14)*. It appears that there are mechanisms to ensure constant supply and quality of nutrients to the breastfed infant. The major difference between a breastfed and a formula-fed infant is that many of the components of human milk also facilitate the absorption of nutrients and have a function beyond nutrient requirements. Adding more of a nutrient to formula is not necessarily as good as having a bioactive component in human milk even if present in small amounts (e.g., lactoferrin for both iron absorption and as a bactericide). There are many properties of human milk that attend to such details for the benefit of the infant.

3. BIOACTIVITY OF HUMAN MILK AND FORMULAS

Human milk is "alive," that is, it has functional components that have a role beyond simply the provision of essential nutrients. Bioactive compounds in human milk can be divided into several broad categories: (1) those compounds involved in milk synthesis, nutritional composition, and bioavailability and (2) those compounds that aid in protection and subsequent development of the infant. To date many bioactive compounds have been identified in human milk including cytokines, immune factors, growth factors, hormones, antimicrobial agents, nucleotides, antioxidants, and enzymes (*see* review *(15)*). Hormones, enzymes, cytokines for immunity, and cells present in milk have physiologically active roles in other tissues so that it is reasonable to assume that they play a role in infant growth and development. Indeed, many bioactive compounds can survive the environment of the neonatal stomach thereby potentially exerting important physiological functions *(15, 16)*.

Early postnatal exposure to flavor passed into human milk from the mother's own diet can predispose the young infant to respond to new foods. The transition from the breastfeeding period to the initiation of a varied solid food diet can be made easier if the infant has already experienced these flavors. Cues from breast milk can influence food choices and make safe new foods with flavors already experienced in breast milk *(17)*. Again, this does not happen with formula feeding.

A variety of cells exist in human milk. Macrophages, polymorphonuclear leukocytes, epithelial cells, and lymphocytes have been identified in human milk and appear to have a dynamic role to play within the infant gut. These cells may offer systemic protection after transport across the "leaky gut," particularly in the first week of life *(18)*. Antiviral and antibacterial factors exist in human milk with secretory IgA produced in the mammary gland being one of the major milk proteins *(6)*. There may even be a pathway from the infant back to the mother, which tailors production of antibodies against microbes to which the infant has been exposed.

Hamosh *(15)* classifies enzymes in human milk into three categories: (1) those that function in the mammary gland, (2) enzymes that might function in the infant, and (3) enzymes whose function are unclear. It is only recently that the physiological significance of enzymes in human milk has started to become appreciated. More than just protein, and not present at all in infant formulas, enzymes are another example of why human milk must be seen as alive. These enzymes appear to have a more highly organized tertiary structure than enzymes from other tissues, which may be to protect function by resisting denaturation in the gut *(15)*. We think that as well as serving an immediate function in the intestine, some enzymes may be transported across the gut or act within the body to offer protection to the infant. Interestingly, amylase digests polysaccharides that are not present in human milk. Amylase is important after the initiation of starch supplements like cereals *(15)*. It is as if the mammary gland is "thinking ahead" and assisting the infant gut in the transition to weaning. Milk digestive lipase assists the newborn whose endogenous lipid digestive function is not well developed at birth.

Recent interest has focused on the antioxidant properties of human milk. Several groups have reported the ability of colostrum *(19)* and mature milk *(20)* to resist oxidative stress using a variety of end points. This feature of human milk appears to be heterogeneous rather than attributable to a specific compound. Infant formulas appear to be less resistive to oxidative stress than human milk. This is noteworthy since formulas always have considerably more vitamin E and vitamin C, considered to be two of the more important antioxidants, than are found naturally in human milk. Some have suggested that the attainment of adult levels of some antioxidants during infancy is dependent on human milk feeding *(16)*.

4. HEALTH BENEFITS OF HUMAN MILK

The health benefits of human milk are significant. Breastfeeding protects against a wide variety of illnesses, particularly incidence and severity of diarrhea, otitis media, upper respiratory illnesses, botulism, and necrotizing enterocolitis *(14, 22)*. Prior to advancements in hygiene, infants who were not breastfed did not fare well and mortality rates could be as high as 90% *(4, 14)*. Even with the use of current formulas, breastfed infants have lower incidences of many illness and are generally sicker for shorter times than formula-fed infants *(21)*. Later in life breastfed infants are reported to have decreased risk of diabetes, cancer, and cardiovascular disease *(22)*.

The most practical measure of overall infant health and well-being is growth. One would expect that with all the advantages of human milk, a breastfed baby would gain more weight. It is a puzzling phenomenon that growth of the exclusively breastfed infant is lower in weight-for-age than a formula-fed infant. Likely there is more energy intake by a formula-fed infant. However, the relevance of less growth in breastfed infants is questionable as no negative effects on functional outcomes have been observed. We found infants who had consumed home formulas made of evaporated milk grew more than either formula-fed or breastfed babies (23), yet they did not perform as well as breastfed infants on tests of visual function (24).

There is controversy in the area of cognitive development as it is difficult to carry out the ideal study. Breastfed infants appear to have enhanced cognitive and neurological outcomes in comparison to formula-fed infants (25). Small differences have been seen even in later childhood (25). Increased duration of breastfeeding and higher verbal IQ scores have been reported. Increasing the period of exclusive breastfeeding appears to enhance infant motor development (26). We found enhanced visual acuity in full-term breastfed infants compared to formula-fed infants; this was related to blood fatty acid levels (24). The explanation for these consistent observations is highly controversial. Possibly, there are components of human milk that enhance cognitive development. Other factors that may be responsible are the act of breastfeeding itself, maternal education, and social class.

A paper by Allan Lucas (25) reporting improved neurological development in breastfed infants sparked a major debate on which factors really explained increased cognitive development. It is reasonable to assume that the long-chain polyunsaturated fatty acids, enzymes, hormones, trophic factors, peptides, and nucleotides present in breast milk may enhance brain development and learning ability. Further, it would be sensible to feed human milk whenever possible if any or all of the above differences turn out to be true. Whether a breastfed infant has better development because of maternal factors or biological factors does not lessen the value of enhanced development to the infant.

5. TRANSITION TO SOLID FOODS

During the second 6 months of infancy, breast milk no longer meets all the nutritional needs of the infant. Therefore, solid foods should be introduced. However, continuation of breastfeeding is recommended for the first year of life and can be continued until the mother and infant decide to cease. The introduction of solid foods is known as complementary feeding. A proper transition between a liquid diet and a diet with solids is crucial for the development of infants. The WHO outlines complementary feeding with four goals: complementary feeding should be timely, adequate, safe, and properly administered (27).

The timely introduction of complementary foods should begin at 6 months. Most infants start consuming complementary foods at 3–4 months of age. Early introduction of complementary foods was once believed to promote a healthy appetite, food acceptance, and a full night of sleep; however, those theories have been discredited. Delaying the introduction of solid foods till 6 months of age and thereby extending formula or breastfeeding has shown to decrease gastrointestinal infections and morbidity rates in infants (14, 22). Delaying complementary feeding allows for the infant to gain more benefits from breast or formula feeding.

Complementary foods need to meet the infants' growing nutritional needs. These foods need to be nutritionally adequate to provide enough energy, macronutrients, and micronutrients to support normal development (27). Traditionally, the first solid foods a baby consumes are cereals and other grain-based products. Fruits and vegetables are normally the next food groups introduced, with meats and other protein-rich foods being introduced later. Breast milk is a poor source of iron and zinc; the ideal complementary food would be rich in both of these micronutrients. Iron-rich foods like meats are being suggested as one of the first solids consumed (28). Currently, meats are not consumed regularly until 7–8 months of age, with other food groups starting at 4–6 months.

The physical act of feeding is important to a developing infant. As they age, infants become more aware of feeding methods and eventually learn how to self-feed by mimicry. Development of gross and fine motor skills is encouraged through self-feeding. Formation of emotional connections with other people is facilitated through feeding. Many of the infant's attitudes about food, hunger, and appetite can be affected by the type of relationship the infant forms with his or her feeder. The frequency of feedings should start with 2–3 meals a day from 6–8 months and then increase to 3–4 meals a day to the end of toddlerhood. Feeding should promote a positive correlation with food, appetite, hunger, and emotional relationships. Food safety is also a concern for infant nutrition. Food must be prepared in a hygienic environment including clean water, utensils, and storage facilities for the food.

The proper transition to solid foods is key to the growth and development of infants. The type of foods and feeding methods presented to the infant have an impact on food preferences and future eating habits (29). There have been correlations made between unbalanced diets in infancy and being overweight or obese later in life (30). The protein content of the infant's diet is of concern for obesity risks. Diets high in protein in infancy have been shown to cause obesity in childhood. A balanced amount of all the macronutrients and micronutrients is critical to the health and growth of the infant. Stunting is often the result of inadequate micronutrient intakes and can result in growth and developmental retardation.

6. SUMMARY

There is no doubt that human milk is the best food for a human infant. The reasons are endless and convincing. Nonetheless, it is a challenge for the formula industry to make the best suitable alternative to human milk. There are, were, and always will be some women who are unable or choose not to follow recommendations to breastfeed for whatever the reason. We have a responsibility to those mothers and their infants to produce a formula that meets their needs. Future changes in infant formulas are likely to be designed to have a positive effect on physical, mental, and immunological outcomes. Our hope is that formula will include bioactive ingredients that perform some of the same functions found in that exemplary fluid, human milk.

When breast milk is no longer adequate, the correct approach needs to be taken for complementary feeding. Incorporating the themes of timely feeding, nutritionally sound and safe meals, and properly administering meals into complementary feeding will prompt appropriate development and growth (27). The importance of proper complementary feeding practices is not normally stressed; however, several incentives have been proposed to address the current practices. The lengthening of exclusive breastfeeding to 6 months and delaying complementary feeding until then is recommended. Benefits for this are similar to the benefits of breastfeeding. Molding the infant's diet to include appropriate amounts of micronutrients, especially iron and zinc, is a primary concern for parents. A suitable transition to a diet of solid foods sets the pace for the rest of the infant's life.

SUGGESTED FURTHER READING

Dewey KG. What is the optimal age for introduction of complementary foods? Nestlé Nutrition Workshop Series. Pediatric Program 2006; 58:161–170; discussion 170–175.

REFERENCES

1. American Academy of Pediatrics. Breastfeeding and the use of human milk. Pediatrics 1997; 100:1035–1039.
2. Canadian Paediatric Society, Dieticians of Canada, Health Canada. Nutrition for Healthy Term Infants. Minister of Public Works and Government Services, Ottawa, 1998.
3. American Academy of Pediatrics. The use of whole cow's milk in infancy. Pediatrics 1992; 89:1105–1107.
4. Fomon SJ. Recommendations for feeding normal infants. In: Nutrition of Normal Infants. Mosby, St. Louis, 1993, pp. 455–458.

5. Jenkins DJA, Wolever TMS, Vinson U, et al. Nibbling vs. gorging: metabolic advantages of increased meal frequency. N Engl J Med 1989; 321:929–934.

6. Lonnerdal B, Atkinson S. Nitrogenous components of milk. A. Human milk proteins. In: Jensen UG, ed. Handbook of Milk Composition. Academic Press, San Diego, 1995, pp. 351–368.

7. Redenials WAN, Chen Z-Y. Trans, n-2, and n-6 fatty acids in Canadian human milk. Lipids 1996; 31:5279–5282.

8. Friel JK, Longerich H, Jackson S, Dawson B, Sutrahdar B. Ultra trace elements in human milk from premature and term infants. Biol Tr Elem Res 1999; 67:225-247.

9. Lonnerdal B. Regulation of mineral and trace elements in human milk: exogenous and endogenous factors. Nutr Rev 2000; 58:223–229.

10. Friel JK, Bessie JC, Belkhode SL, et al. Thiamine, riboflavin, pyridoxine, and vitamin C status in premature infants receiving parenteral and enteral nutrition. J Pediatr Gastroenterol Nutr 2001; 33:64–69.

11. Fomon SJ, Straus UG. Nutrient deficiencies in breast-fed infants. N Engl J Med 1978; 299:355–357.

12. Friel JK, Aziz K, Andrews WL, Harding SV, Courage ML, Adams RJ. A double-masked, randomized control trial of iron supplementation in early infancy in healthy term breast-fed infants. J Pediatr 2003; 143:582–586.

13. Nelson SE, Ziegler EE, Copeland AM, Edwards BB, Fomon SJ. Lack of adverse reaction to iron-fortified formula. Pediatrics1988; 81:360–364.

14. Lonnerdal B. Breast milk: A truly functional food. Nutrition 2000; 16:509–511.

15. Hamosh M. Enzymes in human milk. In: Jensen UG ed. Handbook of Milk Composition. Academic Press, San Diego, CA, 1995, pp. 388–427.

16. L'Abbe MR, Friel JK. Enzymes in human milk. In: Huang V-S, Sinclair A, eds. Recent Advances in the Role of Lipids in Infant Nutrition. AOCS Press, Champaign, IL, 1998, pp. 133–147.

17. Mennella JA, Jagnow CP, Beauchamp GK. Prenatal and postnatal flavor learning by human infants. Pediatrics 2001; 107:E88.

18. Weaver LT, Lalver MF, Nelson R. Intestinal permeability in the newborn. Arch Dis Child 1984; 59:236–241.

19. Buescher ES, McIllherhan SM. Antioxidant properties of human colostrum. Pediatr Res 1988; 24:14–19.

20. Friel JK, Martin SM, Langdon M, Herzberg G, Buettner GR. Human milk provides better antioxidant protection than does infant formula. Pediatr Res 2002; 51:612–618.

21. Dewey KG, Heinig MJ, Nommsen-Rivers LA. Differences in morbidity between breast-fed and formula-fed infants. J Pediatr 1995; 126:696–702.

22. Heinig, MJ, Dewey KG. Health advantage of breast feeding for infants: A critical review. Nutr Res Rev 1996; 9:89–97.

23. Friel JK, Andrews WL, Simmons BS, Mercer C, Macdonald A, McCloy U. An evaluation of full-term infants fed on evaporated milk formula. Acta Paediatr 1997; 86: 448–453.

24. Courage ML, McCloy UR, Herzberg GR, et al. Visual acuity development and fatty acid composition of erythrocytes in full-term infants fed breast milk, commercial formula, or evaporated milk. J Dev Behav Paediatr 1997; 19:9–17.

25. Lucas A, Morley R, Cole TJ, Lister G, Leeson-Payne C. Breast milk and subsequent intelligence quotient in children born preterm. Lancet 1992; 339:261–264.

26. Dewey KG, Cohen RJ, Brown KH, Rivera LL. Effects of exclusive breast feeding for four versus six months on maternal nutritional status and infant motor development. J Nutr 2001; 131:262–267.

27. World Health Organization. Complementary Feeding. Report of the Global Consultation, and Summary of Guiding Principles for Complementary Feeding of the Breast-fed Child. WHO, Geneva, 2003. Available at: http://www.who.int/child_adolescent_health/documents/924154614X/en/index.html. Last accessed November 26, 2008.

28. Krebs NF. Meat as an early complementary food for infants: implications for macro- and micronutrient intakes. Nestlé Nutrition Workshop Series. Pediatric Program. Denver, Colorado 2007; 60:221–229.

29. Fox MK, Pac S, Devaney B, Jankowski L. Feeding infants and toddlers study: What foods are infants and toddlers eating? J Am Diet Assoc 2004; 104:S22–S30.

30. Agostoni C, Riva E, Giovannini M. Complementary food: international comparison on protein and energy requirement/intakes. Nestlé Nutrition Workshop Series. Pediatric Program 2006; 58:147–156.

17 Young Children: Preparing for the Future

Jennifer J. Francis

Key Points

- A carefully chosen diet can provide the energy and nutrients that children need to grow, learn, and play.
- The Centers for Disease Control and Prevention (2000) growth charts are typically used to monitor growth.
- The Dietary Guidelines for Americans and the MyPyramid Food Guidance System are appropriate tools to support healthy food choices for children.
- Childhood overweight is a multifactoral problem which requires approaches that incorporate diet, physical activity, psychological support, behavior modification, and caretaker involvement.
- Food insecurity, iron deficiency anemia, and food allergies are all issues which may affect dietary quality and may require referrals to registered dietitians or food assistance programs.
- Nutritional and vitamin supplements are not necessary for well-nourished children.

Key Words: Child; growth charts; child obesity; dietary guidance; MyPyramid for kids; physical activity; food allergies; iron deficiency anemia; food insecurity

1. INTRODUCTION

The job of children is to grow, play, and learn. To achieve these goals, they need the right fuel – food that provides optimal energy and nutrients. In addition, good nutrition, even in the early years of childhood, can help reduce risk of chronic diseases in adulthood, such as obesity, heart disease, diabetes, and hypertension *(1)*. The eating habits children form will carry over into adulthood, establishing a firm foundation for lifelong health.

From: *Nutrition and Health: Nutrition Guide for Physicians*
Edited by: T. Wilson et al. (eds.), DOI 10.1007/978-1-60327-431-9_17,
© Humana Press, a part of Springer Science+Business Media, LLC 2010

2. MONITORING GROWTH

Typically, practitioners use the Centers for Disease Control and Prevention 2000 growth charts to monitor growth. Children under 2 years of age should be weighed without clothes or diapers and measured in a recumbent position. Children over the age of 2 should be weighed and measured in lightweight clothing without shoes, standing for measure of stature. The growth charts can plot trends in weight for age, height for age, head circumference for age, weight for height, and body mass index (BMI) for age. Trends for these measures should be monitored, rather than relying on single data points.

BMI does not remain constant throughout childhood, typically decreasing from age 2 until age 4–6, and then increasing again as puberty approaches. A BMI less than the 5th percentile for age indicates underweight, while a BMI between the 85th and the 95th percentile indicates elevated risk for overweight, and a BMI greater than the 95th percentile indicates overweight.

3. NUTRITION GUIDANCE

3.1. Energy and Nutrient Needs

Total estimated energy requirements increase throughout the childhood period, from approximately 1000 kcal/day at age 1–3 years to approximately 2000 kcal/day at age 9–13 years. See Table 1 for estimated energy requirements for different age and gender groups.

Macronutrient distribution varies with age as well. For younger children, from age 1 to 3 years, fat should provide 30–40% of calories, from age 4 to 18 years, 25–35% is more appropriate. The fat content of the diet can be provided by whole foods that contain fats, such as dairy, meat, fish, nuts, seeds, and cooking oils, rich in monounsaturated and polyunsaturated fats. Total protein needs increase from 13 g/day at age 3 to 34 g/day at age 9–13 for both sexes; see Table 1.

Carbohydrate needs after age 1 are determined based on the amount of glucose required by the brain, at 130 g/day. For children, a diet rich in fiber provided by fresh fruits and vegetables, whole grains, and legumes is essential for preventing constipation (2). In addition, children who consume high-fiber diets are more likely to consume more nutrient-rich foods (3). For fiber intake, the "age +5 rule" has been replaced by more specific recommendations for total fiber, which includes both dietary fiber and functional fiber (4). See Table 1 for recommended fiber intakes.

Another concern is the volume of sugar-sweetened beverages in the diet, including fruit drinks other than 100% juice and soft drinks. Although a

Table 1

Estimated Energy Requirement (EER), Recommended Dietary Allowance (RDA), and Adequate Intake (AI) for Selected Nutrients in Childhood

Gender and Life Stage (years)	EER Energy (kcal/day)	RDA Protein (g/day)	AI Fiber (g/day)	RDA Iron (mg/day)	AI Calcium (mg/day)	AI Total Fluid (L/day)
Male (1–3)	1046	13	19	7	500	1.3
Male (4–8)	1742	19	25	10	800	1.7
Male (9–13)	2279	34	31	8	1300	2.4
Female (1–3)	992	13	19	7	500	1.3
Female (4–8)	1642	19	25	10	800	1.7
Female (9–13)	2017	34	26	8	1300	2.1

Source: Institute of Medicine. Dietary Reference Intakes: The Essential Guide to Nutrient Requirements. National Academies Press, Washington, DC, 2006.

direct link between *sugar* intake and obesity has not been proven, studies show that children who drink these *beverages* do so in place of milk and juice, consume more total calories, are more likely to be overweight and consume less nutrient-dense diets *(5, 6)*. Many parents believe that there is a link between sugar intake and hyperactive behavior in their children, though the vast majority of research shows no such relationship *(7)*.

Fluids in the diet should be provided by water, milk, and 100% fruit juice. Fluid needs are increased with physical activity; fever; vomiting; diarrhea; and hot, dry, or humid environments. *See* Table 1 for recommended fluid intakes. Note that fluid needs are close to 1 ml of fluid per kilocalorie of energy needs.

Children consuming a diet in compliance with the Dietary Guidelines for Americans (*see* below) are likely to consume adequate vitamins and minerals. However, iron and calcium intakes are often deficient in the diets of children. Recommended intakes are presented in Table 1. Dietary strategies to increase iron intake and absorption include limiting milk intake to less than 24 oz/day, consuming meat products concurrent with a source of vitamin C, and including fortified breakfast cereals in the diet. For calcium, strategies to increase intake can include limiting soft drink consumption and offering a variety of low-fat dairy products and calcium-fortified foods such as cereal and orange juice. Flavored milks may increase intake of calcium without increasing overall intake of sugar in the diet *(8)*. The topic of how nutrition affects calcium homeostasis is also discussed in Chapter 30.

3.2. Dietary Guidance

The Dietary Guidelines for Americans were developed for individuals aged 2 years and older and are applicable to children and adolescents. However, there are also some specific recommendations for younger children *(9)*:

- Physical activity for 60 min on most or all days.
- Half of all grains consumed should be whole grains.
- Children aged 2–8 should consume at least two servings of low-fat or fat-free dairy per day and older children should consume at least three servings of low-fat or fat-free dairy.
- For children aged 2–3 years, fat should comprise 30–35% of calories and for older children fat intake should be reduced to 25–35% of calories, primarily from unsaturated fats.

The MyPyramid Food Guidance System (Chapter 11) can be personalized for children and adolescents by entering their age, gender, and physical activity level *(10)*. Following the personalized recommendations can help children meet their energy and nutrient needs and encourage physical activity. *See* Fig. 1 for a sample plan for a 2-year-old boy who is active for 30–60 min/day.

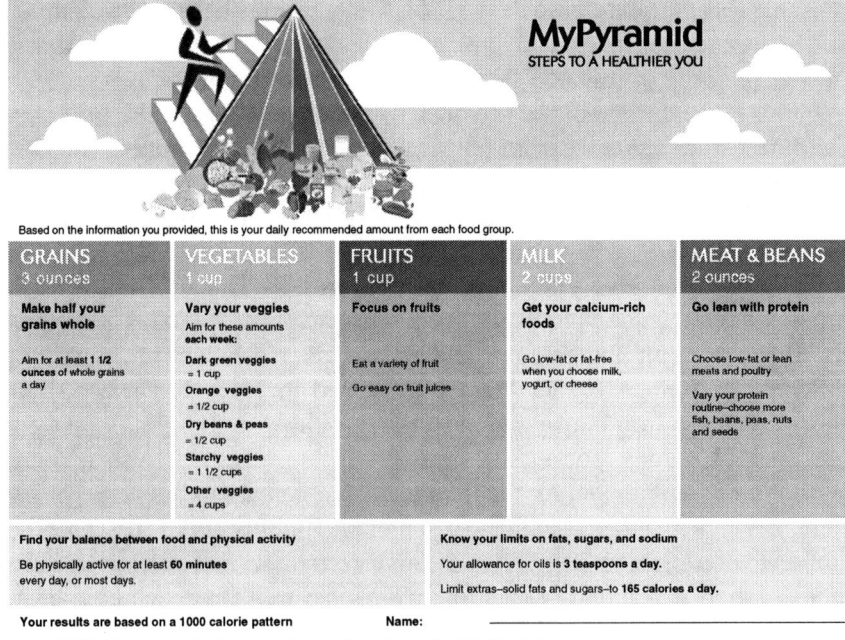

Fig. 1. MyPyramid individual plan for a 2-year-old boy who is physically active for 30–60 min/day *(10)*.

4. HEALTHY EATING BEHAVIORS

As children enter their toddler years, the rate of growth slows and there is a corresponding decrease in appetite. This can be a great source of worry to parents who may become overwhelmed with the task of achieving nutrition recommendations with a toddler who has suddenly become less interested in food.

This decrease in appetite coincides with developmental stages in which asserting independence and establishing self-control are central to the child. Evidence shows that the more pressure parents use to coerce their children to eat or to try new foods, the less likely they are to succeed *(11)*. Likewise, being overly restrictive about certain foods can increase the desirability of those foods. Parental tactics regarding food intake (for example, requiring that a child "clean their plate") can diminish the child's internal cues about hunger and satiety, leading to a decreased capacity for food self-regulation *(12)*.

Ellyn Satter's work on eating competence recommends a division of parental and child responsibility. It is the parent's responsibility to offer a variety of healthy foods at meals and snacks, and the child's responsibility to decide how much they will eat, and even whether they will eat at all. When parents overstep the boundaries of these responsibilities, for example, nagging the child to "eat just one more bite" or offering bribes for finishing their vegetables, the child's sense of independence and self-control is compromised, and struggles arise *(13)*.

The following suggestions may help to encourage children to eat a variety of healthy foods:

- Eat regular mealtimes together as a family as much as possible. Mealtimes should be social and pleasant, not a time for television, arguing, or conducting work.
- Model good food choices, do not expect children to eat a better diet than their parents!
- Discourage "grazing" throughout the day. Rather, offer three meals and two or three snacks each day, giving the child a chance to build up an appetite between eating occasions.
- Snacks should be chosen from the major food groups, i.e., whole grains, fresh fruits and vegetables, low-fat dairy, and lean protein foods.
- Children should be seated and supervised any time that they eat.
- Encourage children to participate in food selection at the grocery store, food preparation, and serving of the meal.
- Serve appropriate portion sizes. A reasonable portion size for children up to 2 years of age is one to two tablespoons of a food. For children up to 4 years, portion sizes are about two-thirds the size of adult portions.

- Be tolerant of infant and toddler-feeding skills. Self-feeding and food exploration allows the child to become familiar with new tastes and textures.
- Serve new foods in small portions, along with familiar foods, at the beginning of the meal when the child is hungry. A new food may need to be offered up to 15 times before it is accepted.
- Never force a child to eat.
- Avoid using foods as rewards, and never withhold food as a punishment.

5. NUTRITION CONCERNS DURING CHILDHOOD

5.1. Childhood Obesity

The prevalence of overweight in children has been rising steadily over the past two decades. According to NHANES data for 2003–2004, 14% of children aged 2–5 and 17.5% of children aged 6–11 are overweight, defined as a BMI for age greater than the 95th percentile *(14)*. Besides the social and emotional problems associated with overweight, these children are also at higher risk for chronic diseases, including hypertension, the beginnings of atherosclerosis, and type 2 diabetes *(1)*.

The causes of overweight are multifactorial, and approaches for prevention and treatment must address not only diet and physical activity, but also psychological support, behavior modification, and caretaker involvement. The goal of treatment is to slow the rate of weight gain and allow growth in height to catch up to weight. In children with severe overweight, moderate weight loss may be advised but should be overseen by a physician and registered dietitian. When calories are restricted, it becomes more difficult to achieve sufficient intake of vitamins and minerals; nutrient-dense foods must therefore be emphasized.

Parents should be encouraged to follow the suggestions outlined above for improving intake of a variety of healthy foods. In addition, three factors have a pronounced impact on overweight in children: physical activity, consumption of sugar-added beverages, and television viewing.

The National Association for Sport and Physical Education recommends that toddlers engage in at least 30 min of structured physical activity per day and at least 60 min of unstructured physical activity. Older children should engage in at least 60 min of structured physical activity per day and at least 60 min of unstructured physical activity. Children of any age should not be sedentary for more than 60 min at a time except when sleeping *(15)*. For children who have difficulty engaging in physical activity because of existing overweight, simply reducing sedentary activities such as television viewing *(see* below) may help *(16)*.

Beverages high in sugar content have been shown to be a significant factor in the development of obesity in children *(5, 6, 16, 17)*. While dairy beverages and fruit juice contribute nutrients to the diet, and should be included in moderate amounts, soda and many fruit drinks offer little or nothing in the way of nutrition and should be offered in child-sized portions on special occasions; they are not appropriate for daily use.

Television viewing (and increasingly Internet use) can contribute to overweight in several ways. Television viewing is a sedentary activity that uses very little energy above basal metabolic rates, and time spent viewing television replaces physical activity in the daily schedules of children. In addition, foods of low nutrient density are promoted during children's programming *(18)*. Lastly, children often snack during television viewing and may consume large portions of the very same foods that they see promoted by television commercials *(16)*. The American Academy of Pediatrics recommends no more than 2 h total screen time for children above the age of 2.

5.2. Food Insecurity

An estimated 17% of all children aged under 17 live in households that are food insecure, that is, households in which there is not access at all times to enough food for active, healthy lives for all family members *(19)*. Characteristics of households more likely to be food insecure include incomes below the poverty level; education of parents less than high school diploma; headed by a single mother; and black, Hispanic descent, or American Indian/Alaska Native descent. Chronic food insecurity can result in poor nutrition, poor academic performance, and behavioral problems. Children from low-income, food-insecure households are at increased risk of iron deficiency anemia (*see* below). Children from food-insecure households should be referred for food assistance programs such as the National School Lunch and Breakfast Programs, Food Stamps, and Special Supplemental Nutrition Program for Women, Infants, and Children (WIC).

5.3. Food Allergies and Sensitivities

True food allergies involve an antibody response to large molecules in the bloodstream; therefore the only way to make a diagnosis is to test for antibodies. The foods that most commonly cause allergies are peanuts, tree nuts, milk, eggs, wheat, soybeans, fish, and shellfish, with peanuts being the most common. Children may outgrow allergies to milk, eggs, and soy. When a true food allergy is present, the only remedy is strict avoidance of the food. Children with food allergies must be taught skills to recognize and refuse foods that they are allergic to and to recognize symptoms of an allergic attack, such as tingling of the mouth and throat. Children who have serious food allergies should carry a supply of epinephrine in case of accidental ingestion of the offending food. If whole food groups, such as dairy, must be eliminated, a dietitian should work with the family to ensure that all nutrient needs are met. *See* Chapter 34 for more about food allergies.

In contrast, children with food sensitivities or intolerances may experience symptoms, including nausea, vomiting, headache, or hives, but without an antibody response. Foods that are commonly implicated in intolerances include monosodium glutamate (MSG) and lactose-containing dairy products.

5.4. Iron Deficiency Anemia

According to the NHANES 1999–2000 data, approximately 5% of children aged 3–5 and 4% of children aged 6–11 have iron deficiency anemia (IDA) *(20)*. Low-income children are at greater risk of IDA *(21)*. Children diagnosed with IDA often lack the energy necessary to sustain their activities of daily living, and their academic performance may also suffer. Strategies to increase iron intake were discussed above. When dietary measures to increase iron intake do not resolve the problem, iron supplements may be necessary.

5.5. Vitamin and Mineral Supplementation

When children consume a carefully selected nutrient-dense diet, vitamin and mineral supplements are not necessary. Some children may benefit from iron supplementation, as noted above. When supplements are given, parents should be cautioned to use supplements specifically formulated for children and to make sure that the doses given do not exceed the tolerable upper intake for the child's age. Care must be taken to keep iron supplements safely out of children's reach, as iron poisoning from supplements is a major cause of poisoning in children. Herbal supplements are not tested for safety in children.

SUGGESTED FURTHER READING

Maternal and Child Health Bureau http://www.mchb.hrsa.gov/.
Center for Disease Control 2000 Growth Charts http://www.cdc.gov/growthcharts/
MyPyramid Food Guidance System http://www.mypyramid.gov
American Association for Physical Activity and Recreation http://www.aahperd.org/naspe
Satter E. Child of Mine. Bull Publishing Company, Boulder, CO, 2000.
Nicklas T, Johnson R. Position of the American Dietetic Association: Dietary guidance for healthy children ages 2–11. JADA 2004; 104:660–677.

REFERENCES

1. Daniels SR. The consequences of childhood overweight and obesity. Future Child 2006; 16:47–67.
2. Corkins MR. Are diet and constipation related in children? Nutr Clin Pract 2005; 20: 536–539.
3. Kranz S, Mitchell DC, Seiga-Riz AM, Smiciklas-Wright H. Dietary fiber intake by American preschoolers is associated with more nutrient-dense diets. J Am Diet Assoc 2005; 105:221–225.
4. Marcason W. What is the "age+5" rule for fiber? J Am Diet Assoc 2005; 105:301–302.
5. Pflugh M. The registered dietitian's role in promoting healthful beverage consumption patterns in young children. J Am Diet Assoc 2007; 107:934–935.
6. Vasanti MS, Schulze MB, Hu FB. Intake of sugar sweetened beverages and weight gain: a systemic review. Am J Clin Nutr 2006; 84:274–278.
7. Wolraich ML, Wilson DB, White JW. The effect of sugar on behavior or cognition in children, a meta-analysis. JAMA 1995; 274:1617–1621.
8. Murphy MM, Douglas JS, Johnson RK, Spence LA. Drinking flavored or plain milk is positively associated with nutrient intake and is not associated with adverse effects on weight status in US children and adolescents. J Am Diet Assoc 2008; 108:631–639.
9. U.S. Department of Health and Human Services and USDA. Dietary Guidelines for Americans, 2005. 6th ed. Government Printing Office, Washington, DC, 2005.
10. USDA. MyPyramidforkids. www.MyPyramid.gov.
11. Wardle J, Carnell S, Cooke L. Parental control over feeding and children's fruit and vegetable intake: how are they related? J Am Diet Assoc 2005; 105:227–232.
12. Fox MK, Devaney B, Reidy K, Razafindrakoto C, Ziegler P. Relationship between portion size and energy intake among infants and toddlers: evidence of self-regulation. J Am Diet Assoc 2006; 106:S77–S83.
13. Satter E. Child of Mine. Bull Publishing Company, Boulder, CO, 2000.
14. National Center for Health Statistics. Health, United States 2007 with Chartbook on trends in the Health of Americans. Hyattsville, MD, 2007.
15. Gunner KB, Atkinson PM, Nichols J, Eissa MA. Health promotion strategies to encourage physical activities in infants, toddlers and preschoolers. J Pediatr Health Care 2005; 19:253–258.
16. Caprio S. Treating child obesity and associated medical conditions. Future Child 2006; 16:209–224.
17. Lindsay AC, Sussner KM, Kim J, Gortmaker S. The role of parents in preventing childhood obesity. Future Child 2006; 16:169–186.
18. Batada A, Seitz MD, Wootan MG, Story M. Nine out of 10 food advertisements shown during Saturday morning children's television programming are for foods high in fat, sodium or added sugars, or low in nutrients. J Am Diet Assoc 2008; 108:673–678.
19. Federal Interagency Forum on Child and Family Statistics. America's Children: Key National Indicators of Well-Being, 2007. Federal Interagency Forum on Child and Family Statistics. US Government Printing Office, Washington, DC, 2007.
20. Center for Disease Control and Prevention. Iron deficiency in the United States, 1999–2000. MMWR 2002; 51:897–899.
21. Skalicky A, Meyers AF, Adams WG, Yang Z, Cook JT, Frank DA. Child food insecurity and iron deficiency anemia in low-income toddlers in the United States. 2006. Matern Child Health J 2006; 10:177–185.

18 Adolescents and Young Adults: Facing the Challenges

Kathy Roberts

Key Points

- Adolescent nutrition is impacted by increased need for energy to support periods of significant growth and development.
- Adolescents are at risk for inadequate intake of specific vitamins and minerals.
- The rate of pediatric overweight and obesity and the risk for other disordered eating patterns are additional challenges present in this population.
- Promoting healthy food habits can have immediate and long-term health implications.

Key Words: Adolescent nutrition; growth; dietary reference intake (DRI); energy needs; nutrition assessment; overweight/obesity; eating disorder; food habits

1. INTRODUCTION

Adolescence, the period of life between 10 and 19 years of age *(1)*, is a time of physical, psychological, and social development as the child transitions into adulthood. Nutritional needs are influenced by increased rate of growth and physical development, sexual maturation, and changing lifestyle that can impact nutrient intake. Promoting healthy food patterns during adolescence is an important consideration as these practices can track into adulthood. Eating patterns established at this time tend also to carry over into adulthood and in part determine a person's risk for overweight, diabetes, cancer, and cardiovascular disease, hence the need to establish what can be called "healthy eating patterns."

From: *Nutrition and Health: Nutrition Guide for Physicians*
Edited by: T. Wilson et al. (eds.), DOI 10.1007/978-1-60327-431-9_18,
© Humana Press, a part of Springer Science+Business Media, LLC 2010

2. GROWTH

Adolescents experience a gain in height and weight at a rate not seen since infancy. During puberty, male and female sex hormones (testosterone and estrogen) promote the periods of accelerated growth (growth spurts) during which 15–25% of final adult height can be gained *(2)*. Because the age of onset of puberty varies considerably, chronological age alone is not useful in assessing growth. Sexual maturation rating, also called Tanner stages, is used to evaluate growth and development based on the degree of development of secondary sexual characteristics, regardless of chronological age. The stages of sexual maturation range from prepubertal (Tanner 1) to adult (Tanner 5) and are based on the development and progression of genitals and pubic hair in boys and of breasts and pubic hair in girls. In general, linear growth in girls starts at an earlier age than boys, with onset typically during stage 2 (ages 9.5–14.5) and peak velocity during stage 3 just prior to menarch (ages 10–16.5) *(3)*. Girls can gain approximately 3.5 inches a year during this growth spurt *(2)*. Peak velocity of growth in boys occurs between stages 3 and 4 *(3)* during which time increase in height can be 2.8–4.8 inches a year *(2)*. Linear growth ends once closure of the epiphyseal plates occurs.

Weight and body composition also change during adolescence and differ between the sexes. Between the ages of 10 and 17 years, girls gain approximately 53 lbs, the equivalent of 42% of adult weight *(4)*. This is accompanied by a change in body composition with lean body mass declining from 80 to 74% of total weight and body fat increasing from 16 to 27% *(2)*. During this same period, boys reach approximately 51% of adult body weight with an average weight gain of 70 lbs *(4)*. Contrary to girls, boys experience an increase in lean body mass from 80 to 90% of total body weight. The difference in rate of growth and accumulation of lean body mass in boys and girls influences nutrient needs. In general, boys will have greater need for energy and the micronutrients needed to support growth.

3. ENERGY AND NUTRIENT REQUIREMENT

Nutritional needs vary depending on velocity of growth, sexual maturation, and degree of physical activity. The dietary reference intakes (DRI) provide a guideline for acceptable macronutrient distribution range (AMDR) and recommended daily allowances (RDA) for micronutrients based on chronological age. Nutrition recommendations should be individualized based on SMR, rate of growth, and estimated energy expenditure.

3.1. Energy

Adequate energy intake is essential to sustain growth and maturation and to support physical activity. The DRI provide equations for calculating estimated energy requirements (EER) based on gender, age, height, weight, and physical activity level, with additional calories added to support growth (Table 1) *(5)*.

Table 1
Calculating Estimated Energy Requirements (EER) of Adolescents

Males	EER = 88.5 – (61.9 × age [year]) + PA × (26.7 × weight [kg] + 903 × height [m]) +25 kcal	Physical activity (PA) coefficient: PA = 1.00 (sedentary) PA = 1.13 (low active) PA = 1.26 (active) PA = 1.42 (very active)
Females	EER = 135.3 – (30.8 × age [year]) + PA × (10.0 × weight [kg] + 934 × height [m]) + 25 kcal	Physical activity (PA) coefficient: PA = 1.00 (sedentary) PA = 1.16 (low active) PA = 1.31 (active) PA = 1.56 (very active)

3.2. Macronutrients

Table 2 shows the Food and Nutrition Board, Institute of Medicine, DRI for acceptable macronutrient distribution range (AMDR). Appropriate distribution of macronutrients within total energy consumed is essential to support overall health and to reduce the risk of developing chronic disease in adulthood *(6)*.

3.3. Micronutrients

The Supplemental Children's Survey to the 1994–1996 Continuing Survey of Food Intakes by Individuals (CSFII 1998) has identified low dietary intakes of some vitamins (A, B_6, C, E, folate) and minerals (calcium, iron, zinc) in 12 to 19-year-olds *(7)*. Inadequate vitamin and mineral intake can have both immediate and long-term impact on the health and development of adolescents *(8, 9)*. Zinc impacts sexual maturation; adequate calcium intake is needed to support skeletal growth and accretion of peak bone mass, decreasing the risk for developing osteoporosis in adulthood. Vitamins A, C, and E are antioxidants that function in inhibiting cellular oxidative damage; inadequate intake during adolescence may increase risk of developing cardiovascular disease and some cancers in adulthood *(9)*. Table 3 provides the

Table 2
Acceptable Macronutrient Distribution Range

	Carbohydrate (g and % total energy)	Fiber (g)	Fat (% total energy)	Protein (g and % total energy)
Males				
9–13 years	130 g/day (45–65%)	31 g/day	25–35%	34 g/day (10–30%)
14–18 years	130 g/day (45–65%)	38 g/day	25–35%	52 g/day (10–30%)
Females				
9–13 years	130 g/day (45–65%)	26 g/day	25–35%	34 g/day (10–30%)
14–18 years	130 g/day (45–65%)	26 g/day	25–35%	46 g/day (10–30%)

Adapted from Dietary Reference Intakes for Energy, Carbohydrate, Fiber, Fatty Acids, Cholesterol, Protein, and Amino Acids (5).

Table 3
DRI (Quantity Per Day) for Vitamins/Minerals at Risk for Inadequate Intake in Adolescents

Vitamin/ Mineral	Males		Females		Function in Adolescence
	9–13 years	14–18 years	9–13 years	14–18 years	
A	600 µg	900 µg	600 µg	700 µg	Growth, bone development, antioxidant
E	11 mg	15 mg	11 mg	15 mg	Antioxidant, tissue maintenance
B$_6$	1.0 mg	1.3 mg	1.0 mg	1.3 mg	Growth, conversion of tryptophan to niacin
Folate	300 µg	400 µg	300 µg	400 µg	Biosynthesis of nucleic acids, maturation of red blood cells
C	45 mg	75 mg	45 mg	65 mg	Enhances absorption of iron, synthesis of collagen
Calcium	1300 mg	1300 mg	1300 mg	1300 mg	Bone growth, bone mass
Iron	8 mg	11 mg	8 mg	15 mg	Oxygen transport, immune function
Zinc	8 mg	11 mg	8 mg	9 mg	Growth, sexual maturation

Adapted from Dietary Reference Intake series, National Academies Press, 2001 (10).

DRI for selected nutrients identified as at risk for inadequate consumption in the adolescent population.

3.4. Nutrition Assessment

Patients should be assessed yearly for indicators of nutritional risk. This should include

- Physical assessment of height, weight, body mass index (BMI).
- Greater than 10% loss of previous weight requires further assessment for possible eating disorder or organic disorder (e.g., celiac, diabetes).
- Blood pressure.
- Assessment of risk behavior: excessive consumption of fat and added sugars, skips meals 3+ times/week, has poor appetite, chronic dieting, bingeing, and purging *(11–13)*.

4. SPECIAL ADOLESCENT NUTRITIONAL CONSIDERATIONS

4.1. Overweight and Obesity

In 2007, the Expert Committee on the Assessment, Prevention, and Treatment of Child and Adolescent Overweight and Obesity recommended the following assessment to determine overweight and obesity in the pediatric population:

- Body mass index (BMI) for age and sex $\geq$85th–94th percentile is overweight.
- BMI for age and sex $\geq$95th percentile is obese.
- BMI for age and sex $\geq$99th percentile is severe obesity.

Treatment for overweight and obesity differs from that in adults in that the treatment plan must accommodate for the nutritional needs to support growth and development. Table 4 provides the recommendations for weight management goals for adolescents aged 12–18 years based on BMI percentiles *(14)*.

Treatment of pediatric overweight is best accomplished with a combination of structured interventions that includes promotion of physical activity, behavioral counseling, and nutrition education for the child and family *(14, 15)*. Based on the level of intervention, this may include referral to an allied health-care provider, such as a registered dietitian (RD) or multidisciplinary team trained in pediatric weight management.

4.2. Eating Disorders

Eating disorders occur most often in adolescents and young adults, especially females. The American Psychiatric Association provides diagnostic

Table 4
Overweight/Obesity Treatment Goals for Adolescents 12–18 years

BMI Percentile	Weight Management Goals	Laboratory Tests
85th–94th	Maintain weight until BMI <85th percentile, or slowing of weight gain demonstrated by downward plotting on curve	No risk factors: fasting lipid profile. Risk factors in history or physical exam:lipids + AST and ALT
95th–98th	Lose weight ($\leq$ 2 lb/week) until BMI $\leq$85th percentile	Fasting lipid profile, AST, ALT, BUN, and creatinine
$\geq$ 99th	Lose weight ($\leq$ 2 lb/week)	Fasting lipid profile, AST, ALT, BUN, and creatinine

criteria for anorexia nervosa, bulimia nervosa, and binge-eating disorder (BED). The topic of eating disorders is also discussed in greater length in Chapter 21.

4.2.1. ANOREXIA NERVOSA

Characterized by eating a severely low amount of energy in order to lose weight; intense fear of weight gain even though underweight; disturbance in body image; amenorrhea in girls and women post-puberty. Health consequences include slow heart rate and low blood pressure, osteoporosis, muscle loss, and severe dehydration that can lead to kidney failure.

4.2.2. BULIMIA NERVOSA

Characterized by regular intake of large amounts of food accompanied by sense of loss of control over behavior; regular use of compensatory measures such as vomiting, laxative use, fasting, and obsessive exercise; extreme concern over body weight and shape. Health consequences include electrolyte imbalance leading to heart arrhythmia, inflammation, and possible rupture of esophagus and/or tooth decay from vomiting.

4.2.3. BINGE-EATING DISORDER

Characterized by frequently consuming large quantities of food in short periods of time with a sense of being out of control over the behavior without the use of compensatory measures and feeling ashamed or disgusted by the behavior. Health risks are usually associated with obesity and include high blood pressure, hyperlipidemia, diabetes, and gallbladder disease.

Diagnosis is based on presenting symptoms such as amenorrhea, GERD, abdominal pain, and palpitations; dietary history that includes discussion of use of laxatives or diuretics; physical exam for weight and BMI and supporting laboratory abnormalities such as hypokalemia, metabolic alkalosis, or elevated salivary amylase. Treatment requires a multidisciplinary team of a physician, registered dietitian (RD), and psychotherapist or social worker and, depending on the severity, may require inpatient treatment.

5. PROMOTING HEALTHY FOOD HABITS

As adolescents transition from child to adulthood, they become more autonomous in their food behavior. Several factors influence food behavior including peer standards, body image, food culture/advertising, constraints of a busy lifestyle that impact time available for meals, and "24/7"availability of high-energy/low nutrient-dense foods.

The 2005 Dietary Guidelines recommends including a variety of nutrient-dense foods and beverages within the basic food groups, while limiting the intake of saturated and trans fats, cholesterol, added sugars, salt, and alcohol. The USDA Food Guide suggests an eating pattern that concentrates on a variety of vegetables, legumes, fruits, whole grains, and low-fat milk and milk products. Results of behavior and food intake surveys indicate that children and adolescents do not follow eating patterns that meet these recommendations, suggesting a need for nutrition intervention and education.

The American Medical Association's Guidelines for Adolescent Preventive Services (GAPS) recommends that "all adolescents should receive health guidance annually about dietary habits, including the benefits of a healthy diet, and ways to achieve a healthy diet and safe weight management" (12). Dietary patterns should be assessed at yearly wellness visits to identify and address risk behavior. Promoting sound nutrition in adolescence can have an immediate effect in supporting growth and development and reducing the risk of obesity and its complications. In addition, it has been suggested that nutrition behaviors can track from adolescence into adulthood so that food choices in adolescence can predict those of adulthood (16).

6. SUMMARY

Adolescence is a period of remarkable physical and psychosocial growth and development that impact nutritional needs. Primary care physicians and allied health professionals can play a critical role in assessing and addressing risk behaviors. Addressing the challenges of adolescent food habits can have immediate and long-term influence on health and wellness.

SUGGESTED FURTHER READING

Appendix: Expert Committee Recommendations on the Assessment, Prevention, and
    Treatment of Childhood and Adolescent Overweight and Obesity. June 6, 2007.
    http://www.ama-assn.org/ama1/pub/upload/mm/433/ped_obesity_recs.pdf.
American Medical Association. Guidelines for Adolescent Preventive Services. American
    Medical Association, Department of Adolescent Health, Chicago, 1997. http://www.ama-
    assn.org/ama/upload/mm/39/gapsmono.pdf.
National Eating Disorders Association. http://www.NationalEatingDisorders.org.

REFERENCES

1. Committee on Nutrition American Academy of Pediatrics. Kleinman RD, ed. Pediatric
    Nutrition Handbook, 4th ed. American Academy of Pediatrics, Elk Grove, IL, 1998.
2. Brown JE. Nutrition through the Lifecycle, 3rd ed. Thomson Wadsworth, Belmont, CA,
    2008.
3. Tanner JM. Growth at Adolescence. Blackwell, Oxford, 1962.
4. Mitchell MK. Nutrition across the Life Span, 2nd ed. Saunders, Philadelphia, PA, 2003.
5. Dietary Reference Intakes for Energy, Carbohydrate, Fiber, Fat, Fatty Acids, Cholesterol,
    Protein, and Amino Acids (Macronutrients). Institute of Medicine, National Academy
    Press, Washington, DC, 2005.
6. Kronsberg SS, Obarzanek E, Affenito SG, et al. Macronutrient intake of black and white
    adolescent girls over 10 years: The NHLBI Growth and Health Study. J Am Diet Assoc
    2003; 103:852–860.
7. USDA, Agricultural Research Service. 1999. Food and Nutrient Intakes by Chil-
    dren 1994–1996, 1998. Available at: http://www.ars.usda.gov/SP2UserFiles/Place/1235
    5000/pdf/scs_all.PDF. Accessed May 24, 2008.
8. Stang J, Taft Bayerl C. Position of the American Dietetic Association: Child and adoles-
    cent food and nutrition program. J Am Diet Assoc 2003; 103:887–893.
9. Stang J, Story M, Harnack L, Neumark-Sztainer D. Relationship between vitamin and
    mineral supplement use, dietary intake, and dietary adequacy among adolescents. J Am
    Diet Assoc 2000; 100:905–910.
10. Dietary Reference Intakes: Applications in Dietary Assessment. Institute of Medicine,
    National Academy Press, Washington, DC, 2002. Available at: http://www.nap.edu/
    catalog.php?record_id=9956. Accessed May 24, 2008.
11. Daniels SR, Greer FR. Committee on Nutrition. Lipid Screening and Cardiovascular
    Health in Childhood. Pediatrics 2008; 122:198–208.
12. American Medical Association. Guidelines for adolescent preventive services. Ameri-
    can Medical Association, Department of Adolescent Health, Chicago, 1997. Available
    online at: http://www.ama-assn.org/ama/upload/mm/39/gapsmono.pdf. Accessed May
    31, 2008.
13. Appendix: Expert Committee Recommendations on the Assessment, Prevention, and
    Treatment of Childhood and Adolescent Overweight and Obesity. June 6, 2007.
    Available at: http://www.ama-assn.org/ama1/pub/upload/mm/433/ped_obesity_recs.pdf.
    Accessed May 31, 2008.
14. Position of the American Dietetic Association: Individual-, Family-, School, and
    Community-Based Interventions for Pediatric Overweight. J Am Diet Assoc 2006;
    106:925–945.

15. National Eating Disorders Association. Available at: http://www.NationalEatingDisorders.org. Accessed May 31, 2008.
16. Lake AA, Mathers JC, Rugg-Gunn AJ, Adamson AJ. Longitudinal change in food habits between adolescence (11–12 years) and adulthood (32–33 years) the ASH30 Study. J Pub Health 2006; 28:10–16.

19 Healthy Aging: Nutrition Concepts for Older Adults

Eleanor D. Schlenker

Key Points

- A lifestyle based on a healthy diet and regular physical activity delays the appearance of age-related changes and slows the development of chronic disease, morbidity, and disability.
- Age-related changes in nutrient requirements follow no general pattern but increase, decrease, or remain unchanged depending on the nutrient; at the same time energy needs continue to decline underscoring the importance of foods high in nutrient density.
- Both inappropriate weight gain and debilitating weight loss increase the risk of chronic disease and disability; loss of muscle leading to frailty and dependence can be prevented or reversed with strength training.
- Nutrient supplements may be needed as energy intake declines but recommendations should take into consideration individual needs, current medications, and food intake to prevent toxicity or dangerous interactions.
- Community nutrition programs providing congregate or home-delivered meals can help older individuals maintain appropriate intakes of important nutrients when loneliness, anorexia, limited resources, or disability make it difficult to obtain or prepare adequate and appropriate food.

Key Words: aging; nutrient requirements; dietary supplements; anorexia of aging; sarcopenia; overweight/obesity; nutritional risk; physiological changes of aging; low body weight

1. INTRODUCTION

By the year 2030, one in five persons in the United States will be aged 65 or over and overall US health-care costs are expected to increase by 25% (1). Our growing diversity is accentuated by an increased prevalence of obesity, hypertension, and diabetes, as well as the desperate need for

From: *Nutrition and Health: Nutrition Guide for Physicians*
Edited by: T. Wilson et al. (eds.), DOI 10.1007/978-1-60327-431-9_19,
© Humana Press, a part of Springer Science+Business Media, LLC 2010

lifestyle intervention in vulnerable race and ethnic groups which make up our graying populations. Optimal nutrition and physical activity represent a golden key to good health in a patient's later years. Appropriate amounts and types of food slow the aging process and improve both short- and long-term outcomes of existing conditions. Optimum nutrient intake in older adults, regardless of age, adds to quality of life and general well-being.

2. PHYSIOLOGIC AGING AND NUTRITION

The aging process leads to changes in physical vigor and strength that may be minor between ages 50 and 60, but become more pronounced at ages 70–80. Age-related changes in body composition, gastrointestinal function, and renal function follow the same progression across the population but occur at different rates such that older persons differ markedly from one another, and these changes influence nutrient needs. Accordingly, this highlights the need for individualizing the nutritional considerations for each patient.

2.1. Body Composition

Loss of lean body mass influences health. Loss of muscle (sarcopenia) and to a lesser extent organ tissue lowers basal metabolism. A sedentary lifestyle accelerates muscle loss and the amount lost is directly related to increased falls and physical disability. Conversely, strength training restores muscle strength in people as old as 98 years, giving renewed ability for self-care *(2)*. Muscle serves as a repository for amino acids to produce immune factors or acute phase proteins or rebuild tissue following a period of stress. Replacing muscle with fat lowers total body water, based on their relative water content (73 vs. 15%). Loss of bone mineral mass contributes to risk of fracture. Increased protein intake (discussed in more detail below) coupled with ongoing physical activity, especially strength training, can help to blunt age-related muscle loss.

2.2. Gastrointestinal Secretions

Gastrointestinal secretions, except for gastric acid, remain adequate to efficiently digest and absorb protein, fat, and carbohydrate. Atrophic gastritis occurs in as many as 30% of people over age 60 but more likely results from *Helicobacter pylori* infestation than normal aging *(3)*. Reduced gastric acid adversely affects the absorption of vitamin B_{12}, folate, iron, and calcium and permits bacterial overgrowth that further lowers availability of vitamin B_{12}.

If fat is poorly absorbed as a result of gallbladder dysfunction, absorption of the fat-soluble vitamins will also decrease.

2.3. Renal System

Loss of nephrons and changes in the renin–angiotensin–aldosterone system lower the ability to conserve water and sodium. Plasma filtration slows and tubular reabsorption and secretion are less efficient. The renal conversion of vitamin D to its active form is reduced, adding to the risk of bone loss. High protein intakes mandate additional fluid to excrete the added nitrogenous waste. Renal changes further heighten the risk of dehydration in elderly patients with reduced thirst and limited fluid intake.

3. NUTRIENT REQUIREMENTS OF THE OLDER ADULT

The aging process coupled with chronic disease and rising use of medications brings uncertainty to the nutrient recommendations for older adults. The dietary reference intakes (DRI) defines two age categories for older adults (51–70 and 71 and over). This is a recognition of the cumulative physiologic and functional changes that occur as a result of the aging process and development of chronic diseases. With advancing age, food intake and energy needs decline while requirements for other nutrients remain the same or even increase, raising further the vulnerability of the patients over 70 years to nutritional deficiency.

3.1. Energy Requirements

Energy intake presents a delicate balance between unwanted weight gain and inappropriate weight loss. Basal calories fall 1–2% per decade over adult life, and for sedentary older adults, basal metabolism may equal 75% or more of total energy expenditure. Energy intake drops by about 800 kcal in women and 1200 kcal in men between the ages of 20 and 80 *(4)*; nonetheless, gradual weight gain can be a problem if activity is low. Estimated energy needs for people aged 60 and over are 2000–2600 kcal for men and 1600–2000 kcal for women, depending on activity level *(5)*, but many fall below 1600 kcal, putting them at risk of nutrient deficiency. At least 130 g of carbohydrate are needed to supply glucose for brain function *(6)*. Fat should provide 20–35% of total calories; the higher level, with emphasis on unsaturated fat, may help prevent weight loss if food intake declines. While some patients may need to be reminded to reduce fat and energy intake, other elderly patients should be reminded that some dietary fat is needed to ensure an adequate supply of essential fatty acids and absorption of fat-soluble vitamins.

3.2. Protein

Dietary protein provides for tissue repair and replacement to counter muscle loss. Studies suggest the current RDA of 0.8 g/kg is not sufficient to prevent muscle loss in older populations and an intake of 1.0 g/kg is more appropriate (7). For those doing strength training, 1.2 g/kg may be beneficial, and because resistance weight training is becoming recognized as increasingly important for the elderly, this higher intake level may well be justified. Two servings (about 6 oz) of good quality protein combined with three servings from the milk group provide about 60 g of protein, easily meeting the RDA. Protein intakes over two times the RDA are best avoided.

3.3. Micronutrients

Mounting evidence indicates that micronutrients play a significant role in aging and the etiology of chronic disease. In this section we discuss selected new aspects and functions of these nutrients.

3.3.1. FAT-SOLUBLE VITAMINS (A, E, D, AND K)

Vitamin A is supplied preformed in animal foods such as milk and butter or as provitamin A in fruits and vegetables. Traditionally associated with vision, vitamin A also supports immune function, giving it a role in both health and aging. Preformed vitamin A (retinol) is highly absorbed and toxicity can occur with high potency supplements and high intakes of fortified foods. Provitamin A (beta-carotene), by contrast, is nontoxic. Excessive vitamin A may accelerate bone mineral loss (6).

Vitamin E helps prevent the oxidation of LDL cholesterol, known to worsen atherosclerosis; however, excessive vitamin E is not beneficial and indeed daily intakes over 400 IU may be harmful (8). Those anticipating surgery need to be warned of the anticlotting action of vitamin E supplements.

Vitamin K-dependent proteins help form bone matrix and facilitate its mineralization. Older adults eating more lettuce, high in vitamin K, have lower risk of hip fracture (9). Patients taking anticoagulants should monitor their intake of vitamin K to avoid neutralizing the action of the drug.

Roles of vitamin D – the "sunshine" vitamin – have expanded to include cancer prevention, insulin action, and muscle metabolism, but over 50% of community-living older adults are reported to be vitamin D-deficient (10). Normally, skin synthesis can meet body needs, although age-related changes in skin cells, use of sunscreen, and limited sun exposure put older adults at risk. Those with darker skin produce vitamin D at about one-sixth the rate of white people. Vitamin D-fortified dairy products, soy products, juices, and cereals supply about 100 IU (2.5 μg) per serving but portions are often inadequate to meet the recommended intakes, creating need for a supplement (see Table 1). Some experts recommend 800 IU per day to prevent bone loss and lower frequency of falls. Such doses pose no risk of toxicity (10). The reader may also wish to consult Chapter 30 on bone health for additional information on vitamin D, especially with regard to the suggestions that larger than previously recommended vitamin D intake levels may be beneficial.

Table 1
Dietary Reference Intakes for Vitamin D and Calcium

Age	Vitamin D	Calcium
30–50	200 IU (5 μg)	1000 mg
51–70	400 IU (10 μg)	1200 mg
Over 70	600 IU (15 μg)	1200 mg

From Ref. (6)

3.3.2. WATER-SOLUBLE VITAMINS

The elderly also have special needs for water-soluble vitamins. Poor vitamin C status comes from low intake rather than increased need. As an antioxidant it may help prevent senile cataract and preserve immune function. Thiamin, riboflavin, and niacin control carbohydrate, fat, and protein metabolism. Requirements do not change with age; still, thiamin deficiency is not uncommon in frail elderly with low food intake. Alcohol interferes with thiamin absorption and long-term use of diuretics can result in thiamin depletion. Milk and cereals are major sources of riboflavin and intake is low if these foods are not consumed regularly. Increased physical activity raises the need for riboflavin. Protein intakes are generally adequate among older adults, supplying niacin and tryptophan for niacin synthesis if needed.

Vitamin B_6 requirements increase after age 50 and inadequate intake adversely affects immune function and synthesis of neurotransmitters. Vitamin B_6 acts with folate and vitamin B_{12} to modulate plasma homocysteine. Megadoses of B_6 (2000-fold the RDA) impair muscle coordination and neural damage is permanent if prolonged.

Current folate (folic acid) fortification policies have implications for older adults. Folate added to grain foods is better absorbed than naturally occurring folate in plant foods (85 vs. 50%) which requires acid for best absorption. High folate, however, compensates for a lack of vitamin B_{12}. As a result it delays the appearance and diagnosis of pernicious anemia and B_{12} deficiency as neural damage continues *(4)*.

Vitamin B_{12} status is precarious for those with low stomach acid, as acid is needed to release B_{12} from animal food proteins and make it available for absorption. Vitamin B_{12} added to fortified foods, such as juice or cereal, does not require acid for absorption. It is suggested, therefore, that fortified foods be included in the diet two to three times a week. Older adults are especially vulnerable to the harmful effects of B_{12} deficiency based on its insidious effect on cognitive function.

3.4. Minerals

Calcium remains a problem nutrient for older adults, with average intakes well below what is recommended. Dairy foods and calcium-fortified juices, cereals, and soy milk supply 300 mg per serving. Fortified foods supplying both calcium and vitamin D are good choices. However, supplements may still be needed to reach optimum intake (Table 1). Older adults should avoid aluminum-containing antacids that bind with phosphorus, leading to phosphate depletion and adult rickets (osteomalacia). The DASH (Dietary Approaches to Stop Hypertension) study reported that calcium may help to control blood pressure *(11)*, yet another reason to meet calcium recommendations.

Based on the effect of potassium in controlling blood pressure, the RDA was set at 4700 mg; however, low food intake, limited resources, or chewing problems can make it difficult to include five to nine servings of fruits and vegetables recommended to reach this goal. Unless kidney function is severely compromised, added consumption of potassium in the form of food does not add to risk.

Many older adults consume well over the recommended upper limit of 2300 mg/day sodium. About 77% of sodium intake comes from processed foods, including fast foods; about 11% is added in home preparation or at the table; and only 12% is naturally occurring *(6)*. Those unable to shop for fresh ingredients or prepare meals from scratch depend on canned or frozen items that are often high in sodium. Products with no-added salt often cost more, putting them out of reach for those with limited resources. Salt substitutes often exchange sodium for potassium.

Magnesium has an important role in forming bone mineral crystals. Dairy products are a major source and persons avoiding those foods can have a low intake. Poor magnesium status has been associated with renal wasting related to diuretic therapy. Hypermagnesemia is a threat for those abusing magnesium-containing antacids or cathartics.

Iron needs are minimal in the older adult but risk of deficiency may be increased by poor absorption, chronic use of aspirin, or pathological conditions resulting in blood loss through the gastrointestinal tract. Once iron is absorbed, it is poorly excreted, so iron overload is a danger with high potency supplements. Highly fortified cereals containing 18 mg of iron per serving pose a risk when multiple servings are eaten frequently. Alcohol enhances iron absorption and alcohol users have higher iron stores.

Zinc deficiency is related to loss of taste and impaired wound healing which are sometimes reported in older people. Normal function is dependent on an adequate supply of zinc and zinc deficiency may contribute, but age-related changes or other nutrient deficiencies may also play a part.

3.5. Fluid Homeostasis

Changes in hormonal secretion and receptor sensitivity coupled with cardiovascular disease and related medications can upset a delicate fluid balance, thereby increasing the risk of dehydration or excessive fluid retention. Decreases in total body water, reduced ability of the kidneys to conserve fluid, and changes in the "thirst center" of the hypothalamus that lowers voluntary fluid intake increase risk of dehydration. Various medications interfere with thirst and incontinent elderly may self-limit fluid intake. Dehydration can result in drug toxicity and heat stroke in uncontrolled environments. Conversely, inappropriate secretion of vasopressin can lead to water intoxication or hyponatremia. Current recommendations call for 9 cups of fluid, including water, for women and 13 cups for men with the caveat that thirst should drive fluid intake (6). The debilitated older adult following the mandate to "drink eight cups of water a day," in addition to other fluids such as milk, tea, or soup, is at risk of fluid imbalance.

3.6. Special Benefits of Plant Foods

The dietary fiber found in whole grains, fruit, and vegetables helps lower blood cholesterol, prevents constipation, and improves intestinal health. Older adults with diets low in fiber should be encouraged to *gradually* increase their fiber along with additional fluid. Phytochemicals (plant chemicals), such as lycopene, carotenoids, and polyphenols, act as antioxidants and offer some protection against a variety of chronic diseases. Phytochemicals must be consumed as food not supplements in order to provide benefit, suggesting that they interact with other unidentified substances also found in food.

3.7. Dietary Supplements

Individual needs and circumstances govern the selection and use of dietary supplements. When energy intake falls below 1600 kcal, it is unlikely that all vitamin and mineral requirements will be met from food alone.

In that situation a multivitamin–mineral supplement, with a composition approximating the DRI, is helpful *(12)*. Supplements containing more than 100% of the DRI are best avoided to prevent adverse interactions among nutrients or total intakes that exceed the tolerable upper intake levels. Older adults with good diets may still need supplemental calcium and vitamins B_{12} and D. Vitamin B_{12} can be provided in fortified foods or a multivitamin supplement. Calcium supplements with added vitamin D are readily available. Iron and folate supplements require medical supervision. To the extent possible, food is the preferred way to supply nutrients: a poor diet with added vitamins and minerals is still a poor diet. Older adults are vulnerable to advertisements promoting dubious supplements, such as herbs and botanicals, and need to be made aware of potential benefits or dangerous interactions with medications. The problem of dishonest marketing of supplements is discussed by Temple in Chapter 13.

4. BODY WEIGHT IN THE OLDER ADULT

Body weight management poses particular problems for older people. Involuntary weight loss and decreasing muscle mass lower functional capacity whereas ill-advised weight gain aggravates any existing disability and worsens chronic disease. Changes in food intake regulation prevent appropriate responses to short-term changes in food intake that would bring about a return to the former weight *(13)*. Consequently, weight lost during serious illness or emotional distress is unlikely to be regained.

4.1. Low Body Weight

The anorexia of aging leading to unwanted weight loss and frailty is complex in nature. Age-related changes in the hypothalamus (which controls the feeding drive), reduced stomach elasticity, and delayed gastric emptying lead to early satiety. Many commonly prescribed medications influence appetite and reduce food intake (Table 2). Cachexia arising from chronic inflammation and the subsequent release of cytokines can be resistant to even aggressive nutritional intervention. Involuntary loss of 10 lb within a 6-month period or a body mass index (BMI) below 22 is cause for intervention in the older adult *(14)*.

4.2. Overweight/Obesity

The effect of moderate overweight on mortality beyond age 65 remains unclear. Studies reveal a J-shaped curve with higher mortality at the extremes of underweight and overweight *(15)*. Mortality was lowest and disability-free life expectancy highest among older white, African-

Table 2
Examples of Medications Influencing Food Intake

Loss of appetite	Digoxin
	Diuretics
	Levodopa
	Methotrexate
Loss of taste or bad taste	ACE inhibitors
	Digoxin
	Levodopa
	Methocarbamol
	Propranolol
	Quinidine
Dry mouth	Antianxiety agents
	Anticholinergics
	Antihypertensive agents
	Antiinflammatory agents
	Bronchodilators
	Congestive heart failure medications
	Diuretics
Difficulty with swallowing	Alendronate
	Anticholinergics
	NSAIDs
	Quinidine

American, and Mexican-American adults with a BMI of 25–29 (representing moderate overweight), although a BMI above 34 was associated with higher mortality or disability *(16)*. Weight-loss interventions should balance the possible functional benefits with the need for appropriate intakes of essential nutrients. Chair exercises, strength training, and walking programs increase energy expenditure and contribute to gradual weight loss, or even more importantly, help prevent unwanted weight gain. Rapid weight loss in the elderly may reflect an occult medical problem rather than a successful weight-loss regimen *(14)*.

4.3. Factors Influencing Food Intake in Older Adults

4.3.1. SOCIOECONOMIC FACTORS

Changes in social relationships influence food intake as we age. Eating alone can be a new and difficult adjustment for a widow(er). Loss of close friends or nearby family, changes in the neighborhood, or fear about the future take away interest in eating. Financial losses and rising prices present difficult choices when a fixed income must be stretched to cover food, home heating and air conditioning, and medications. Although only 10% of those above age 60 have incomes below the poverty line, food choices can still be dictated more by money available than need for nutrients. Many older adults are eligible for the Supplemental Nutrition Assistance Program (formerly referred to as the food stamp program) which extends food dollars, but relatively few apply.

4.3.2. HEALTH FACTORS

Poor health and chronic disease affect food intake in various ways. Physical infirmity makes food shopping challenging, and if available transportation or food delivery is infrequent, access to fresh fruits, vegetables, or milk is curtailed. Severe arthritis makes food preparation difficult and interferes with opening packages of pre-prepared foods. Highly restrictive diets to manage chronic conditions can be counterproductive if comfort foods or cultural favorites are discouraged. Familiar diets with attention to portion control may have more success. Chewing is often painful for edentulous elderly with ill-fitting or no dentures, or with periodontal disease; left untreated this can lead to systemic infection.

Multiple medications and medical treatments can exacerbate age-related changes to make eating less enjoyable. Loss of taste and smell or distorted taste related to normal aging, radiation therapy, or common medications lower food intake (Table 2). Bitter medications delivered to the taste receptors via the blood result in unpleasant tastes in the saliva and affect appetite. The interaction of nutrition and drugs is discussed more completely in Chapter 35, while Chapter 14 looks at the interactions of taste and food intake.

Dry mouth and the more serious condition, xerostomia, make eating and swallowing difficult. Loss of saliva to lubricate the oral tissues enables rapid bacterial growth with ulceration if left unchecked. Dysphagia and fear of choking influence both the amount and types of food that can be handled comfortably. Swallowing can be particularly troublesome for those with neurological impairment as may occur in Parkinson's disease, diabetes, or following radiation treatment; a speech pathologist may be helpful in those cases.

4.3.3. EVALUATING NUTRITIONAL RISK

Community programs that provide congregate meals in a social environment or deliver meals to the homebound provide nutritional support and promote independent living. Most are subsidized with local and federal funds and are accessible to elderly people with limited resources. Various individ-

Table 3
Identifying Risk Factors for Inadequate Food Intake

Do you sometimes have problems obtaining the food you need?

(could relate to problems with shopping or lack of money to buy food)

Do you have any problems that make it difficult to eat?

(may involve chewing, loss of taste, problems with swallowing)

Do you eat at least two meals every day?

(amount of food eaten)

Have you gained or lost 10 pounds over the last 6 months?

(involuntary weight loss or unwanted weight gain)

Adapted from Nutrition Screening Initiative. *DETERMINE Your Health Check List.* A project of the American Academy of Family Physicians, the American Dietetic Association, and the National Council on the Aging and funded in part by Ross Products Division of Abbott Laboratories, Inc. Available from www.eatright.org. Accessed April 17, 2008.

ual circumstances can assist health professionals in identifying older adults at risk of poor nutrition who could benefit from such programs (Table 3). Contact information for local nutrition programs can be found on web sites or telephone listings of county or state departments for the aging.

5. HEALTH PROMOTION FOR THE OLDER ADULT

Positive changes in the quality or amount of food consumed are never without benefit, regardless of age or physical status. Increased intakes of fruits, vegetables, whole grains, and good sources of calcium and protein add important nutrients and phytochemicals for resisting chronic disease and enhancing immune response. Regular physical activity to the extent possible, including walking and strength training, helps maintain bone and muscle mass and extend independence. Small changes add up to make a significant difference in the well-being of the aging adult.

SUGGESTED FURTHER READING

Centers for Disease Control and Prevention and the Merck Company Foundation. The State of Aging and Health in America 2007. Merck Company Foundation, Whitehouse Station, NJ, 2007. Available from   www.cdc.gov/aging

Evans WJ. Protein nutrition, exercise and aging. J Am Coll Nutr 2004; 23(suppl):601S–609S.

Holick MF. Vitamin D deficiency. N Engl J Med 2007; 357:266–281.

Lichtenstein AH, Russell RM. Essential nutrients: Food or supplements? JAMA 2005; 294:351–358.

Thomas DR. Loss of skeletal muscle mass in aging: Examining the relationship of starvation, sarcopenia and cachexia. Clin Nutr 2007; 26:389–399.

REFERENCES

1. Centers for Disease Control and Prevention and the Merck Company Foundation. The State of Aging and Health in America 2007. The Merck Company Foundation, Whitehouse Station, NJ, 2007. Available from www.cdc.gov/aging . Accessed April 17, 2008.
2. Fiatarone MA, O'Neill EF, Ryan ND, et al. Exercise training and nutritional supplementation for physical frailty in very elderly people. N Engl J Med 1994; 330:1769–1775.
3. Russell RM. Factors in aging that effect the bioavailability of nutrients. J Nutr 2001; 131(suppl): 1359S–1361S.
4. Lichtenstein AH, Rasmussen H, Yu WW, et al. Modified MyPyramid for older adults. J Nutr 2008; 138:5–11.
5. United States Department of Agriculture. MyPyramid Food Intake Pattern Calorie Levels. Center for Nutrition Policy and Promotion, Washington, DC, April 2005. Available from www.MyPyramid.gov . Accessed April 17, 2008.
6. Institute of Medicine. Dietary reference intakes. The Essential Guide to Nutrient Requirements. National Academies Press, Washington, DC, 2006.
7. Campbell WW, Carnell NS, Thalacker AE. Protein metabolism and requirements. In: Chernoff R, ed. Geriatric Nutrition: The Health Professional's Handbook, 3rd ed. Jones & Bartlett, Sudbury, MA, 2006, pp. 15–22.
8. Miller ER III, Pastor-Barriuso R, Dalal D, et al. Meta-analysis: high-dosage vitamin E supplementation may increase all-cause mortality. Ann Intern Med 2005; 142:37–46.
9. Feskanich D, Weber P, Willett WC, et al. Vitamin K intake and hip fractures in women: A prospective study. Am J Clin Nutr 1999; 69:74–79.
10. Holick MF. Vitamin D deficiency. N Engl J Med 2007; 357:266–281.
11. Champagne CM. Dietary interventions on blood pressure. The Dietary Approaches to Stop Hypertension (DASH) trials. Nutr Rev 2006; 64(part 2): S53–56.
12. American Dietetic Association. Position of the American Dietetic Association: Fortification and nutritional supplements. J Am Diet Assoc 2005; 105:1300–1311.
13. Roberts SB. A review of age-related changes in energy regulation and suggested mechanisms. Mech Ageing Dev 2000; 116:157–167.
14. Thomas DR. Loss of skeletal muscle mass in aging: Examining the relationship of starvation, sarcopenia and cachexia. Clin Nutr 2007; 26:389–399.
15. Adams KF, Schatzkin A, Harris TB, et al. Overweight, obesity, and mortality in a large prospective cohort of persons 50–71 years old. N Engl J Med 2006; 355:763–778.
16. Al Snih S, Ottenbacher KJ, Markides KS, et al. The effect of obesity on disability vs. mortality in older Americans. Arch Intern Med 2007; 167:774–780.

20 Nutritional Status: An Overview of Methods for Assessment

Catherine M. Champagne and George A. Bray

Key Points

- Obesity is increasing and needs assessment.
- Dietary intake and consumption patterns are a very challenging area to evaluate accurately.
- Body mass index (BMI), body composition, and routine laboratory testing add to the information obtained from dietary history.
- Poor diets are observed at various ages, particularly in adolescents and the elderly, often for very different reasons due to the aging process.

Key Words: Nutrition assessment; obesity; body mass index; dietary intake

1. INTRODUCTION

This chapter focuses on the whole area of nutritional assessment and may involve a wide spectrum of testing to determine the health of an individual. This process typically entails in-depth evaluation of both subjective data and objective evaluations of an individual's food and associated nutrient intake, components of lifestyle, and medical history. It is essentially an overview of nutritional status focusing on nutrient intake analysis of diet, blood tests, and physical examination.

These data are organized so that the physician can conduct the most precise estimate of that person's nutritional status. With this information, decisions can be made as to an appropriate plan of action to either maintain

From: *Nutrition and Health: Nutrition Guide for Physicians*
Edited by: T. Wilson et al. (eds.), DOI 10.1007/978-1-60327-431-9_20,
© Humana Press, a part of Springer Science+Business Media, LLC 2010

current health or referral to counseling or other interventions that would enable the individual to reach a more healthy state. Only with sufficient anthropometric, biochemical, clinical, and dietary information can an appropriate plan be prepared.

Many years ago, one of the main objectives of assessing nutritional status was to improve nutritional status of malnourished individuals suffering from protein and micronutrient deficiencies, in addition to caloric deficiencies. Now the tables have somewhat turned to the overweight and obese individuals who may also suffer micronutrient deficiencies based on the poor nutrient content of what many perceive as a high-calorie diet.

The worldwide epidemic of obesity increases health concerns for both men and women. The body mass index (BMI), which is defined as weight in kilograms divided by height in meters squared (kg/m^2), is the current criterion for assessing overweight and obesity. Overweight is commonly defined as a BMI greater than or equal to 25, and obesity is defined as a BMI greater than or equal to 30. Use of the waist circumference to gauge the degree of central adiposity is also recommended.

More than 30% of adult Americans are now obese, and the prevalence of obesity is higher in women than in men (33.4% vs. 27.5%). The prevalence of obesity in children and adults has increased more than 50% in the past decade. This epidemic also has led to concerns regarding the widespread development of diabetes, heart disease, and complications associated with these disorders. A recent report estimates that obesity causes more than 100,000 deaths each year in the United States *(1)*.

2. PRINCIPLES OF NUTRITIONAL ASSESSMENT

There are a number of instruments and questionnaires that can help to identify potential areas of concern regarding caloric intake and perhaps a lack of essential nutrients for health.

2.1. Food Frequency Questionnaires

Currently there are very extensive validated diet history questionnaires available from the National Cancer Institute, but they are long and burdensome. Shorter dietary questionnaires focused on targeted intakes (fruits, vegetables, dietary fats) are less burdensome. The food frequency questionnaire – often referred to simply as FFQ – is one means of establishing what usual intakes are and, depending on the care taken by the patient in filling out this information and how carefully it is reviewed with the person, can provide valuable insight into his or her usual diet.

2.2. Diet and Lifestyle History

An example of a basic nutrition and lifestyle history is included in Box 1. Sample questions can be used depending on the information desired. The first couple of questions solicit information about the previous day's food intake. Other questions devoted to specific foods, lifestyle, and behaviors can be helpful in providing information that may be predictive of successful weight management and disease risk. Most likely this involves more time than the physician has available.

Box 1 Sample Questions for Basic Nutrition and Lifestyle History

I would like to know everything you ate and drank yesterday.

When did you first have something to eat or drink, and what did you have? _____

When was the next time you ate or drank something? _____

(continue)

Do you avoid any foods for any reason (religious, cultural, likes/dislikes, food sensitivity, or allergy)?

Yes __ No ___ Which ones? _____

How often do you eat away from home? _____

Do you drink alcoholic beverages? Yes ___ No ___ How often? _____

How much? _____

Do you take any vitamin, mineral, or other supplements? Yes _____ No _____

What kind? _____ How much? _____

Do you exercise? Yes ___ No ___ What kind? _____ How often? _____

Do you smoke cigarettes? Yes _____ No ____

Has your weight changed in the past 5 years? Yes ___ No ___ How? _____ Why? _____

Are you trying to lose (or gain) weight? Yes ___ No ___ How? _____ Why? _____

Are you on a special diet? Yes ____ No ____ What kind? _____ Why? _____

Do you have problems with planning and preparing meals for yourself or your family?

2.3. Assessing Current Dietary Intake

Several options exist for collecting current dietary intake and eating patterns. The 24-h recall is a simple method that can be very helpful in focusing on real foods consumed. If the food consumption was representative of usual intake, the method can be especially valuable. Currently, the methodology promoted in this type of research is known as a multiple pass method *(2)*. Using this procedure, one obtains a quick listing of foods from the individual, probes for foods commonly forgotten (condiments, common foods added to other foods, etc.), and collects the time and information about the eating occasion, which may further prompt the individual's memory. A more detailed cycle follows and the description, portion size, and additions to foods are collected; omitted food probes are used for foods eaten between main meals (e.g., snacks). The final step in the process is a question that asks whether anything else has come to the individual's memory, even in very small amounts.

The 24-h recall may be helpful in targeting behaviors with a link to possible disease risk. Where weight control is of concern, information on intakes of fat, sugar, and unhealthy food options (fast-food restaurants and foods high in sugars or high-fructose corn syrup [HFCS]) may enable the physician to counsel the patient more effectively. This recall is most efficiently collected by a registered dietitian.

A helpful, although perhaps less attractive, option might be to have the patient keep a record or diary of foods consumed over a specified period of time. If the physician opts to do this, it would mean an additional return visit with the patient in a week or two following the initial visit. Another option would be to have the patient keep a longer record and return it to the physician's office without the additional visit. In this way, the dietitian can review it at a more convenient time and then discuss the information collected with the physician. One of the problems with this might be that the patient does not record accurately what foods are consumed or may choose to modify intakes with the realization that the dietitian and/or physician will review their diary.

2.4. Underreporting of Dietary Intake

Since the issue of self-reporting of dietary intake has been discussed, it is important to realize that the underreporting of actual food eaten is one of the major problems facing dietetic professionals *(3)*. Misreporting of energy intake has been routinely observed in surveys of the US population *(4)*, among overweight/obese individuals *(5)*, in elderly low socioeconomic status populations *(6)*, and even in developing nations *(7)*. Consequently, it is essential to keep in mind that the occurrence of underreporting is to be expected.

2.5. Physical Examination

As part of measuring the patient's vital signs, the physician needs to determine height and weight along with waist circumference. The measurement of height and weight is necessary for calculation of BMI (Table 1). For details on the exact meaning of the BMI the physician can refer to the guidelines of the National Heart, Lung, and Blood Institute and the North American Association for the Study of Obesity. The BMI has a curvilinear relation to the risks related to excess weight and provides one of the "vital signs" needed to assess any patient. A BMI between 18.5 and 25 is considered normal for most Americans, although for Asian populations a normal BMI is considered to be less than 23. The BMI is divided into 5-unit intervals that are used to define overweight and various levels of obesity (Table 1).

The BMI must be interpreted in an ethnically sensitive context because the amount of body fat for a given BMI differs among ethnic groups. For Japanese Americans and other Asians, a BMI greater than 23 has the same association with disease as a BMI greater than 25 for Caucasians. For African Americans and probably for Hispanics and descendants of Polynesians, a BMI of 27 is probably equivalent to a BMI of 25 in Caucasians. Once the BMI has been determined, assessment should include central fat distribution measured as waist circumference. The rate of weight gain (greater than 1 kg [2.2 lb]/year is high) and level of physical activity are additional criteria for determining the risk from a given BMI.

Table 1
BMI Classification of Obesity and the Impact of Waist Circumference on Overall Risk

| | | | Overall Risk Waist Circumference | |
| | | *Obesity* | | |
	BMI	*Class*	*Low*	*High*
Overweight	25.0 – 29.9		Increased	High
Obesity	30.0 – 34.9	I	High	Very high
Obesity	35.0 – 39.9	II	Very high	Very high
Extreme obesity	≥40	III	Extremely high	Extremely high

High waist circumference: Men > 40 in. Women >35 in.
National Institutes of Health. *Obes Res* 1998; 6(suppl 2):51S–209S.

Fat located in the abdominal and visceral fat depots carries a higher risk for diseases associated with obesity than does extra fat on the hips and thighs. The challenge for clinicians is to estimate fat distribution with reasonable accuracy while also doing this quickly and cheaply. Several studies have suggested that waist circumference provides a reasonable surrogate for the more precise measurements provided by computed tomography or magnetic resonance imaging. A waist circumference greater than 88 cm (35 in.) in women or 102 cm (40 in.) in men signifies a high risk. A very large international trial, the International Day for the Evaluation of Abdominal Obesity (IDEA) study, has shown that waist circumference is a stronger predictor of cardiovascular disease (CVD) outcomes than BMI. First results of this large international study in over 170,000 people indicate that waist circumference is associated with CVD, independently of the relationship that BMI has with CVD risk, and regardless of age or geography *(8)*.

A steady weight gain exceeding 1.0 kg (2.2 lb) per year over a number of years and a sedentary lifestyle are additional clues to a future risk of heart disease, diabetes, or hypertension. Measuring body fat can be valuable in some populations, such as athletes, who may be overweight but not overfat.

2.6. Body Composition Analyses

Dual X-ray absorptiometry (DXA) has replaced underwater weighing as the gold standard for determining body fat and lean body mass. DXA's advantages are that it is safe, easy to use, and very accurate with the use of appropriate standards. The disadvantages are the generally high cost and the need for regular cross-standardization of the instrument, as well as the weight limits of the table (e.g., for assessment of very obese people) *(9)*.

Bioelectric impedance analysis (BIA) has also been used to determine body composition and, with proper training and careful placement of electrodes, very reproducible measurements can be obtained. Compared to DXA, BIA is relatively low cost, easy to use, and measures body water, which is then used to estimate body fat *(9)*.

In children, Lazzer and colleagues *(10)* found that DXA and BIA were not interchangeable for the assessment of percent fat mass in severely obese children and adolescents; they offered a new predictive equation for estimation of body composition for use in such subjects. Researchers at the Children's Nutrition Research Center in Houston *(11)* have claimed that DXA has not achieved the reliability in children to be considered the "gold standard" for body composition assessment in pediatric studies. Nichols and colleagues *(12)* concluded that the relatively low cost and minimal time required for training make the BIA a useful and appropriate technique for the assessment of body composition in adolescent girls.

Völgyi and colleagues *(13)* found that BIA methods systematically produced lower values for fat mass than did DXA, further suggesting that the difference depends on gender and body weight, which should be important considerations when identifying people with excess fat mass. DXA was found to be a reliable tool in assessing skeletal muscle mass in older women *(14)*. Others have suggested that BIA underestimates total and truncal fatness compared to DXA and, furthermore, that the discrepancies increase with degree of adiposity, an indication that accurate BIA measures are negatively affected by level of obesity *(15)*.

Waist circumference is a measurement that is relatively easy to determine using a tape measure and locating the important strategic points to take the reading. Since waist circumferences of >102 cm (>40 in.) for men and of >88 cm (>35 in.) for women are the defining levels of risk factors for diagnosis of the metabolic syndrome, this is valuable to collect on a routine office visit with a physician *(9)*.

2.7. *Laboratory Tests*

Routine blood testing is necessary for the evaluation of nutrient status. Anemia is one of the most frequently detected abnormalities in women of postmenopausal age. Protein status based on a low albumin can also be assessed in both sexes. Routine laboratory testing should include lipid profiles to enable the physician to diagnose the potential risk for CVD among both male and female patients. Laboratory examinations also are important to assess whether the patient has the metabolic syndrome. These laboratory examinations should include measurements of fasting plasma glucose, triglyceride, and HDL-C levels.

3. SPECIAL CONCERNS BY AGE

3.1. *Obesity and Age*

Individuals can become overweight at any age, but obesity is more common at certain ages. Several surveys have suggested that 75–80% of individuals will become overweight at some time in their life. Between 20 and 25% of individuals will become overweight before age 20 years, and 50% will do so after age 20. One-third of overweight adults became overweight before age 20.

Therefore, individuals can be divided into four subgroups. The first group includes individuals who will never become overweight, although this group can be identified only in retrospect. The second group includes pre-overweight or pre-obese individuals who have a BMI of less than

25. The third group includes "pre-clinically overweight" individuals, who become overweight without clinically significant problems. As these individuals age or gain weight, they may show clinical signs of diabetes and develop complications such as hypertension, gallbladder disease, dyslipidemia, or the metabolic syndrome. This is the fourth group of individuals; they are considered "clinically overweight."

3.2. Adolescents

Obesity is becoming a significant health problem among adolescents. In 2004, 17% of US adolescents aged 12–19 years were overweight (16), triple the prevalence of two decades earlier. The prevalence of type 2 diabetes, previously considered an adult disease, has increased substantially in children and adolescents.

Weight in adolescence becomes a progressively better predictor of weight in adulthood. Adolescents who are above the 95th percentile for weight have a 5- to 20-fold greater risk for overweight in adulthood than other adolescents. During adolescence, parental overweight is a less important predictor than it is for children at younger ages, or it has already had its effect. Although 70–80% of overweight adolescents with an overweight parent will be overweight as young adults, the numbers are only modestly lower (54–60%) for overweight adolescents without overweight parents. Despite the importance of childhood and adolescent weight status, most overweight adults develop the condition only after they become adults.

Adolescence is a unique period in life during which there is intensive physical, psychosocial, and cognitive development. Nutritional needs are greatest during this period, when adolescents gain up to 50% of their adult weight, more than 20% of their adult height, and 50% of their adult skeletal mass. Many establish lifelong eating habits during this period. Although young people from low socioeconomic backgrounds are at greatest risk for poor dietary patterns, many adolescents rely on high-fat, high-fructose (sugar or HFCS) foods for much of their intake or skip meals, as many women do, as a method of weight control. The diets of adolescents often lack adequate fruits and vegetables and sufficient amounts of vitamins A and C, folate, calcium, iron, and fiber.

Because most bone deposition occurs during adolescence, adequate calcium and vitamin D intake is important. Many teenagers do not consume the daily requirement of 1,300 mg of calcium. It is important to recognize that adolescents who drink more soft drinks consume less milk and thus get less calcium. Dairy products, calcium-enriched orange juice, and calcium supplements can help to overcome this problem. Iron deficiency as a result of growth, menses, and poor diet is also common in adolescent girls. For more details regarding nutrition and adolescence, *see* Chapter 18 by Roberts.

3.3. Elderly

Elderly individuals often have poor dietary intakes; major causes include inadequate finances, ill-fitting dental appliances, or the inability or lack of desire to prepare healthful foods and a loss of sense of smell, which makes food seem tasteless. Older people often find that their tastes have changed, and sweet, easy-to-eat foods rich in refined carbohydrates (breads, cereals, sweet rolls) are favored over more healthful items.

The elderly often lack vitamins A and C, folate, and potassium because of inadequate intake of fruits and vegetables. Vitamin B_{12} status may be poor because of inadequate consumption of protein-rich foods and because of declining vitamin B_{12} absorption, which occurs with aging. Calcium may be inadequate because of low intake of dairy foods and leafy green vegetables or because of lactose intolerance. Many elderly people spend a considerable amount of time indoors, and vitamin D synthesis and activation decrease with age, often resulting in inadequate vitamin D. This depends on geography, with those living in northern locales at greater risk. Although clinical zinc deficiencies are uncommon, older individuals often have marginal zinc levels because of low intake of protein-rich foods. *See* also Chapter 19 on aging by Schlenker.

Reduced physical activity and a decrease in metabolic rate with aging require that older patients often choose foods with high nutrient density and low energy density. If the caloric intake for an elderly patient is less than 1,600 kcal/day, the patient is at risk of inadequate intake of vitamins and minerals. A multiple vitamin and mineral supplement can provide nutritional insurance to older patients, especially if there are concerns about appropriate meal planning and/or problems consuming certain types of foods.

Walking and weight training can improve an older person's balance and endurance and should be encouraged. A full exercise regimen allows older individuals to feel more independent and lessens the likelihood of falls and injuries. Exercise also has a positive effect on mental attitude and helps control weight and maintain bone health.

3.4. Food Access and/or Food Security

As mentioned briefly, an energy-dense diet does not necessarily equate to a nutrient-dense diet. However, energy-dense, nutrient-poor foods are the cheapest sources of calories. As a result of this, findings from both

America and France have indicated that economic factors may be pressuring poor people to select an unhealthy diet. However, other factors may also be at work. Taste and convenience of added sugar and fats may be more appealing and further influence the consumer into selecting less healthy foods *(17, 18)*.

Another factor that pressures poorer people to eat an unhealthy diet is that for millions of Americans there is limited availability locally of healthy foods (i.e., with a low energy density and a high nutrient density). Poorer people are often faced with barriers regarding both the available choices in their local stores combined with a lack of transportation which limits their access to foods that are healthier. This is common in rural areas of America where foods may oftentimes not be classified as healthy *(19, 20)*.

3.5. Other Areas of Concern

In addition to the issue of obesity, it is important to remember that specific areas of concern that need to be addressed pertain to essential nutrients. Indeed, much of the population suffers from specific deficiencies. Key to women and in particular those who are vegetarian is iron deficiency. Obviously, in all women it is necessary to test for iron status and address the problem if the diagnosis is anemia. Another mineral of concern is calcium because of osteoporosis and bone health.

Fiber is an issue in practically all American diets, since the reported intake of dietary fiber is about half of the recommended intake which is 30–38 g/day for men and 21–25 g/day for women. (*See* Chapter 2 on dietary fiber by Slavin and Jacobs.) Males reportedly consume about 17 g/day and women about 12.5 g/day. Focusing on increasing fruit and vegetable intake and switching from refined carbohydrates to whole grains is a simple and easy way to begin addressing how to increase fiber intake and should be a standard message disseminated by physicians.

Emerging evidence on the beneficial effects of vitamin D and *n*–3 fatty acids can also be a take-home message from the physician to his patient population. *n*–3 fats may be obtained from fish oil supplements. Lower vitamin D levels are more likely to be seen in northern climates due to the lesser exposure to sun which activates vitamin D in the skin. The risk is also higher in persons with a darker skin color.

4. HEALTHY EATING INDEX

In assessing the adequacy of the diet of the patient, it may be helpful to utilize a tool such as the healthy eating index or HEI *(21)*. This tool measures diet quality based on conformance to federal dietary guidance. The

HEI-2005 is a standardized tool that can be used to monitor nutrition interventions, consumer education, and research and could be adapted for use in the physician's office. Scores are given for all dietary components then expressed on a 1,000-kcal basis. In order to complete the evaluation, there needs to be an analysis of dietary intake of the individual, either by a 24-h recall, food frequency, or analyzed food records.

5. CONCLUSION

The physician plays a crucial role in assessing the nutritional status of the patient. Using the instruments available to evaluate dietary intake along with appropriate biological testing and physical evaluation, the physician will receive insight to assess the diet and environmental factors that weigh in on the health status of the patient. The evaluation of weight status is, by far, the most pressing of diagnoses to aid in the prevention of obesity. Counseling during the visit could help an overweight individual begin a program to lose weight, especially if this occurs at a very early age. As the primary health-care provider for many, the routine office visit presents an opportunity to encourage proper diet and weight control and to help manage underlying organic disorders that cause obesity. Research continues to elucidate the pathologic process of obesity. However, because of the alarming increase in obesity in the United States, the rapid increase in type 2 diabetes (especially in children), and the limited effectiveness of even the best treatments, prevention will remain the best way to avoid the morbidity and mortality associated with obesity. The health-care provider needs to recognize that dietary behavior is modified by economic factors – the cost of food. As long as cheap, energy-dense, nutrient-poor foods are available, it will be difficult to prevent obesity.

SUGGESTED FURTHER READING

Food and Nutrition Board, Institute of Medicine – FNB, available at http://www.healthfinder.gov/orgs/HR0139.htm

Handbook of Obesity. Clinical Applications, 3rd Ed. Bray GA, Bouchard C, eds. Informa Healthcare, New York, 2008.

Krause's Food, Nutrition, and Therapy, 12th Ed. Mahan LK, Escott-Stump S, eds. W.B. Saunders Co., Philadelphia, 2007.

NHANES Laboratory Methods, available at http://www.cdc.gov/nchs/about/major/nhanes/nhanes2003-2004/lab_methods_03_04.htm

Schlenker E, Roth SL. Williams' Essentials of Nutrition & Diet Therapy – Text and E-Book Package. Mosby, Philadelphia, 2006.

USDA, National Agricultural Library, Food and Nutrition Information Center, available at http://fnic.nal.usda.gov/nal_display/index.php?info_center=4&tax_level=2&tax_subject=256&topic_id=1325

REFERENCES

1. Flegal KM, Graubard BI, Williamson DF, Gail MH. Excess deaths associated with underweight, overweight, and obesity. JAMA 2005; 293:1861–1867.
2. Blanton CA, Moshfegh AJ, Baer DJ, Kretsch MJ. The USDA automated multiple-Pass method accurately estimates group total energy and nutrient intake. J Nutr 2006; 136:2594–2599.
3. Bray GA. Review of: Good Calories, Bad Calories by Gary Taubes. AA Knopf, New York, 2007. Obes Rev 2008; 9:251–263.
4. Yanetz R, Kipnis V, Carroll RJ, et al. Using biomarker data to adjust estimates of the distribution of usual intakes for misreporting: application to energy intake in the US population. J Am Diet Assoc 2008; 108:455–464; discussion 464.
5. Abbot JM, Thomson CA, Ranger-Moore J, et al. Psychosocial and behavioral profile and predictors of self-reported energy underreporting in obese middle-aged women. J Am Diet Assoc 2008; 108:114–119.
6. Tooze JA, Vitolins MZ, Smith SL, et al. High levels of low energy reporting on 24-hour recalls and three questionnaires in an elderly low-socioeconomic status population. J Nutr 2007; 137:1286–1293.
7. Scagliusi FB, Ferriolli E, Lancha AH, Jr. Underreporting of energy intake in developing nations. Nutr Rev 2006; 64(7 Pt 1):319–330.
8. Balkau B, Deanfield JE, Despres JP, et al. International Day for the Evaluation of Abdominal Obesity (IDEA): a study of waist circumference, cardiovascular disease, and diabetes mellitus in 168,000 primary care patients in 63 countries. Circulation 2007; 116: 1942–1951.
9. Bray GA. Contemporary Diagnosis and Management of Obesity. 3rd ed. Handbooks in Health Care Co, Newtown, PA, 2003.
10. Lazzer S, Bedogni G, Agosti F, De Col A, Mornati D, Sartorio A. Comparison of dual-energy X-ray absorptiometry, air displacement plethysmography and bioelectrical impedance analysis for the assessment of body composition in severely obese Caucasian children and adolescents. Br J Nutr 2008; 18:1–7.
11. Shypailo RJ, Butte NF, Ellis KJ. DXA: can it be used as a criterion reference for body fat measurements in children? Obesity (Silver Spring) 2008; 16:457–462.
12. Nichols J, Going S, Loftin M, Stewart D, Nowicki E, Pickrel J. Comparison of two bioelectrical impedance analysis instruments for determining body composition in adolescent girls. Int J Body Compos Res 2006; 4:153–160.
13. Volgyi E, Tylavsky FA, Lyytikainen A, Suominen H, Alen M, Cheng S. Assessing body composition with DXA and bioimpedance: effects of obesity, physical activity, and age. Obesity (Silver Spring) 2008; 16:700–705.
14. Chen Z, Wang Z, Lohman T, et al. Dual-energy X-ray absorptiometry is a valid tool for assessing skeletal muscle mass in older women. J Nutr 2007; 137:2775–2780.
15. Neovius M, Hemmingsson E, Freyschuss B, Udden J. Bioelectrical impedance underestimates total and truncal fatness in abdominally obese women. Obesity (Silver Spring) 2006; 14:1731–1738.
16. Ogden CL, Carroll MD, Curtin LR, McDowell MA, Tabak CJ, Flegal KM. Prevalence of overweight and obesity in the United States, 1999–2004. JAMA 2006; 295: 1549–1555.
17. Drewnowski A. Obesity and the food environment. Dietary energy density and diet costs. Am J Prev Med 2004; 27(3S):154–162.
18. Kant AK, Graubard BI. Energy density of diets reported by American adults: association with food group intake, nutrient intake, and body weight. Int J Obes 2005; 29:950–956.

19. Champagne CM, Casey PH, Connell CL, et al. Lower Mississippi Delta Nutrition Intervention Research Initiative. Poverty and food intake in rural America: diet quality is lower in food insecure adults in the Mississippi Delta. J Am Diet Assoc 2007; 107: 1886–1994.
20. Stuff JE, Casey PH, Connell CL, et al. Household food insecurity and obesity, chronic disease, and chronic disease risk factors. J Hunger Environ Nutr 2006; 1(2):43–62.
21. http://www.cnpp.usda.gov/healthyeatingindex.htm. Last accessed June 20, 2008.

21 Eating Disorders: Disorders of Under- and Overnutrition

Kelly C. Allison

Key Points

- Eating disorder diagnoses consist of anorexia nervosa (restricting type and binge-eating/purging type); bulimia nervosa (purging and nonpurging types); and eating disorder, not otherwise specified (including binge-eating disorder, night eating syndrome, and purging disorder).
- Physical complications of anorexia nervosa affect most major systems in the body and are caused by starvation and the effects of purging. Most physical complications of bulimia nervosa are due to purging.
- Overweight and obesity are linked with binge-eating disorder and night eating syndrome. Patients typically request that weight loss be addressed with treatment.
- Anorexia nervosa is difficult to treat and may need initial inpatient treatment for refeeding. Subsequently, family therapy is recommended for patients still living with their families.
- Cognitive behavioral therapy is the first line of therapy recommended for bulimia nervosa, binge-eating disorder, and night eating syndrome. Interpersonal therapy has also been shown effective for bulimia nervosa and binge-eating disorder with similar efficacy as cognitive behavioral therapy at 12 months post-treatment.
- Selective serotonin reuptake inhibitors have been shown effective for treating bulimia nervosa, binge-eating disorder, and night eating syndrome, as has topiramate. Sibutramine is also effective for binge-eating disorder. Medication trials have not identified a drug that effectively addresses the refusal to maintain a healthy body weight, the core symptom of anorexia nervosa.
- Prevention studies are in their infancy, but dissonance-based programs have shown promise.

Key Words: Anorexia nervosa; bulimia nervosa; binge-eating disorder; night eating syndrome; therapy for eating disorders

From: *Nutrition and Health: Nutrition Guide for Physicians*
Edited by: T. Wilson et al. (eds.), DOI 10.1007/978-1-60327-431-9_21,
© Humana Press, a part of Springer Science+Business Media, LLC 2010

1. INTRODUCTION

Eating disorders represent extremes in nutrition. These extremes of under- and overnutrition can exist within the same person, as in anorexia nervosa, binge-eating/purging type, where an individual severely restricts daily caloric intake while periodically consuming extremely large amounts of food. Alternatively, the extremes can be found by definition, as in anorexia nervosa, restricting type, and binge-eating disorder. Current diagnostic criteria for eating disorders are outlined in the Diagnostic and Statistical Manual IV - TR (DSM-IV-TR) from the American Psychiatric Association (1) and include anorexia nervosa, bulimia nervosa, and eating disorder – not otherwise specified (ED-NOS). Binge-eating disorder is currently included as a disorder in need of further research and may be included as a formal eating disorder category in the next DSM. There are also other forms of disordered eating that are included in the ED-NOS category that are growing in recognition, including night eating syndrome and purging disorder.

This chapter will provide diagnostic criteria for each of these forms of disordered eating and a brief overview of prevalence, assessment issues, treatment, and prevention efforts.

2. ANOREXIA NERVOSA

Anorexia nervosa was first noted in the scientific community in the late 17th century and first appeared in the DSM-III in 1980 as a diagnostic entity. By the DSM-IV-TR definition there are four key attributes. The first, a core feature, is a refusal to maintain a minimally normal body weight for age and height. While there is variability across individuals by body type, ethnicity, and gender for what is a "minimally acceptable weight," it is generally defined as weighing less than 85% of expected weight for height, or at or below a body mass index (BMI) of 17.5 kg/m^2. For adolescents and children, lack of weight gain, rather than active weight loss, would also be an appropriate measure of this criterion. Centers for Disease Control growth charts (2) should be reviewed to assess if a child or adolescent has fallen significantly below his or her original weight trajectory.

The second criterion describes an intense fear of gaining weight despite being underweight. The third requires a distortion in the way that body weight and shape are viewed or a denial of the seriousness of the condition. Persons with anorexia nervosa evaluate their self-worth almost entirely by their perceptions of their body weight and shape, and these distorted beliefs help maintain the severe caloric deficits necessary to sustain their low weight. Finally, among postmenarcheal females, menstrual cycles must have been absent for at least 3 months. If women are on hormonal birth control, a retrospective account of menstrual cyclicity is recommended; otherwise this criterion cannot be assessed. This criterion would also not apply to men, but they typically experience lowered testosterone levels accompanied by a diminished sex drive and sexual functioning.

There are two subtypes of anorexia nervosa. The restricting type is classified by the strict use of caloric restriction and excessive exercise as a means of controlling their weight. The binge-eating/purging subtype describes those who engage in binge eating or inappropriate compensatory measures, such as vomiting or misuse of laxatives, diuretics, or enemas. Those with the anorexia nervosa, binge-eating/purging subtype differ from persons with bulimia nervosa who binge and purge because of their extremely low body weight and amenorrhea. Thus, a diagnosis of anorexia nervosa supersedes a diagnosis of bulimia nervosa.

Almost every physical system is negatively impacted by anorexia nervosa; this is due to starvation and, when present, the effects of purging. Resulting abnormalities include bradycardia, arrhythmia, hypothyroidism, low bone density, constipation, infertility, and perinatal complications. Gray matter volume in the brain is decreased. Atrophied neural networks may maintain sufferers' psychological delusions regarding their fears of fat and beliefs that they are not thin enough, as well as obsessions and compulsive rituals with food. Despite the gravity of their symptoms, those with anorexia nervosa do not typically complain of their ailments and deny the seriousness of their physical and psychological states.

Paradoxically, excessive exercise and movement are observed in anorexia nervosa, perhaps due to lowered leptin levels that increase the drive for movement once associated food-finding behaviors to avoid starvation. With this denial, many sufferers refuse medical treatment until they have been seriously medically compromised. When excessive movement subsides and fatigue sets in, this may indicate severe depression, electrolyte imbalance, or severe dehydration. Cardiac functioning may also be poor at that point. For these reasons, along with high rates of suicide, anorexia nervosa is considered the deadliest psychiatric disorder.

3. BULIMIA NERVOSA

The core features of bulimia nervosa are binge eating and subsequent use of inappropriate compensatory behaviors. These behaviors are used in an attempt to attain a low body weight or prevent weight gain. As with anorexia nervosa, there is undue influence of weight and shape on self-evaluation and self-concept. Diagnosis requires that the binge-eating episodes and inappropriate compensatory behaviors occur at least twice per week for at least 3 months.

There are two subtypes of bulimia nervosa: purging type and nonpurging type. Purging behaviors most often consist of vomiting, used in 80–90% of cases *(1)*, followed by laxative abuse. Many persons with bulimia nervosa become skilled at inducing vomiting so that they no longer need to use their fingers or another instrument and can vomit at will. Four common signs associated with vomiting include "Russell's sign" (scarring on the back of the knuckles due to self-induced vomiting), swollen cheeks associated with parotid gland enlargement, dental enamel erosion, and receding gums. Laxative abuse is commonly associated with peripheral edema and bloating. Constipation results when laxatives abuse is discontinued, but it generally resolves in less than a month with exercise and gradual increases in fluids and fiber. Both vomiting and laxative use are associated with electrolyte imbalance, fatigue, heart arrhythmias, and gastrointestinal problems, such as gastroesophageal reflux disease (GERD).

Most persons with bulimia nervosa have a BMI in the healthy weight range, with some in the overweight and obese ranges. Individuals with bulimia nervosa feel free of their binge food after purging and consequently experience psychological relief (if only temporarily), but, in reality, many of the calories from their binge episodes are absorbed and metabolized. They may also restrict between binge episodes and exercise, but not to the extent that is observed with anorexia nervosa, binge-eating/purging subtype. Malnutrition may still occur in bulimia nervosa, but most of the medical complications in this disorder are caused by the purging behaviors. While these medical complications are not as severe as those observed in anorexia nervosa, persons with bulimia nervosa generally are less tolerant of their physical symptoms. Those with bulimia nervosa typically have more insight into their disorder than those with anorexia nervosa, often feeling guilt and shame related to their binge-eating and purging behaviors.

4. EATING DISORDER – NOT OTHERWISE SPECIFIED

There are many forms of disordered eating that are serious and cause psychological and physical distress that do not fit the diagnostic criteria for bulimia nervosa or anorexia nervosa. These are captured in the ED-NOS category. The most prominent of these is binge-eating disorder, which will be considered for inclusion as its own diagnosis for the next edition of the DSM. Two other disorders also gaining more attention are night eating syndrome and purging disorder. Each of these is described below.

4.1. Binge-Eating Disorder

The hallmark of binge-eating disorder is eating large amounts of food, accompanied by a loss of control. Additionally, at least three of five of the following signs must be present during binge-eating episodes: (1) eating more rapidly than normal; (2) eating until uncomfortably full; (3) eating when not physically hungry; (4) eating alone due to embarrassment; and (5) feeling disgusted, depressed, or markedly guilty after an episode. Diagnosis requires that distress regarding the binge eating must be present, and the episodes must occur, on average, at least twice per week for 6 months *(1)*.

Most individuals with binge-eating disorder are overweight or obese, and many present primarily for weight loss. Persons with bulimia nervosa typically restrict more consistently between binges than do persons with binge-eating disorder, but in laboratory studies those with bulimia nervosa consume more energy during binges than those with binge-eating disorder. Persons with binge-eating disorder typically engage in binge eating in addition to eating normal to large-sized meals throughout the day. This general pattern of overeating coupled with the lack of compensatory behaviors contributes to weight gain.

4.2. Night Eating Syndrome

The night eating syndrome was first described in 1955 as a disorder of morning anorexia, evening hyperphagia, and insomnia, usually accompanied by a depressed mood and stressful life circumstances *(3)*. Night eating syndrome did not receive much research or clinical attention until the 1990s. This renewed attention was likely influenced by the rise of the prevalence of obesity and the search for correlates and contributors of excessive weight gain. In 1999, awakenings with ingestions (*nocturnal ingestions*) were added to the provisional set of criteria *(4)*. However, as research advanced our understanding of night eating syndrome, different criteria sets were increasingly used, making comparisons across studies difficult.

The following diagnostic criteria were reached by consensus at the First International Night Eating Symposium in 2008 *(5)*. First, the daily pattern of eating must show greatly increased intake in the evening and/or night time, as manifested by one or both of the following: (a) at least 25% of food intake is consumed after the evening meal and/or (b) at least two eating episodes occur upon awakening during the night per week. Second, the clinical picture is characterized by at least three of five of the following features: (a) a lack of desire to eat in the morning and/or breakfast is omitted on four or more mornings per week; (b) the presence of a strong urge to eat between dinner and bedtime and/or during the night; (c) sleep onset and/or sleep maintenance insomnia are present four or more nights per week; (d) presence of a belief that one must eat in order to get to sleep; and (e) mood is frequently depressed and/or mood worsens in the evening.

Persons who meet these criteria must also have awareness and recall of the evening and nocturnal eating episodes to distinguish the behavior from sleep-related eating disorder, which is a parasomnia marked by impaired consciousness and the consumption of unusual food or nonedible objects. Diagnosis requires that the night eating behaviors must be present for at least 3 months, and there must be distress or impairment of functioning present in relation to the night eating.

One epidemiological and two clinical studies have shown a link between night eating syndrome and obesity. However, other studies have failed to verify this. Average caloric intake consumed during nocturnal ingestions is similar to regular snacks (approximately 300–400 kcal). An early report *(4)* suggested that carbohydrates dominate nocturnal food choices but a subsequent report has shown no difference in the proportion of macronutrient content of foods consumed during the night vs. the day *(6)*. However, the repeated and persistent nature of the disorder likely contributes to weight gain among its sufferers.

4.3. Purging Disorder

Purging disorder is generally defined as the regular occurrence of inappropriate compensatory behaviors (e.g., vomiting, laxative use, or diuretic misuse) in the absence of regular binge-eating episodes and with a body weight greater than 85% of that expected *(7)*. The frequency used for the purging criterion has varied between greater than once per week to greater than twice per week. Some studies have also included undue influence of weight and shape on self-evaluation. Thus, persons with purging disorder generally feel distressed after eating anywhere from a typical meal to a small snack and have an overwhelming urge to purge afterward.

The effects of purging are the same as those presented for bulimia nervosa. Thus, the impact of purging disorder can be dangerous and debilitating. A feeding study has shown that women with the disorder reported more postprandial fullness and gastrointestinal discomfort after a standardized meal than those with bulimia nervosa, and greater release of cholecystokinin (CCK) *(8)*, suggesting that physiological cues may contribute to the purging behavior.

5. PREVALENCE

A recent study provided comprehensive lifetime prevalence estimates: anorexia nervosa had occurred in 0.9% of women and 0.3% of men; bulimia nervosa in 1.5% of women and 0.5% of men; and binge-eating disorder in 3.5% of women and 2.0% of men *(9)*. Furthermore, subthreshold binge-eating disorder, which did not include the five descriptors (e.g., eating more rapidly than usual) or the distress criteria, was assessed, yielding prevalence estimates of 0.6% of women and 1.9% of men.

Estimates of night eating syndrome in the general population of the United States are 1.5% *(10)*. Epidemiological studies among women of purging disorder reveal rates of 5.3% in an Australian twin cohort, 1.1% in an Italian cohort, and 0.85% in an adolescent Portuguese cohort [for review *see* Keel, *(7)*]. The relative frequency of these rates, as compared to the other eating disorders, has varied, with some studies finding purging disorder more common and others less common than bulimia nervosa and anorexia nervosa.

6. TREATMENT

Much progress has been made in treating bulimia nervosa, binge-eating disorder, and night eating syndrome. However, treatments for anorexia nervosa that have long-term effectiveness are still sorely lacking. Table 1 provides an overview of effective treatment modalities. The first step in assigning treatment is to assess how medically compromised a patient may be. With anorexia nervosa, inpatient hospitalization may be

Table 1
Effective Treatments for Eating Disorders

Disorder	Cognitive Behavioral Therapy	Interpersonal Therapy	SSRIs	Other
Anorexia nervosa	Mixed	Mixed	No	Inpatient/residential multidisciplinary treatment; family therapy; no medications proven effective
Bulimia nervosa	Yes	Yes	Yes	Not buproprion
Binge-eating disorder	Yes	Yes	Yes	Topiramate, sibutramine, behavioral weight loss
Night eating syndrome	Yes	Not tested	Yes	Topiramate (case reports only)

Note: Purging disorder is not included because specific treatment studies have not been reported.

warranted for refeeding. The next step down is residential treatment, followed by partial-hospitalization or day-treatment programs. These treatments typically involve a multidisciplinary team of professionals, including physicians, dietitians, psychologists, and, in some cases, art therapists and occupational therapists. Interventions include both group and individual treatments. Therapeutic meals are included where patients are challenged to eat nutritionally balanced meals and snacks at regular intervals each day, typically every 3–4 h. Patients are encouraged to gain approximately 1–2 lb/week, at an initial intake of about 1,500 kcal/day (30–40 kcal/kg/day), increasing up to 70–80 kcal/kg/day (11). Liquid meal supplements are often used to help patients reach this goal. Patients must be carefully monitored after meals, particularly in the bathroom and their rooms, to prevent purging. Bulimia nervosa can typically be treated on an outpatient basis, but persistent or very severe cases require residential or partial treatment.

6.1. Psychotherapy

The most effective outpatient psychotherapy approach for eating disorders is cognitive behavioral therapy (CBT). A 20-session course of treatment is effective for bulimia nervosa and binge-eating disorder (12). Sessions occur twice weekly for the first 2 weeks of treatment, followed by weekly sessions. Maintenance sessions are encouraged after the initial 20-week course. Cognitive behavioral therapy produces abstinence from binge-eating and purging behaviors in varying proportions of study participants with bulimia nervosa, ranging from 24 to 71% (13). Similarly, cognitive behavioral therapy in binge-eating disorder produces abstinence in binge eating ranging from 37 to 79% of study participants (14). However, weight is not significantly reduced among persons with binge-eating disorder, despite large reductions in binge episodes. Less impressive results have been reported for treatment of active anorexia nervosa, although cognitive behavioral therapy may be helpful in maintaining treatment gains. Only an uncontrolled study among patients with night eating syndrome has been tested to date with significant reductions in nocturnal ingestions and evening eating.

Interpersonal psychotherapy has been tested by several groups of researchers and applied successfully to bulimia nervosa and binge-eating disorder. Anorexia nervosa has not responded as robustly as bulimia nervosa and binge-eating disorder. As persons with eating disorders typically experience interpersonal or social dysfunction, interpersonal therapy for eating disorders focus on how these social deficits contribute to binge-eating and purging behaviors. Interpersonal therapy focuses on one of four areas of interpersonal functioning, including unresolved grief, role transition (e.g., graduating high school or college), role dispute (e.g., problems in communicating with a boyfriend or parent), and interpersonal deficit. Interpersonal psychotherapy is not generally recommended as a first-line approach because it relieves symptoms at a slower pace than cognitive behavioral therapy. However, at 1-year follow-up, the treatment outcomes are equivalent (13,14).

Family therapy has been shown to be the only effective psychotherapeutic approach for anorexia nervosa (15), and it is also effective among those with bulimia nervosa (16). It works particularly well for younger patients living with their families. The Maudsley Approach, or family-based treatment, is the most well-validated family therapy approach for anorexia and is intended to reduce the need for inpatient treatment and to help parents successfully refeed their child, which is the first goal. The second goal is for the adolescent to start to take control again of eating and weight gain, at a level appropriate to maturational status. Finally, an overview of normal adolescent development is covered with the family, and the therapist helps to identify any other outstanding social–emotional issues for which the family may still need help.

Finally, behavioral weight-loss therapy reduces binge eating and produces weight loss in persons with binge-eating disorder [see Ref. (17) for review]. However, abstinence rates from binge eating are not as high as those produced through cognitive behavioral therapy. Thus, if weight loss is strongly desired by a patient and their other psychiatry comorbidities, such as major depression, substance abuse, or an anxiety disorder, are not causing noticeable impairments in functioning, then a behavioral weight-loss program may suit those patients best.

6.2. Psychotropic Medications

Antidepressants are widely prescribed for the treatment of eating disorders for two reasons: they are effective in reducing binge-eating and purging behaviors, and they improve comorbid mood and anxiety symptoms. Unfortunately, they have not been shown to reduce the core symptom of anorexia nervosa, i.e., refusal to maintain a healthy body weight. Thus, there are currently no efficacious medications used for the treatment or maintenance of anorexia nervosa. However, antidepressants may still relieve comorbid depression or anxiety, when present.

Tricyclic antidepressants, monoamine oxidase inhibitors (MAOIs), and selective serotonin reuptake inhibitors (SSRIs) have all shown efficacy over placebos in reducing binge eating and purging (13,14). SSRIs are now most commonly used, with typical reductions of 45–65% in binge eating. The SSRI, sertraline, has also been shown to reduce evening hyperphagia and nocturnal ingestions significantly among those with night eating syndrome. Topiramate successfully decreases binge eating and purging as compared to placebo treatment and is associated with weight loss; however, cognitive side effects may be intolerable for some users. Case reports of topiramate in the treatment of night eating syndrome have also shown significant reductions in evening hyperphagia, nocturnal ingestions, and weight. Sibutramine effectively reduces binge eating and produces weight loss among those with binge-eating disorder, but blood pressure should be monitored, particularly in those with hypertension. Buproprion is not indicated for those with eating disorders as it has been associated with increased risk of seizures.

7. PREVENTION

Prevention programs aimed at reducing the incidence of eating disorders have been designed for children, adolescents, and college students. Dissonance-based interventions have been tested most rigorously and have been shown to have the greatest effect on reduction of eating disorder risk factors, symptoms, risk of onset, and future risk of development of obesity *(18)*. Cognitive dissonance programs involve having participants speak or behave in a manner that is opposite to their beliefs. As applied to eating disorders, women would be challenged to voice active criticism of the thin ideal; this is because internalization of the thin ideal is a risk factor for developing anorexia nervosa and bulimia nervosa. Among college students, peer-led dissonance-based interventions have been shown effective among women considered at high and low risk for developing anorexia nervosa or bulimia nervosa.

Other approaches have focused on media literacy and advocacy, but more evidence is needed, particularly in light of the superior effectiveness of the dissonance-based programs. In peer-led programs, the media advocacy intervention is effective in reducing risk for disordered eating among high-risk women, but not those at low risk *(19)*. One trial of a cognitive behavioral therapy-based prevention program delivered through the Internet showed reductions in the onset of eating disorders in two subgroups, those who were overweight and a subset of those who reported pre-existing purging behaviors *(20)*. Finally, programs that focus on body shape and weight acceptance for children and adolescents have also been used in school programming, but little to no formal testing of these programs' effects has been reported. As with other prevention approaches, more controlled studies are needed to confirm these results and to compare their efficacy with the dissonance-based and media advocacy approaches.

8. CONCLUSION

Eating disorders range from severe caloric restriction to severe overeating. Extreme dissatisfaction with weight and shape is present across the different diagnoses. In most diagnoses, there is also an uncontrollable urge to binge-eat. When medical complications are severe, inpatient treatment is warranted, particularly in anorexia nervosa. For most cases of bulimia nervosa, binge-eating disorder, night eating syndrome, and purging disorder, outpatient psychotherapy is the first line of treatment. Psychotropic medications, most recently SSRIs, have also been proven effective in treating bulimia nervosa, binge-eating disorder, and night eating syndrome. Prevention programs using dissonance-based interventions are promising for decreasing the incidence of eating disorders among college-age students, but other programs that target children and adolescents need to be formally evaluated.

SUGGESTED FURTHER READING

Fairburn CG, Wilson GT, eds. Binge eating: Nature, Assessment and Treatment. Guilford Press, New York, 1993.

Mitchell JE, Devlin MJ, de Zwaan M, Crow SJ, Peterson CB. Binge-Eating Disorder: Clinical Foundations and Treatment. Guilford Press, New York, 2008.

Allison KC, Stunkard AJ, Thier SL. Overcoming Night Eating Syndrome: A Step-By-Step Guide to Breaking the Cycle. New Harbinger, Oakland, CA, 2004.

Yager J, Powers PS. Clinical Manual of Eating Disorders. American Psychiatric Publishing, Washington, DC, 2007.

REFERENCES

1. American Psychiatric Association. Diagnostic and Statistical Manual of Mental Disorders (4th ed., text rev.). American Psychiatric Association, Washington, DC, 2000.

2. 2000 Centers for Disease Control Growth Charts for the United States. Available at: www.cdc.gov/growthcharts/. Last accessed June 9, 2008.

3. Stunkard AJ, Grace WJ, Wolff HG. The night-eating syndrome: A pattern of food intake among certain obese patients. Am J Med 1955; 19:78–86.

4. Birketvedt G, Florholmen J, Sundsfjord J, et al. Behavioral and neuroendocrine characteristics of the night-eating syndrome. JAMA 1999; 282:657–663.

5. Allison KC, Lundgren JD, O'Reardon JP, et al. Proposed diagnostic criteria for night eating syndrome. Int J Eat Disord 2009 Apr 17, Epub ahead of print.

6. Allison KC, Ahima RS, O'Reardon JP, et al. Neuroendocrine profiles associated with energy intake, sleep, and stress in the night eating syndrome. J Clin Endocr Metab 2005; 90:6214–6217.

7. Keel PK. Purging disorder: subthreshold variant or full-threshold eating disorder? Int J Eat Disord 2007; 40:589–594.

8. Keel PK, Wolfe BE, Liddle RA, DeYoung KP, Jimerson DC. Clinical features and physiological response to a test meal in purging disorder and bulimia nervosa. Arch Gen Psychiatry 2007; 64:1058–1066.

9. Hudson JI, Hiripi E, Pope HG, Kessler RC. The prevalence and correlates of eating disorders in the National Comorbidity Survey replication. Biol Psychiatry 2007; 61; 348–358.

10. Rand CSW, MacGregor AM, Stunkard AJ. The night eating syndrome in the general population and among post-operative obesity surgery patients. Int J Eat Disord 1997; 22:65–69.

11. Halmi KA. Management of anorexia nervosa in inpatient and partial hospitalization settings. In: Yager J, Powers PS, eds. Clinical Manual of Eating Disorders. American Psychiatric Publishing, Washington, DC, 2007, pp. 113–125.

12. Fairburn CG, Marcus MD, Wilson GT. Cognitive-behavioral therapy for binge eating and bulimia nervosa: a comprehensive treatment manual. In: Fairburn CG, Wilson GT, eds. Binge Eating: Nature, Assessment, and Treatment. Guilford Press, New York 1993, pp. 361–404.

13. Mitchell JE, Steffen KJ, Roerig JL. Management of bulimia nervosa. In: Yager J, Powers PS, eds. Clinical Manual of Eating Disorders. American Psychiatric Publishing, Washington, DC, 2007, pp. 171–193.

14. Mitchell JE, Devlin MJ, de Zwaan M, Crow SJ, Peterson CB. Psychotherapy for binge eating disorder. Binge-Eating Disorder: Clinical Foundations and Treatment. Guilford Press, New York, 2008, pp. 58–69.

15. Dare C, Eisler I. Family therapy for anorexia nervosa. In: Garner DM, Garfinkel P. Handbook of Treatment for Eating Disorders. Guilford Press, New York, 1997, pp. 307–324.

16. le Grange D, Lock J, Dymek M. Family-based therapy for adolescents with bulimia nervosa. Am J Psychother 2003; 57:237–251.

17. Stunkard AJ, Allison KC. Binge eating disorder: disorder or marker? Int J Eat Disord 2003; 34:S107–S116.

18. Stice E, Shaw H, Becker CB, Rohde P. Dissonance-based interventions for the prevention of eating disorders: using persuasion principals to promote health. Prev Sci 2008; 9: 114–128.

19. Becker CB, Bull S, Schaumberg K, Cauble A, Franco A. Effectiveness of peer-led eating disorders prevention: a replication trial. J Consult Clin Psychol 2008; 76:347–354.

20. Taylor CB, Bryson S, Luce KH, et al. Prevention of eating disorders in at-risk college-age women. Arch Gen Psychiatry 2006; 63:881–888.

22 Obesity: Understanding and Achieving a Healthy Weight

George A. Bray and Catherine M. Champagne

Key Points

- Obesity is a chronic problem that is increasing in prevalence, affecting both adults and children.
- A small positive energy imbalance causes the problem, but focusing on calories may not be as productive as modulating some of the economic and societal factors.
- Obesity increases risk of death and many diseases; weight loss provides benefits in reducing health risks and improving the quality of life.
- Treatments must redress the energy imbalance. Diet, lifestyle modification, and exercise are the cornerstones of treatment.
- Two drugs are approved by the FDA for long-term treatment, and they can effectively improve health-related risks.
- Bariatric surgery has become a major treatment strategy and has proven that it can reduce long-term health risks from obesity.

Key Words: Obesity; body mass index; drug treatment; bariatric surgery; diet treatment

1. INTRODUCTION

Either increased body weight, as expressed in the body mass index [BW (kg)/Ht (m)^2], or waist circumference can be used to assess the degree of obesity, and both indices have been rising steadily as the epidemic of obesity has spread over the past 20 years *(1)*. Although obesity results from an imbalance between energy intake and expenditure, it is the connections between these two components of the first law of thermodynamics that can provide the clues about how we should understand, prevent, and treat this

From: *Nutrition and Health: Nutrition Guide for Physicians*
Edited by: T. Wilson et al. (eds.), DOI 10.1007/978-1-60327-431-9_22,
© Humana Press, a part of Springer Science+Business Media, LLC 2010

problem *(1)*. While nutrition is of course the ultimate "source" of a positive energy balance, improper nutrition may not be as critical to the treatment of obesity as was once believed.

The pathology of obesity can best be understood as an enlargement of fat cells, and in some individuals an increased number of them *(2, 3)*. These large fat cells release more fatty acids and a variety of cytokines that can provide a basis for understanding how obesity produces insulin resistance and changes in the inflammatory, thrombotic, and coagulation systems. There is a large industry offering various forms of treatment. Although we can treat obesity with some success, we rarely cure it, and a plateau in body weight during treatment with subsequent relapse when treatment is terminated is the common experience. Surgical intervention with gastric bypass or gastric restriction is the most effective treatment but at an increased risk of mortality and with substantial morbidity. Only two pharmacologic agents are currently approved for long-term use, and they produce only modest weight loss.

Let us start with the premise that all of us want to have a healthy weight. Interest in obesity has taken a sharp upturn in recent years, as the prevalence has increased. Obesity can be viewed as a chronic, stigmatized, neurochemical disease *(1)*. In this context, the goal is to return weight to a healthy level and to remove the stigma associated with the use of the word "obesity." To consider it in the context of a neurochemical derangement has the advantage of focusing on the underlying mechanisms that produce the distortion in energy balance resulting in an unhealthy state *(1)*.

2. DEFINITION AND PREVALENCE OF OBESITY

2.1. Body Mass Index

Over the past 50 years there has been a steady upward shift in the distribution curve for body weight. This trend can most effectively be traced using the BMI which provides a useful operating definition of overweight and obesity. A normal BMI is between 18.5 and 24.9 kg/m^2. A BMI between 25 and 29.9 is operationally defined as overweight, and individuals with BMI >30 are obese, after taking into consideration other factors such as muscle builders, who have a high BMI, which may not be the most appropriate measure of weight status due to muscle. BMI also provides the risk measure for obesity *(1)*.

2.2. Central Adiposity

The waist circumference is a practical measure of central adiposity that is a surrogate for more precise measures of visceral fat, such as a CT or MRI scan of the abdomen at the L4-5 position. Risk for disease increases with a higher waist circumference. In the United States, a waist of more than 40 in. in men and more than 35 in. in women is a high-risk category, but most of the rest of the world uses considerably lower cut-points (80 cm [31.5 in.] for women and 90–94 cm [35.5–37 in.] for men). When BMI and waist circumference were used to predict the risk of hypertension, dyslipidemia, and the metabolic syndrome, the waist circumference was shown to be a better predictor than the BMI *(1)*.

2.3. Prevalence

Using the BMI, it is clear that there is an epidemic of obesity that began in the 1980s and that continues, although it may be slowing down *(4)*. It affects children as well as adults. We are now seeing a rise in the prevalence of type 2 diabetes in adolescents that is directly related to obesity. Obesity has a higher prevalence in Latino and African-American populations. Both height and weight have increased in adults aged 20–74 years between 1960 and 2000 but may have leveled off in adults between 2000 and 2004 *(4)*.

2.4. Cost of Obesity

Obesity is expensive, costing between 3 and 8% of health-care budgets *(5)*. Hospital costs and use of medication also increase with increasing BMI. In a large health-maintenance organization, mean annual costs were 25% higher in participants with a BMI between 30 and 35, and 44% higher in those with a BMI greater than 35, than in individuals with a BMI between 20 and 25. Costs for lifetime treatment of hypertension, hypercholesterolemia, type 2 diabetes, heart disease, and stroke in men and women with a BMI of 37.5 were $10,000 higher than for men and women with a BMI of 22.5 according to data from the National Center for Health Statistics and the Framingham Heart Study (*see* Ref. *(1)*).

3. ETIOLOGY

3.1. Energy Imbalance

We become obese because, over an extended period of time, we ingest more carbon- and nitrogen-containing compounds from food than we expend for energy. We and other animals thus obey the first law of thermodynamics. Voluntary overeating (by subjecting individuals to repeated ingestion of energy exceeding daily energy needs) can increase body weight. When these individuals stop overeating, they invariably lose most or all of the excess weight. The use of overeating protocols to study the consequences of food ingestion has shown the importance of genetic factors in the pattern of weight gain.

3.2. Epidemiologic Model

An epidemiologic model may be a better way than the energy-balance model to conceptualize obesity as a disease *(1)*. In an epidemiologic model, environmental agents act on a host to produce a disease. Disease is a function of the virulence of the agent and the susceptibility of the host. For obesity, the environmental agents include food, medications, toxins, physical inactivity, and viruses. In Western affluent societies, foods, particularly foods high in fat, are abundant. In addition, portion sizes have increased, providing more energy to people with each portion. Toxins are an interesting potential group of agents where more research is needed. Viruses are known to produce obesity and their potential role in obesity needs to be studied further. Physical activity within the general population has gradually been reduced, thereby decreasing energy expenditure. Some have described the current "environment" as a "virulent" or "toxic" environment that has heightened the risk for obesity. For the genetically susceptible host, this excess of food energy, environmental toxins, and viruses, along with the reduced level of physical activity, may lead to an accumulation of fat in fat cells. Genetics loads the gun, environment pulls the trigger (*see* Ref. *(1)*).

3.3. Environmental Agents

3.3.1. INTRAUTERINE FACTORS

Several intrauterine events influence postnatal weight and lifetime weight gain and fatness. These include maternal diabetes, maternal smoking, and intrauterine undernutrition, all of which heighten the individual's risk for increased body weight and diabetes later in life.

3.3.2. DRUG-INDUCED WEIGHT GAIN

In our current medicated society, it would not be surprising if drugs cause weight gain. Table 1 is a list of medications that produce weight gain when used to treat various diseases such as psychosis, depression, allergies, and diabetes. Also listed in the table are alternative treatments that can be used to avoid the weight gain. In most instances there are alternative strategies that can be used to treat a patient when weight gain is closely associated with the initiation of a new medication for one of these conditions. Several receptors, especially the H_1, α_{1A}, and serotonin (5-HT)-2C and -6 (5-HT$_{2C}$ and 5-HT$_6$) receptors, explain much of the weight gain associated with atypical antipsychotic drugs (*see* Ref. *(1)*).

3.4. Diet

Many aspects of the diet may contribute to obesity. Portion size and consumption of high-fructose corn syrup (HFCS) in beverages have all been

Table 1
Drugs That Produce Weight Gain and Alternatives

Category	Drugs That Cause Weight Gain	Possible Alternatives
Neuroleptics	Thioridazine, olanzapine, quetiapine, risperidone, clozapine	Molindone Haloperidol Ziprasidone
Antidepressants Tricyclics Monoamine oxidase inhibitors Selective serotonin reuptake inhibitors	Amitriptyline, nortriptyline Imipramine Mirtazapine Paroxetine	Protriptyline Bupropion Nefazodone Fluoxetine Sertraline
Anticonvulsants	Valproate, carbamazepine Gabapentin	Topiramate Lamotrigine Zonisamide
Antidiabetic drugs	Insulin Sulfonylureas Thiazolidinediones	Acarbose Miglitol Metformin Sibutramine
Antiserotonin Antihistamines	Pizotifen Cyproheptidine	Inhalers Decongestants
β-Adrenergic blockers α-Adrenergic blockers	Propranolol Terazosin	ACE inhibitors Calcium channel blockers
Steroid hormones	Contraceptives Glucocorticoids Progestational steroids	Barrier methods Nonsteroidal anti-inflammatory agents

implicated in the current obesity epidemic. Consumption of soft drinks predicted future weight gain in children and adults.

3.4.1. INFANT AND CHILD ENVIRONMENT

Infants who are breastfed for more than 3 months may have a reduced risk of future obesity. In addition, children who sleep less have a higher risk for weight gain during school years.

3.4.2. FAT INTAKE

Epidemiologic data suggest that a high-fat diet is associated with obesity *(1)*. For example, the relative weights in several populations are directly related to the percentage of fat in the diet. A high-fat diet provides high energy density (i.e., more calories for the same weight of food), which makes overconsumption more likely. Differences in the storage capacity for various macronutrients may also be involved. The capacity to store glucose as glycogen in the liver and muscle is limited, so glucose must be continually replenished. In contrast, fat stores contain more than 100 times as many calories as in the daily intake of fat. This difference in storage capacity makes eating carbohydrates a more important physiologic need that may lead to overeating when dietary carbohydrate is limited and carbohydrate oxidation cannot be reduced sufficiently.

3.4.3. GLYCEMIC INDEX

The rate at which glucose is absorbed can be expressed as the glycemic index (GI). The GI is a way of describing the ease with which starches are digested in the intestine with the release of glucose that can be readily absorbed. A food with a high GI is readily digested and produces a large and rapid increase in plasma glucose levels. Conversely, a food with a low GI is digested more slowly and is associated with a slower and lower increase in glucose levels. Foods with a high GI suppress food intake less than foods with a low GI. Foods with a low GI include whole fruits and vegetables that tend to have fiber (but not juices) plus legumes and whole wheat. Potatoes, white rice, and white bread have a high GI.

In a review of six studies, investigators documented that the consumption of foods with a high GI is associated with higher energy intake *(6)*. This confirms that the high-fiber foods with a low GI stimulate less food intake than foods with a high GI. In addition to the role of the GI, research has shown that high-fiber diets are associated with decreased weight.

3.4.4. CALCIUM INTAKE

Inverse relationships have been reported between calcium intake and the risk of having a BMI in the highest quartile *(7)*. Others have reported similar inverse associations between body fat gain and calcium intakes in children and young women *(8)*. It has been suggested that a difference in calcium intake of 1000 mg is associated with an 8 kg difference in mean body weight, and, furthermore, that calcium intake explains roughly 3% of the variance in body weight *(8)*. These data suggest that low calcium intake has a role in the current epidemic of obesity.

Most clinical trials, however, do not support a relation of dietary calcium to body weight. Researchers suggest that diets high in dairy calcium do not necessarily translate into weight loss beyond that achieved in behavioral interventions. Thompson et al. *(9)* did not find that diets high in dairy products enhanced weight loss, stating that high-dairy (as opposed to moderate-dairy) and other specialized diets (e.g., low GI) should not be viewed as more effective without additional data from long-term randomized trials.

3.4.5. FREQUENCY OF EATING

The relationship between the frequency of meals and the development of obesity is not known. However, the frequency of eating does affect lipid and glucose metabolism. When normal-weight individuals eat several small meals per day, serum cholesterol concentrations are lower than when they eat a few large meals per day. Similarly, mean blood glucose concentrations are lower when meals are eaten frequently. One explanation for the difference between eating frequent small meals and a few large meals may be the greater insulin secretion associated with eating larger meals. One mechanism leading to weight gain caused by irregular meal patterns might occur from the lower thermic effect of food and higher energy intake associated with irregular meal frequencies *(10)*.

3.4.6. RESTRAINED EATING

A pattern of conscious limitation of food intake is called "restrained" eating. It is a common practice in many, if not most, middle-aged women of normal weight. Higher restraint scores in women are associated with lower body weights. Weight loss is associated with an increase in restraint, indicating that higher levels of conscious control can maintain lower weight. Greater increases in restraint were correlated with greater weight loss but also with a higher risk of lapses, loss of control, and overeating.

3.5. Physical Activity

Low levels of physical activity correlate with weight gain. In a 10-year study of individuals aged 20–74 years in the National Health and Examination Survey (NHANES I), those with low levels of recreational activity gained more weight than did those with higher levels. Low levels of baseline energy expenditure predicted weight gain in Pima Indians. Exercise capacity and body composition predict mortality among men with diabetes. Time spent watching television correlates with percent of overweight children *(see* Ref. *(1))*.

3.6. Smoking

Smokers have a lower body weight, and cessation of smoking is generally associated with weight gain.

3.7. Host Agents

3.7.1. GENETIC CAUSES

There are several other rare clinical forms of obesity. The Prader–Willi syndrome is the most common. This disease is transmitted as a chromosome/gene abnormality on chromosome 15 and is characterized by a "floppy" baby who has difficulty feeding. These children are mentally slow, short in stature, and obese *(11)*. The Bardet–Biedl syndrome is due, in at least one pedigree, to a defect in the chaperonin-like gene *(11)*.

The leptin gene, the melanocortin-4 receptor gene, the proopiomelanocortin (POMC) gene, and agouti gene have significant effects on body fat and fat stores. MC4-receptor defects may account for up to 6% of obesity in early-onset, severely obese children *(11)*. Treatment of leptin-deficient children with leptin decreased body weight and hunger, indicating the importance of leptin for modulation of these processes in normal subjects. Heterozygotes for leptin deficiency have low but detectable serum leptin and have increased adiposity, indicating that low levels of leptin are associated with increased hunger and gain in body fat. Leptin can also increase energy expenditure and during reduced calorie intake, leptin attenuates the fall in thyroid hormones and the fall in 24-h energy expenditure.

The epidemic of obesity is occurring on a genetic background that does not change as fast as the epidemic has been exploding. It is nonetheless clear that genetic factors play an important role in the development of obesity and over 90 genes have so far been implicated (*see* Ref. *(1)*).

3.7.2. PHYSIOLOGIC FACTORS

The discovery of leptin in 1994 opened a new window on the control of food intake and body weight. The response of leptin-deficient children to leptin indicates the critical role that this peptide plays in the control of energy balance. Leptin enters the brain, probably by transport across the blood–brain barrier. It then acts on receptors in the arcuate nucleus to regulate in a conjugate fashion the production and release of at least four peptides. Leptin inhibits the production of neuropeptide Y (NPY) and agouti-related peptide (AGRP), both of which increase food intake, while enhancing the production of proopiomelanocortin (POMC), the source of α-melanocyte-stimulating hormone (α-MSH), which reduces food intake.

Two other brain peptide systems have also been linked to the control of feeding. Melanin-concentrating hormone (MCH) is found in the lateral hypothalamus and decreases food intake when injected into the ventricular system of the brain. Orexin (also called hypocretin) was identified in a search of G protein-linked peptides that affect food intake. It increases food intake and plays a role in sleep.

Endocannabinoids are derived from membrane fatty acids. The endogenous cannabinoids (anandamide and arachidonoyl 2-glycerol) increase food intake by acting on CB-1 receptors. Antagonists to the CB-1 receptor are a new class of potential anti-obesity drug *(12)*.

Gut peptides, including glucagon-like peptide-1, polypeptide YY oxyntomodulin, and cholecystokinin, reduce food intake, whereas ghrelin, a small peptide produced in the stomach, stimulates food intake.

Metabolism of fatty acids in the brain may be another important control point. A drug that blocks fatty acid synthase leads to significant weight loss. Malonyl-CoA accumulates in this setting and has been suggested to be a molecule that modulates food intake.

4. PATHOLOGY OF OBESITY

Enlarged fat cells are the hallmark of obesity, and in some individuals there is also an increased number of fat cells. It is the increased size of fat cells that is the characteristic pathology for obesity *(2)*.

5. PATHOPHYSIOLOGY

5.1. The Fat Cell as an Endocrine Cell

Two mechanisms can explain the pathophysiology of obesity: the first is increased fat mass, which can explain the stigmatization of physically obvious obesity, and the accompanying osteoarthritis and sleep apnea (Fig. 1; Ref. *(2)*). The second mechanism is the increased amount of peptides that are produced by the enlarged fat cells that act on distant organs. The discovery of leptin catapulted the fat cell into the arena of endocrine cells. In addition to leptin, there are increased amounts of cytokines, angiotensinogen, adipsin (complement factor D), etc., and metabolites such as free fatty acids and lactate. In contrast to the other fat cell products, adiponectin release is decreased in obesity. The products of the fat cell in turn modify the metabolic processes in other organs of the host. For the susceptible host, these metabolic changes lead in turn to a variety of other processes, including hyperinsulinemia, atherosclerosis, hypertension, and physical stress on bones and joints.

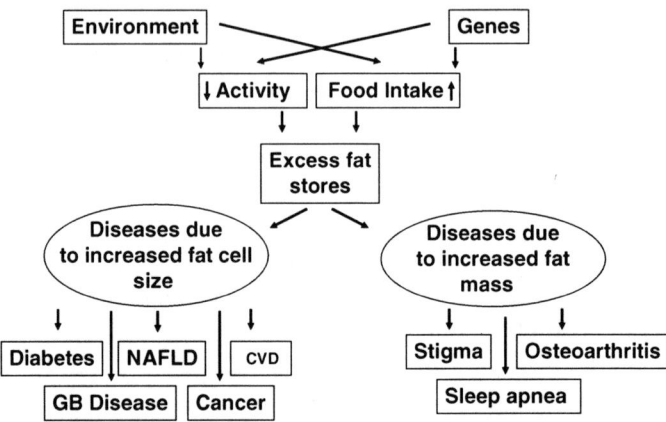

Fig. 1. Pathogenesis of health problems associated with obesity. The mass of fat and the responses to products produced by fat cells can explain most of the diseases that result from prolonged obesity. NAFLD = nonalcoholic fatty liver disease; CVD = cardiovascular disease; GB = gall bladder. Adapted from Ref. *(2)*.

5.2. Visceral Fat

A considerable body of data suggest that visceral fat has a stronger relationship with the complications associated with obesity than does total body fat *(13)*. Moreover, central adiposity is one of the key components of the metabolic syndrome, whose diagnostic criteria based on the recommendation of the National Cholesterol Education Program Adult Treatment Panel III *(14)* are shown in Table 2.

Table 2
National Cholesterol Education Program Adult Treatment Panel III Criteria for the Metabolic Syndrome[a]

Risk Factor	Defining Level
Waist circumference (central adiposity)	
Males	>40 in. (102 cm)
Females	>35 in. (88 cm)
HDL cholesterol	
Males	<40 mg/dL
Females	<50 mg/dL
Triglycerides	>150 mg/dL
Blood pressure (SBP/DBP)	>130/>85 mm Hg
Glucose (fasting)	100–126 mg/dL

[a]Modified criteria from the National Cholesterol Education Program Adult Treatment Panel III. The metabolic syndrome is present when three of these five criteria are abnormal. Adapted from Ref. *(14)*.

6. COMPLICATIONS OF OBESITY

6.1. Death

Obesity is associated with shortened life span and contributes between 100,000 and 400,000 excess deaths per year. Both the NCHS data and the Framingham data showed that a BMI of 30 or more decreases life span by 3–5 years compared to normal weight.

6.2. Diseases

The curvilinear "J"-shaped relationship of BMI to risk of complications has been known for 100 years. Among Asians the risk for diabetes at the same BMI is increased compared to Caucasians. The prevalence of diabetes increases with a high BMI in all ethnic groups. Many kinds of cancer are also increased in obese people.

7. PREVENTION

A number of epidemiologic studies have used change in body weight as an end point in the intervention. A reduction in TV watching by children slows the gain in BMI. In children, decreasing the consumption of "fizzy" beverages, primarily soft drinks, was associated with slower weight gain than in children who were not given this advice (*see* Ref. *(1)*). In adults, there are unfortunately few successful programs, but some individuals do lose weight and maintain it as demonstrated by the National Weight Control Registry of individuals who are "successful" weight losers for at least a year.

8. TREATMENT

8.1. Realities of Treatment

The National Heart, Lung, and Blood Institute has provided an algorithm for evaluating the overweight patient *(15)*. It is a useful framework on which to hang the information that is collected during the evaluation of obese patients (Fig. 2).

Realism is one important aspect of treatment for obesity. For most treatments, including behavior therapy, diet, and exercise, the weight loss (measured as percentage loss from the baseline weight) plateaus at less than 10%. For many patients this is a frustrating experience as their dream weight requires a weight loss of nearly 30%. A loss of less than 17% can be a disappointment to women entering a weight-loss program. It is important for the patient and physician to realize that an initial weight loss of 10% should be considered a success; it produces health benefits.

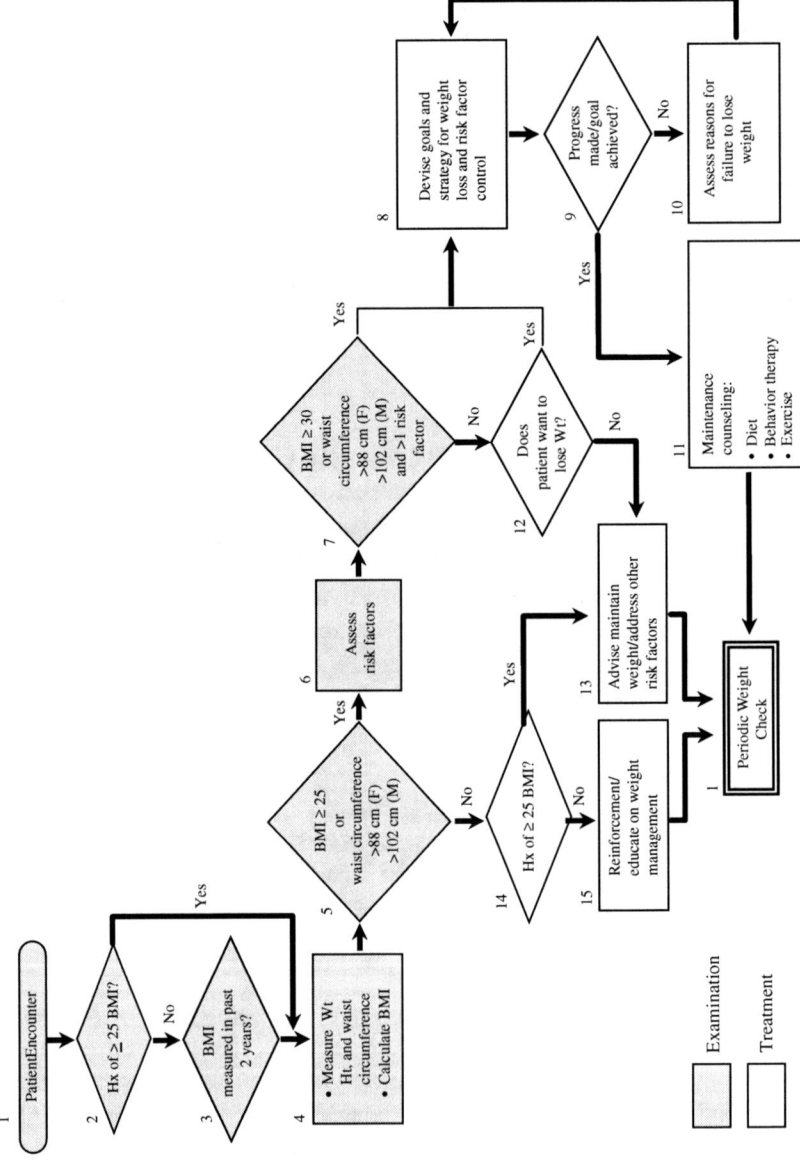

Fig. 2. NHLBI algorithm for diagnosis and treatment of obesity. Adapted from Ref. *(10)*.

8.2. Diet

8.2.1. DIETS LOW IN FAT AND LOW IN ENERGY DENSITY

A variety of diets, including low-fat foods, low-carbohydrate food, or a balanced reduction of all macronutrients, have been used to treat obesity. Table 3 is a compilation of several of these. A meta-analysis of low-fat vs. conventional studies identified five studies lasting up to 18 months. In comparing the weight loss at 6, 12, and 18 months, there was no statistically significant differences from control, leading the authors to conclude that low-fat diets produce weight loss, but not more so than other diets.

Fat is an important component of energy density. If the diet is high in fat or low in water content, then it will have a high energy density (i.e., more calories per gram). In a recent trial Ello-Martin et al. *(17)* reported a weight loss of 7.9 kg after 1 year by feeding a diet with a low energy density. The diet was low in fat diet and rich in fruits and vegetables with a high water content. This underscores the role of energy density of the diet as a factor in weight loss. It is important to appreciate that little weight loss will occur unless the diet induces an energy deficit, but there may be a number of different ways to do that.

8.2.2. LOW-CARBOHYDRATE DIETS

Several controlled trials showed more weight loss with a low-carbohydrate diet than the control diet in the first 6 months but no difference at 12 months. In two head-to-head comparisons of four popular diets, the average weight loss at 6 and 12 months was the same *(18, 19)*. The best predictor of weight loss for each of the diets was the degree of adherence to the diet *(18, 20)*.

8.2.3. PORTION-CONTROLLED DIETS

Portion control is one dietary strategy with promising long-term results. A trial in diabetic patients using portion-controlled diets as part of the lifestyle intervention (Look AHEAD Program) found more weight loss than a lifestyle intervention in another large clinical trial in prediabetic patients that did not include portion control *(21)*.

8.3. Behavior Modification and Lifestyle Interventions

Behavioral modification in lifestyle programs has been an important part of programs for weight loss for more than a quarter of a century. Weight losses have been in the 5–10% range. The newest innovation in the use of lifestyle intervention is to implement it over the Internet. This has shown promising results *(22)*. Behavior modification has a number of components.

Table 3
Comparison of Diet Programs and Eating Plan to Typical American Diet

Type of Diet	Example	General Dietary Characteristics	Comments
Typical American diet		Carb: 50% Protein: 15% Fat: 35% Average of 2200 kcal/day	Low in fruits and vegetables, dairy, and whole grains. High in saturated fat and unrefined carbohydrates
Balanced nutrient, moderate-calorie approach	DASH Diet or diet based on MyPyramid food guide; Commercial plans such as Diet Center, Jenny Craig, NutriSystem, Physician's Weight Loss, Shapedown Pediatric Program, Weight Watchers, Setpoint Diet, Sonoma Diet, Volumetrics	Carb: 55–60% Protein: 15–20% Fat: 20–30% Usually 1200–1700 kcal/day	Based on set pattern of selections from food lists using regular grocery store foods or prepackaged foods supplemented by fresh food items. Low in saturated fat and ample in fruits, vegetables, and fiber. Recommended reasonable weight-loss goal of 0.5–2.0 lb/week. Prepackaged plans may limit food choices. Most recommend exercise plan. Many encourage dietary record keeping. Some offer weight-maintenance plans/support

Very low-fat, High-carbohydrate approach	Ornish Diet (Eat More, Weigh Less), Pritikin Diet, T-factor Diet, Choose to Lose, Fit or Fat	Carb: 65% Protein: 10–20% Fat: ≤10–19% Limited intake of animal protein, nuts, seeds, other fats	Long-term compliance with some plans may be difficult because of low level of fat. Can be low in calcium. Some plans restrict healthful foods (seafood, low-fat dairy, poultry). Some encourage exercise and stress management techniques
Low-carbohydrate, high-protein, high-fat approach	Atkins New Diet Revolution, Protein Power, Stillman Diet (The Doctor's Quick Weight Loss Diet), the Carbohydrate Addict's Diet, Scarsdale Diet	Carb: ≤20% Protein: 25–40% Fat: ≥55–65% Strictly limits carb to less than 100–125 g/day	Promote quick weight loss (much is water loss rather than fat loss). Ketosis causes loss of appetite. Can be too high in saturated fat. Low in carbohydrates, vitamins, minerals, and fiber. Not practical for long term because of rigid diet or restricted food choices
Moderate-carbohydrate, high-protein, moderate-fat approach	The Zone Diet, Sugar Busters, South Beach Diet	Carb: 40–50% Protein: 25–40% Fat: 30–40%	Diet rigid and difficult to maintain. Enough carbohydrates to avoid ketosis. Low in carb; can be low in vitamins and minerals

(Continued)

Table 3
(Continued)

Type of Diet	Example	General Dietary Characteristics	Comments
Novelty diets	Immune Power Diet, Rotation Diet, Cabbage Soup Diet, Beverly Hills Diet, Dr. Phil	Most promote certain foods, or combinations of foods, or nutrients as having unique (magical) qualities	No scientific basis for recommendations
Very low-calorie diets	Health Management Resources (HMR), Medifast, Optifast	Less than 800 kcal/day	Requires medical supervision. For clients with BMI $\geq$30 or BMI $\geq$27 with other risk factors; may be difficult to transition to regular meals
Weight-loss online diets	Cyberdiet, DietWatch, eDiets, Nutrio.com	Meal plans and other tools available online	Recommend reasonable weight loss of 0.5–2.0 lb/week. Most encourage exercise Some offer weight-maintenance plans/support

Adapted from Ref. (16).

First, it is a strategy designed to help people understand their eating behavior, from the triggers that start it to the location, speed, and type of eating, through the consequences of eating and the rewards that can change it. In addition, it consists of strategies to help people develop assertive behavior, learn cognitive techniques for handling their internal discussions, and ways of dealing with stress.

8.4. Exercise

Exercise is important for maintaining weight loss, but when used alone has not been very successful *(23)*. Comparison of people who successfully maintain weight loss and those who do not shows a critical role of exercise. More than 200 min/week provides much more likelihood of maintaining weight loss than lower levels of exercise. Using a pedometer allows counting of steps. Working toward 10,000 steps per day is a good goal.

8.5. Medications

A list of the currently approved medications for the treatment of obesity is shown in Table 4. At present only two medications are approved for long-term treatment, namely sibutramine and orlistat *(1, 24)*, but several others are approved for short-term use.

8.5.1. NORADRENERGIC DRUGS

Phentermine, diethylpropion, phenmetrazine, and phendimetrazine are approved by the FDA for short-term use, usually considered to be up to 12 weeks. All of these drugs probably work by blocking reuptake of norepinephrine into neurons. Phentermine is among the most widely prescribed appetite suppressants. Clinical trials with these drugs are usually short term, which is why they are only approved for short-term use. Phentermine, a noradrenergic drug, has been used in combination with fenfluramine, a drug that blocks reuptake of serotonin and enhances its release. This combination proved to have serious side effects, producing left ventricular atrial regurgitation in up to 25% of the patients *(1)*.

8.5.2. SIBUTRAMINE

Sibutramine significantly reduces the uptake of norepinephrine, serotonin, and dopamine by the pre-ganglionic nerve endings and produces dose-dependent weight loss. The major drawback has been the small increase of blood pressure in some subjects. Two recent trials using sibutramine did not increase blood pressure in overweight hypertensive patients (they were treated for their hypertension with calcium channel blockers in one trial and

Table 4

Drugs That Have Been Approved by the Food and Drug Administration for Treatment of Obesity

Drug	Trade Names	Dosage	DEA Schedule	Cost ($) per Day
Pancreatic Lipase Inhibitor Approved for Long-Term Use				
Orlistat	Xenical	120 mg tid before meals	–	3.56
Norepinephrine–Serotonin Reuptake Inhibitor Approved for Long-Term Use				
Sibutramine	Meridia Reductil	5–15 mg/day	IV	2.98–3.68
Noradrenergic Drugs Approved for Short-Term Use				
Diethylpropion	Tenuate Tepanil	25 mg tid	IV	1.27–1.52
	Tenuate Dospan	75 mg q AM		
Phentermine	Adipex Fastin	15– 37.5 mg/day	IV	0.67–1.60
	Oby-Cap Ionamin slow release	15–30 mg/day		1.75–2.01
Benzphetamine	Didrex	25–50 mg tid	III	1.19–2.38
Phendimetrazine	Bontril Plegine Prelu-2 X-Trozine	17.5–70 mg tid 105 mg qd.	III	1.20–5.25

beta blockers in the other). In a 2-year trial, patients were randomized to sibutramine or placebo after a 6-month lead-in period of weight loss with sibutramine and diet. During the 18-month placebo-controlled period, the patients on sibutramine maintained essentially all of their weight loss. The placebo-treated group, on the other hand, regained nearly 80% of the weight they initially lost *(1, 24)*.

8.5.3. ORLISTAT

Orlistat blocks intestinal lipase and thus enhances fecal loss of fat. There are now four trials with orlistat, each lasting 2 years, and a recent trial lasting

4 years. During the treatment period, patients on orlistat reached a maximum of 10% weight loss compared to about 5% with placebo. At the end of 4 years, there was still a 2.5% difference in favor of orlistat. In the subgroup that had impaired glucose tolerance, conversion to diabetes was reduced by nearly 40%. Orlistat blocks triglyceride digestion and reduces the absorption of cholesterol from the intestine; this accounts in part for the reduced plasma cholesterol found in patients treated with this drug *(1, 24)*.

One clinical trial added orlistat to patients who had been treated with sibutramine for 1 year, but there was no additional weight loss *(see* Ref. *(1))*.

8.5.4. DRUGS NOT APPROVED BY THE FDA FOR TREATING OBESITY

Clinical trials are available for several drugs that are not approved for treatment of obesity. Metformin produced a 1–3 kg weight loss over an average of 2.8 years in the randomized, double-blind, placebo-controlled Diabetes Prevention Program *(21)*.

Bupropion, which is marketed as an anti-depressant and anti-smoking drug, produced significantly more weight loss in a randomized 6-month clinical trial than did placebo; weight loss was maintained for an additional 6 months.

Topiramate, a drug approved for the treatment of epilepsy and migraine headaches, produced significant weight loss and significant side effects during clinical trials. Zonisamide, another anti-epileptic drug, also produced significant weight loss in a 4-month randomized clinical trial. Finally, rimonabant, an antagonist to the CB-1 receptor, administered to patients with dyslipidemia during a 1-year trial produced significant dose-related weight loss, decrease in triglycerides, increase in HDL cholesterol, and reduction in blood pressure. It also showed promise as an anti-smoking drug *(1)*.

8.6. Surgery

Surgical intervention for obesity has become ever more popular *(25, 26)*. The Swedish Obese Subjects Study offered a gastrointestinal operation for obese patients. The control group comprised obese patients who were treated with the best alternatives. Weight loss for many patients exceeded 50 kg; those that were greater than 50% loss of excess weight were considered a success. There was a graded effect of weight change, measured at 2 years and 10 years after the operation, on HDL cholesterol, triglycerides, systolic and diastolic blood pressure, insulin, and glucose. Extrapolating from the degree of improvement in these comorbidities among the patients who lost weight, it cannot be long before this operated group will show a statistically significant improvement in longevity resulting from a treatment aimed specifically at reducing the mass of body fat.

To maintain successful weight loss after bariatric surgery requires that calorie intake remains low. Failure rates, that is, weight regain or inadequate initial weight loss, can occur in up to 40% of some series indicating the importance of commitment to the goals of bariatric surgery – maintaining weight loss.

9. CONCLUSION

The challenge is to provide nonsurgical treatments that have dose-dependent effects on body fat stores, and thus the size of individual fat cells, as a treatment strategy aimed at reducing the complications of the disease of obesity. A comparison of surgically treated and nonsurgically treated patients shows that weight loss improves long-term health outcomes, but at a cost of significant short-term health problems. Effective medications for treatment of obesity, however, are few in number. With a disease that is affecting upward of 30% of the adult population and reducing life expectancy, there would appear to be a bright future for medicinal agents aimed squarely at treating this epidemic.

SUGGESTED FURTHER READING

The following Web sites contain good information or handouts to determine whether following a particular diet will be harmful or not:

The Federal Trade Commission, www.ftc.gov, which includes "Weighing the Evidence in Diet Ads"

The American Heart Association's *Fad Diets*, at www.americanheart.org

REFERENCES

1. Bray GA. The Metabolic Syndrome and Obesity. Humana Press, Totowa, NJ, 2007.
2. Bray GA. Medical consequences of obesity. J Clin Endocrinol Metab 2004; 89: 2583–2589.
3. Spalding KL, Arner E, Westermark PO, et al. Dynamics of fat cell turnover in humans. Nature 2008; 453:783–787.
4. Ogden CL, Carroll MD, Flegal KM. High body mass index for age among US children and adolescents, 2003–2006. JAMA 2008; 299:2401–2405.
5. Finkelstein EA, Fiebelkorn IC, Wang G. State-level estimates of annual medical expenditures attributable to obesity. Obes Res 2004; 12:18–24.
6. Roberts SB, Pi-Sunyer FX, Dreher M, et al. Physiology of fat replacement and fat reduction: effects of dietary fat and fat substitutes on energy regulation. Nutr Rev 1998; 56 (5 Pt 2):S29–41; discussion S-9.

7. Zemel MB, Shi H, Greer B, Dirienzo D, Zemel PC. Regulation of adiposity by dietary calcium. FASEB J 2000; 14:1132–1138.

8. Davies KM, Heaney RP, Recker RR, et al. Calcium intake and body weight. J Clin Endocrinol Metab 2000; 85:4635–4638.

9. Thompson WG, Rostad Holdman N, Janzow DJ, Slezak JM, Morris KL, Zemel MB. Effect of energy-reduced diets high in dairy products and fiber on weight loss in obese adults. Obes Res 2005; 13:1344–1353.

10. Farshchi HR, Taylor MA, Macdonald IA. Beneficial metabolic effects of regular meal frequency on dietary thermogenesis, insulin sensitivity, and fasting lipid profiles in healthy obese women. Am J Clin Nutr 2005; 81:16–24.

11. Goldstone AP, Beales PL. Genetic obesity syndromes. Front Horm Res 2008; 36:37–60.

12. Pagotto U, Marsicano G, Cota D, Lutz B, Pasquali R. The emerging role of the endo-cannabinoid system in endocrine regulation and energy balance. Endocr Rev 2006; 27:73–100.

13. Klein S, Burke LE, Bray GA, Blair S, Allison DB, Pi-Sunyer X, Hong Y, Eckel RH. American Heart Association Council on Nutrition, Physical Activity, and Metabolism. Clinical implications of obesity with specific focus on cardiovascular disease: a statement for professionals from the American Heart Association Council on Nutrition, Physical Activity, and Metabolism: endorsed by the American College of Cardiology Foundation. Circulation 2004; 110:2952–2967.

14. Executive Summary of the Third Report of the National Cholesterol Education Program (NCEP) Expert Panel on Detection, Evaluation, and Treatment of High Blood Choles-terol in Adults (Adult Treatment Panel III). JAMA 2001; 285:2486–2497.

15. Clinical Guidelines on the Identification, Evaluation, and Treatment of Overweight and Obesity in Adults–The Evidence Report. National Institutes of Health. Obes Res 1998; 6(Suppl 2):51S–209S.

16. Boyle MA, Long S. Personal Nutrition. Wadsworth/Cengage Learning, Florence, KY, 2009.

17. Ello-Martin, Roe LS, Ledikwe JH, Beach AM, Rolls BJ. Dietary energy density in the treatment of obesity: a year-long trial comparing 2 weight-loss diets. Am J Clin Nutr 2007; 85:1465–1477.

18. Dansinger ML, Gleason JA, Griffith JL, Selker HP, Schaefer EJ. Comparison of the Atkins, Ornish, Weight Watchers, and Zone diets for weight loss and heart disease risk reduction: a randomized trial. JAMA 2005; 293:43–53.

19. Gardner CD, Kiazand A, Alhassan S, et al. Comparison of the Atkins, Zone, Ornish, and LEARN Diets for change in weight and related risk factors among overweight premenopausal women. JAMA 2007; 297:969–977.

20. Cassady BA, Charboneau NL, Brys EM, Crouse KA, Beitz DC, Wilson T. Comparison of low-carbohydrate diets rich in either red meat or poultry, fish and shellfish on weight loss and plasma lipids. Nutr Metab 2007; 4:23.

21. Knowler WC, Barrett-Connor E, Fowler SE, Hamman RF, Lachin JM, Walker EA, Nathan DM; Diabetes Prevention Program Research Group. Reduction in the incidence of type 2 diabetes with lifestyle intervention or metformin. N Engl J Med 2002; 346: 393–403.

22. Tate DF, Jackvony EH, Wing RR. Effects of Internet behavioral counseling on weight loss in adults at risk for type 2 diabetes: a randomized trial. JAMA 2003;289: 1833–1836.

23. Jakicic JM, Marcus BH, Gallagher KI, Napolitano M, Lang W. Effect of exercise dura-tion and intensity on weight loss in overweight, sedentary women: a randomized trial. JAMA 2003; 290:1323–1330.

24. Rucker D, Padwal R, Li SK, Curioni C, Lau DC. Long term pharmacotherapy for obesity and overweight: updated meta-analysis. BMJ 2007; 335:1194–1199.
25. Buchwald H, Avidor Y, Braunwald E, Jensen MD, Pories W, Fahrbach K, Schoelles K. Bariatric surgery: a systematic review and meta-analysis. JAMA 2004; 292: 1724–1737.
26. Sjostrom L, Narbro K, Sjostrom CD, et al.; Swedish Obese Subjects Study. Effects of bariatric surgery on mortality in Swedish obese subjects. N Engl J Med 2007; 357: 741–752.

23 Nutrition Therapy Effectiveness for the Treatment of Type 1 and Type 2 Diabetes: *Prioritizing Recommendations Based on Evidence*

Marion J. Franz

Key Points

- Medical nutrition therapy for diabetes using a variety of nutrition interventions and multiple encounters can lower hemoglobin A1c by ~1–2% depending on the type and duration of diabetes.
- For persons with type 1 diabetes

  - Identify a usual or convenient schedule of foods/meals and physical activity
  - Integrate insulin therapy into the patient's lifestyle
  - Determine insulin-to-carbohydrate ratios, calculate insulin correction factors, and review goals
  - Provide ongoing support and education

- For persons with type 2 diabetes

  - Focus on metabolic control – glucose, lipids, and blood pressure
  - Implement nutrition interventions for glucose control
  - Encourage physical activity
  - Monitor outcomes to determine if goals are being met or if medications need to be added or changed
  - Provide ongoing support and education

- Research supports consistency in total amount of carbohydrate eaten, fiber intake for lowering of total and LDL cholesterol, no change in protein intake with normal renal function, and reduction in saturated and *trans* fatty acids and dietary cholesterol.
- Research on the glycemic index/load and micronutrient supplementation is controversial.

From: *Nutrition and Health: Nutrition Guide for Physicians*
Edited by: T. Wilson et al. (eds.), DOI 10.1007/978-1-60327-431-9_23,
© Humana Press, a part of Springer Science+Business Media, LLC 2010

Key Words: Type 1 diabetes; type 2 diabetes; nutrition therapy; insulin therapy; glycemic index

1. INTRODUCTION

Based on 2007 data, approximately 24 million people in the United States have diabetes, an increase of more than 3 million in 2 years *(1)*. Up to 25% of people with diabetes are undiagnosed, which is down from 30% 2 years ago. Diabetes prevalence increases with age, affecting approximately 25% of those 60 years and older. The disease is particularly prevalent in ethnic populations, such as African Americans, Hispanic populations (Latinos and Mexican Americans), Native Americans and Alaska Natives, Asian Americans, and Pacific Islanders. While much of the rise in the prevalence of type 2 diabetes is seen in the middle-aged and elderly, there is a trend to an earlier age of onset of diabetes. Evidence shows a rise in type 2 diabetes among younger adults and in recently diagnosed diabetes in the young, between 8 and 45%, is now due to type 2 diabetes *(2)*.

Studies have shown that medical nutrition therapy (MNT) can play an important role in assisting persons with diabetes to meet their glucose, lipid, and blood pressure goals and, therefore, should be a major component in the medical management of diabetes *(3, 4)*.

2. MEDICAL NUTRITION THERAPY FOR DIABETES

Prior to 1994, nutrition recommendations for diabetes attempted to define an "ideal" nutrition prescription that would apply to all persons with the disease. The nutrition prescription was based on a theoretical calculation of required calories and an identified ideal percentage of carbohydrate, protein, and fat. Individualization, although recommended, needed to be done within the confines of this prescription, which did not allow for much, if any, individualization. Not surprisingly, persons with diabetes often found it difficult, if not impossible, to adhere to these recommendations.

In 1994, the American Diabetes Association (ADA) recommended a different approach. The nutrition prescription, instead of being rigid, was to be based on an assessment of lifestyle changes that will assist the individual in achieving and maintaining therapeutic goals and changes that he or she is willing and able to make. For example, if an individual with type 2 diabetes has been eating 3000 kcal, it is unlikely that the individual would adhere for long to a 1200 kcal weight-reduction diet. A more realistic approach would be to negotiate manageable lifestyle changes that lowers energy intake and that are of the individual's choosing. This approach has continued with subsequent ADA recommendations.

Recently, both the ADA and the American Dietetic Association published updated nutrition recommendations and interventions (5, 6) which are similar. Research supports medical nutrition therapy (MNT) as a very effective therapy in reaching treatment goals. Randomized controlled trials and observational studies of diabetes MNT provided by registered dietitians (RDs) have demonstrated decreases in hemoglobin A1c (A1C) of approximately 1–2%, depending on the type and duration of diabetes (4). MNT outcomes are similar to those from anti-diabetic medications. Although MNT has been shown to be effective at any time in the disease process, it appears to have its greatest impact at diagnosis of diabetes. Outcomes of MNT interventions are evident by 6 weeks to 3 months and at that time it should be determined if additional MNT encounters or medication changes, such as the addition of anti-diabetic medications or insulin therapy in type 2 diabetes or changes in insulin regimens in type 1 or type 2 diabetes, are needed.

Central to MNT interventions are multiple encounters to provide education and counseling initially and on a continued basis. Although attempts are often made to identify one approach to diabetes MNT, a single approach does not exist, just as there is no one medication or insulin regimen that applies to all persons with diabetes. A variety of interventions, such as reduced energy/fat intake, carbohydrate counting, simplified meal plan, healthy food choices, individualized meal-planning strategies, exchange lists, insulin-to-carbohydrate ratios, physical activity, and behavioral strategies were implemented in the 16 studies reviewed by the American Dietetic Association (6). Table 1 is a summary of the mean expected metabolic outcomes from MNT on glucose, lipids, and blood pressure (4).

3. PRIORITIZING NUTRITION INTERVENTIONS FOR TYPE 1 AND TYPE 2 DIABETES

Improving health through food choices and physical activity is the basis of all nutrition therapy recommendations for diabetes. However, a primary goal of medical nutrition therapy (MNT) is to attain and maintain blood glucose levels in the normal range or as close to normal as is safely possible. Because changes in lifestyle can have an immediate impact on glycemia, this is often the first focus of MNT. But MNT must also focus on the effect of lifestyle modifications on lipid and lipoprotein profiles and blood pressure so as to prevent and treat the cardiovascular complications associated with diabetes. Table 2 lists the ADA goals for glucose, lipids, and blood pressure (7).

Table 1
Effectiveness of Medical Nutrition Therapy

Endpoint	Expected Outcome	When to Evaluate
Glycemic Control		6 wk to 3 mo
A1C	1–2% (15–22%) decrease	
Plasma fasting glucose	50 mg/dL (2.78 mmol/L) decrease	
Lipids		6 wk; if goals are
Total cholesterol	24–32 mg/dL	not achieved,
LDL cholesterol	(0.62–0.82 mmol/L)	intensify medical
Triglycerides	[10–16%] decrease	nutrition therapy
HDL cholesterol	19–25 mg/dL	and evaluate
With no exercise	(0.46–0.65 mmol/L)	again in 6 wk
With exercise	[12–16%] decrease	
	15–17 mg/dL	
	(0.17–0.19 mmol/L)	
	[8%] decrease	
	3 mg/dL (0.08 mmol/L)	
	[7%] decrease	
	No decrease	
Blood Pressure (in hypertensive patients)	Decrease of 5 mm Hg in systolic and 2 mm Hg in diastolic	Measured at every medical visit

Source: Reprinted from Ref. (4) with permission.

3.1. Type 1 Diabetes Nutrition Interventions

3.1.1. IDENTIFY A USUAL OR CONVENIENT SCHEDULE OF FOOD/MEALS AND PHYSICAL ACTIVITY

The first priority for persons requiring insulin therapy is to integrate an insulin regimen into the patient's lifestyle. The food/meal plan is developed first and is based on the individual's appetite, preferred foods, and usual schedule of meals and physical activity. After the RD, working with the patient, develops a food plan, this information is shared with the professional determining the insulin regimen.

3.1.2. INTEGRATE INSULIN THERAPY INTO THE PATIENT'S LIFESTYLE

The preferred type of insulin regimen duplicates the normal physiological responses of insulin. Generally this consists of a basal insulin such as

Table 2
Glucose, Lipids, and Blood Pressure Recommendations for Adults with Diabetes

Glycemic Control	
A1C	<7.0%[a]
Preprandial plasma glucose	5.0–7.2 mmol/L (90–130 mg/dL)
Postprandial plasma glucose	<10.0 mmol/L (180 mg/dL)
Blood Pressure	<130/80 mm Hg
Lipids	
LDL cholesterol	<2.6 mmol/L (<100 mg/dL)
Triglycerides	<1.7 mmol/L (<150 mg/dL)
HDL cholesterol	>1.1 mmol/L (>40 mg/dL)[b]

[a]Referenced to a nondiabetic range of 4.0–6.0% using a DCCT-based assay.
[b]For women, it has been suggested that the HDL goal be increased by 10 mg/dL.
Source: From Ref. *(7)*

glargine or determir and a mealtime bolus insulin such as a rapid-acting insulin (lispro, aspart, or aprida) or insulin pump therapy. These types of therapy provide increased flexibility in timing and frequency of meals, amounts of carbohydrate eaten at meals, and timing of physical activity *(8)*.

3.1.3. DETERMINE INSULIN-TO-CARBOHYDRATE RATIOS

Insulin-to-carbohydrate ratios are used to adjust the bolus insulin doses based on the planned carbohydrate content of the meals. Insulin-to-carbohydrate ratios can be determined by either having the individual *(1)* eat a consistent amount of carbohydrate in a meal, adjust the bolus insulin to obtain postmeal glucose goals, and then determine the ratio, or *(2)* start with an estimated ratio (often 1 unit of rapid-acting insulin for every planned 15 g carbohydrate intake) and adjust it based on resulting postmeal glucose results. The insulin-to-carbohydrate ratio can also be determined by a statistically established formula: 500 divided by the daily total insulin dose *(8)*. For example, an individual taking 50 units of insulin per day would have an insulin-to-carbohydrate ratio of 10 (1 unit of insulin per 10 g carbohydrate). Usually the insulin-to-carbohydrate ratio is the same for all meals but may be slightly higher at breakfast.

3.1.4. CALCULATE INSULIN CORRECTION FACTOR

Individuals with type 1 diabetes also need a correction bolus algorithm to correct out-of-range glucose values *(8)*. The insulin correction or insulin sensitivity factor is defined as the estimated number of mg/dL (mmol/L) 1 unit of a rapid-acting insulin will lower blood glucose over 2–4 h. To determine the correction factor 1700 is divided by the daily total insulin dose. For example, an individual taking 50 units of insulin per day would have a correction factor of 35 (1700 divided by 50 = 35). In this case, 1 unit of insulin lowers the patient's blood glucose by approximately 35 mg/dL (2 mmol/L). The correction factor is added to the premeal bolus dose to optimize postmeal glucose levels. Because of overlapping dosing effects, at least 4 h should elapse between correction factor doses.

3.1.5. REVIEW GOALS

For most people, a mid-target premeal glucose is often 100 mg/dL (5.5 mmol/L). However, individuals prone to hypoglycemia may have a higher target (120 mg/dL [6.7 mmol/L]), and pregnant women may have a lower target (80 mg/dL [4.4 mmol/L]) (7). And although carbohydrate counting is emphasized, total energy intake cannot be ignored. Weight gain is common as treatment intensifies; therefore, individuals must also be knowledgeable about the protein, fat, and calorie content of foods.

3.2. Type 2 Diabetes Nutrition Interventions

3.2.1. FOCUS ON METABOLIC CONTROL

Type 2 diabetes is characterized by insulin resistance and insulin deficiency. In most individuals, insulin resistance begins and progresses many years before the development of diabetes. However, as long as the beta cells produce adequate insulin to overcome the resistance, the blood glucose level remains normal. Impaired beta-cell function must be present before hyperglycemia develops. By the time diabetes develops as much as 50% of beta-cell function has been lost (9). Therefore, it is essential that effective therapy lower elevated blood glucose concentrations as early as possible to slow beta-cell exhaustion and to prevent the deleterious effects of hyperglycemia. As a consequence of the progressive loss of beta-cell secretory function, persons with diabetes usually require more medication(s) over time to maintain the same level of glycemic control and eventually exogenous insulin will be required. Medical nutrition therapy (MNT) continues to be an important component of diabetes management but changes over the natural progression of the disease.

Whereas one of the goals for prevention of diabetes is weight loss, for treatment the goal of nutrition therapy shifts to control of glucose, lipid, and blood pressure. Although moderate weight loss may be beneficial for some individuals, especially after new diagnosis of type 2 diabetes (10), for many it is too late for weight loss to dramatically improve hyperglycemia

(11, 12). Furthermore, it is noteworthy that not all individuals with type 2 diabetes are overweight or obese. As medications – including insulin – need to be combined with nutrition therapy, weight gain often occurs and thus preventing this weight gain becomes important. However, glycemic control must still take precedence over concern about weight.

3.2.2. IMPLEMENT NUTRITION INTERVENTIONS FOR GLUCOSE CONTROL

Teaching individuals how to make appropriate food choices (often by means of carbohydrate counting) and using data from blood glucose monitoring to evaluate short-term effectiveness are important components of successful MNT for type 2 diabetes. Many individuals with type 2 diabetes also have dyslipidemia and hypertension, so decreasing intakes of saturated and *trans* fats, cholesterol, and sodium should also be a priority.

Persons with diabetes can benefit from basic information about carbohydrates – what foods contain carbohydrates and how many servings to select for meals (and snacks if desired). For purposes of carbohydrate counting foods are placed into three groups: carbohydrate, meat and meat substitutes, and fat. The carbohydrate list is composed of starches, fruits, milk, and sweets; one serving is the amount of food that contains 15 g of carbohydrate. Table 3 lists some examples of a carbohydrate serving. Carbohydrate

Table 3
Carbohydrate Servings[a]

Starch	Milk
1 slice of bread (1 oz)	1 cup skim/reduced-fat milk
1/3 cup cooked rice or pasta	2/3 cup fat-free fruited yogurt
3/4 cup dry cereal	sweetened with nonnutritive
4–6 crackers	sweetener (6 oz)
$\frac{1}{2}$ large baked potato with skin (3 oz)	
$\frac{3}{4}$ oz pretzels, potato, or tortilla chips	
Fruit	*Sweets and Desserts*
1 small fresh fruit (4 oz)	2 small cookies
$\frac{1}{2}$ cup fruit juice	1 tablespoon jam, honey, syrup
$\frac{1}{4}$ cup dried fruit	$\frac{1}{2}$ cup ice cream, frozen yogurt, or sherbet

[a]One serving contains 15 g of carbohydrate.

counting does not mean that meat and fat portions can be ignored. Individuals with diabetes must also know the approximate number of meat and fat servings they should select for meals and snacks. Weight control is important as is the maintenance of a healthy balance of food choices.

The first decision for food and meal planning is the total number of carbohydrate servings the person with diabetes chooses to eat at meals or for snacks. Women with type 2 diabetes often do well with three or four carbohydrate servings per meal and one to two for a snack. Men with type 2 diabetes may need four to five carbohydrate servings per meal and one to two for a snack.

Learning how to use Nutrition Facts on food labels is also useful. First, individuals should take note of the serving size and the total amount (grams) of carbohydrate. The total grams of carbohydrate are then divided by 15 to determine the number of carbohydrate servings in the serving size.

When insulin is required, consistency in timing of meals and of their carbohydrate content becomes important. The administration of basal insulin once or twice a day may suffice for persons with type 2 diabetes who still have significant endogenous insulin. Once-daily glargine, determir, or NPH at bedtime or a premixed insulin before the evening meals are commonly used regimens *(13)*. The rationale is that supplementing with overnight insulin will control fasting hyperglycemia. However, a concern with evening NPH is nocturnal hypoglycemia. Oral agents may be continued during the day to prevent worsening of daytime glycemia. Many individuals with type 2 diabetes will eventually require an insulin regimen that better mimics the release of endogenous insulin in response to food intake in persons without diabetes.

3.2.3. Encourage Physical Activity

Low cardiorespiratory fitness and physical inactivity are independent predictors of all-cause mortality in type 2 diabetes, regardless of weight *(14)*. Indeed, it was reported that increased body mass index and body fatness did not increase mortality risk in fit men with type 2 diabetes *(15)*. This highlights the importance of clinicians giving greater attention to counseling for increasing physical activity and improving fitness in persons with diabetes, primarily for the benefits associated with enhanced cardiorespiratory fitness that are independent of weight.

At least 150 min/week of moderate-intensity aerobic physical activity is recommended. In the absence of contraindications, performing resistance training three times per week is also encouraged *(7)*.

3.2.4. MONITOR OUTCOMES

Outcomes must be identified and the effectiveness of nutrition therapy measured. Individuals with diabetes need to have identified target goals. Blood glucose monitoring is done to determine if progress is being made or achieved toward these goals. The A1C test is done at least twice a year in patients who are meeting treatment goals and quarterly in patients whose therapy has changed or who are not meeting glycemic goals *(7)*. Lipids are generally measured annually and blood pressure at every routine diabetes visit. If goals are not being achieved, medications may need to be added or adjusted.

4. SUPPORT AND CONTINUING EDUCATION

Successful self-management of diabetes by the patient is an ongoing process of problem solving, adjustment, and readjustment. Individuals must be able to anticipate and deal with the wide variety of decisions they face on a daily basis. And just as support from family and friends is important, continuing education and support from professionals is also essential. Structured programs with consistent follow-up contacts assist individuals to achieve lifestyle goals and to maintain what are often challenging lifestyle changes *(16)*.

5. MACRO- AND MICRONUTRIENTS

5.1. Carbohydrate

Carbohydrates are addressed first as it is the balance between carbohydrate intake and available insulin that determines postprandial glucose response and because carbohydrate is the major determinant of mealtime insulin doses. Foods containing carbohydrate – grains, fruits, vegetables, legumes, low-fat/skim milk – are important components of a healthful diet and should be included in the food/meal plan of persons with diabetes. This recommendation reflects the concern that low-carbohydrate diets eliminate many foods that are important for all persons to eat as part of a healthy lifestyle.

5.1.1. AMOUNT AND TYPE OF CARBOHYDRATE

There is strong evidence to suggest that in regard to the effects of carbohydrate on glucose concentrations, the total amount of carbohydrate in meals (or snacks) is more important than the source (starch or sugar) or the type (low or high glycemic index). Numerous studies have reported that when subjects are allowed to choose from a variety of starches and sugars, the glycemic response is similar, as long as the total amounts of carbohydrate is kept constant. Consistency in carbohydrate intake is also associated with glycemic control *(5, 6)*.

Research does not support any ideal percentage of energy from macronutrients for persons with diabetes *(6)* and it is unlikely that one such combination of macronutrients exists *(5)*. Macronutrient intake should be based on the Dietary Reference Intakes (DRI) for healthy adults.

5.1.2. GLYCEMIC INDEX

Although different carbohydrates do have different glycemic responses (glycemic index, GI), there has been limited evidence to show long-term glycemic benefit when low GI diets versus high GI diets are implemented. Benefits of a low GI diet are complicated by differing definitions of "high GI" or "low GI" foods or diets, and short-term studies comparing high versus low GI diets report mixed effects on A1C *(6)*. However, Wolever et al. *(17)* conducted a multicenter, 12 mo, randomized controlled trial comparing the effects of a high-GI, low-GI, or low-carbohydrate, high-monounsaturated fat diet in subjects with type 2 diabetes managed by nutrition therapy. At study end, A1C, lipids, and body weight did not differ significantly between diets. Previous meta-analyses of studies showing benefit were based primarily on studies lasting less than 3 months. The Wolever study also found a temporary reduction in A1C with the low GI diet which was not sustained long term.

Interindividual variability and intra-individual reproducibility of GI is a concern. For example, mean ± standard deviation GI after white bread in 23 subjects for the first test was 78 ± 73; coefficient of variation (CV) 94% *(18)*. In subjects who completed three tests ($n = 14$) the GI was 78 ± 39 (CV of 50%) with GI values for white bread ranging from 44 to 132.

Furthermore, GI measures the incremental area under the curve (AUC) for blood glucose response over a 2 h period, not how rapidly blood glucose levels increase as emphasized in diet books promoting the use of low GI foods. Peak glucose responses for single foods or meals occur at similar times whether they are high or low GI.

5.1.3. FIBER

Recommendations for fiber intake for people with diabetes are similar to the recommendations for the general public (DRI: 14 g/1000 kcal). Diets containing 44–50 g fiber daily are reported to improve glycemia, but more usual fiber intakes (up to 24 g/day) have not shown beneficial effects on glycemia. It is unknown if free-living individuals can daily consume the amount of fiber needed to improve glycemia. However, diets high in total and soluble fiber, as part of cardioprotective nutrition therapy, have been shown to reduce total cholesterol by 2–3% and LDL cholesterol up to 7% *(6)*. Therefore, foods containing 25–30 g/day of fiber, with special emphasis on soluble fiber sources (7–13 g) are to be encouraged.

5.2. Protein

There is no evidence to suggest that usual intake of protein (15–20% of energy intake) be changed in people who do not have renal disease *(5, 6)*. Although protein has an acute effect on insulin secretion, usual protein intake in long-term studies has minimal effects on glucose, lipids, and insulin concentrations.

In persons with diabetic nephropathy, a protein intake of 1 g or less per kg body weight per day is recommended. It is interesting to note that in persons with diabetes and nephropathy, diets with less than 1 g protein/kg/day have been shown to improve albuminuria but have not been shown to have significant effects on glomerular filtration rates *(6)*. For persons with late-stage diabetic nephropathy, a protein intake of ~ 0.7 g/kg/day has been associated with hypoalbuminemia (an indicator of malnutrition). Therefore, hypoalbuminemia and energy intake must be monitored and changes in protein and energy intake made to correct deficits.

Protein is probably the most misunderstood nutrient with inaccurate advice frequently given to persons with diabetes. Although patients are often told that 50–60% of protein becomes glucose and enters the bloodstream 3–4 h after it is eaten, research documents the inaccuracy of this statement. Although nonessential amino acids undergo gluconeogenesis in subjects with controlled diabetes, the glucose produced does not enter the general circulation *(19)*. It is often suggested to patients that adding protein to a meal or snack will slow the absorption of carbohydrate but several studies show that this is not the case. If differing amounts of protein are added to meals or snacks, the peak glucose response is not affected by the addition of protein. There is also no evidence that adding protein to bedtime snacks is helpful or will assist in the immediate treatment of hypoglycemia or prevent blood glucose levels from dropping again after the initial treatment.

5.3. Dietary Fat

Cardioprotective nutrition interventions for prevention and treatment of cardiovascular disease include reduction in saturated and *trans*fats and dietary cholesterol. This topic is discussed in more detail in Chapter 25. Nutrition goals for persons with diabetes are the same as for persons with preexisting CVD, as the two groups have equivalent cardiovascular risk. Thus, saturated fats <7% of total energy, minimal intake of *trans* fats, and cholesterol intake <200 mg/day are recommended *(5)*. Either polyunsaturated or monounsaturated fats can be substituted for saturated fats. Consumption of *n*–3 fats from fish or from supplements has been shown to reduce adverse CVD outcomes *(5)*. Therefore, two or more servings of fish per week (with the exception of commercially fried fish fillets) are recommended. In persons with type 2 diabetes, intake of ~2 g/day of plant sterols and stanols has been shown to lower total and LDL cholesterol. If products containing plant sterols are used, they should displace, rather than be added to, the diet to avoid weight gain.

5.4. Micronutrients

There is no evidence of benefit from vitamin or mineral supplementation in persons with diabetes (compared with the general population) who do not have underlying deficiencies *(5)*. It is recommended that health professionals focus on nutrition counseling for acquiring daily vitamin and mineral requirements from natural foods sources and a balanced diet rather than micronutrient supplementation. Research including long-term trials is needed to assess the safety and potentially beneficial role of chromium, magnesium, and antioxidant supplements and other complementary therapies in the management of diabetes. In select groups such as the elderly, pregnant or lactating women, strict vegetarians, or those on calorie-restricted diets, a multi-vitamin supplement may be needed. Routine supplementation with antioxidants, such as vitamins E and C and carotene, has not proven beneficial and is not advised because of concern related to long-term safety *(5)*.

5.5. Alcohol

Recommendations for alcohol intake are similar to those for the general public. This topic is discussed in Chapter 9. If individuals with diabetes choose to use alcohol, daily intake should be limited to one drink per day or less for women and two drinks per day or less for men *(7)*. One drink is defined as a 12 oz beer, 5 oz wine, or 1.5 oz of distilled spirits, each of which contains ~15 g alcohol. Moderate amounts of alcohol when ingested with food have minimal, if any, effect on blood glucose and insulin concentrations and the type of beverage consumed does not appear to make a difference. For individuals using insulin or insulin secretagogues, if alcohol is consumed, it should be consumed with food to prevent hypoglycemia.

Observational studies suggest a U- or J-shaped association with moderate consumption of alcohol (~15–30 g/day). Moderate alcohol consumption is associated with a decreased incidence of heart disease in persons with diabetes *(20)*. However, chronic excessive ingestion of alcohol (>3 drinks/day) can cause deterioration of glucose control with the effects from excess alcohol being reversed after abstinence for 3 days. In epidemiological studies moderate alcohol intake is associated with favorable changes in lipids, including triglycerides.

Because the available evidence is primarily observational, it does not support recommending alcohol consumption to persons who do not currently drink. Occasional use of alcoholic beverages can be considered an addition to the regular meal plan, and no food should be omitted.

6. SUMMARY

There have been major changes in nutrition recommendations and therapy for diabetes over the past decade. MNT is essential for effective management of diabetes, but to be successful it involves an ongoing process. Monitoring of glucose, A1C, lipids, and blood pressure is essential in order to assess the outcomes of nutrition therapy interventions and/or to determine if changes in medication(s) are necessary. It is important that all health-care providers understand nutrition issues and guide the individual's efforts by promoting and reinforcing the importance of lifestyle modifications, and by providing support for the lifestyle intervention process.

SUGGESTED FURTHER READING

American Diabetes Association. MyFoodAdvisor^{TM}. Available at: www.diabetes.org/food-nutrition-lifestyle/nutrition/my-food-advisor.jsp.

Franz MJ, Bantle JP, Beebe CA, et al. Evidence-based nutrition principles and recommendations for the treatment and prevention of diabetes and related complications (Technical Review). Diabetes Care 2002; 25:148–198.

Sigal RJ, Kenny GP, Wasserman DH, et al. Physical activity/exercise and type 2 diabetes (Technical Review). Diabetes Care 2004; 27:2518–2539.

Klein S, Sheard NF, Pi-Sunyer X, et al. Weight management through lifestyle modification for the prevention and management of type 2 diabetes: rationale and strategies: a statement of the American Diabetes Association, the North American Association for the Study of Obesity, and the American Society for Clinical Nutrition. Diabetes Care 2004; 27: 2067–2073.

Clement S, Braithwaite SS, Magee MF, et al. The American Diabetes Association Diabetes in Hospitals Writing Committee. Management of diabetes and hyperglycemia in hospitals. Diabetes Care 2004; 27:553–591.

REFERENCES

1. Centers for Disease Control and Prevention. National Diabetes Fact Sheet, 2008. Atlanta, GA: Department of Health and Human Services, Centers for Disease Control and Prevention, 2008. Available at: www.cdc.gov/diabetes. Accessed October 21, 2008.

2. Alberti G, Zimmet P, Shaw J, et al. Type 2 diabetes in the young: the evolving epidemic. Diabetes Care 2004; 27:1798–1811.

3. Franz MJ, Boucher JL, Green-Pastors J, Powers MA. Evidence-based nutrition practice guidelines for diabetes and scope and standards of practice. J Am Diet Assoc 2008; 108:S52–S58.

4. Pastors JG, Franz MJ, Warshaw H, et al. How effective is medical nutrition therapy in diabetes care? J Am Diet Assoc 2003; 103:827–831.
5. American Diabetes Association. Nutrition recommendations and interventions for diabetes (Position Statement). Diabetes Care 2008; 31(suppl 1):S61–S78.
6. American Dietetic Association. Diabetes Type 1 and Type 2 Evidence-Based Nutrition Practice Guidelines for Adults. Available at: http://www.adaevidencelibrary.com/topic.cfm?cat=3252. Accessed August 18, 2008.
7. American Diabetes Association. Executive summary: standards of medical care in diabetes – 2008. Diabetes Care 2008; 31(Suppl 1):S5–S54.
8. Kaufman FR. Medical Management of Type 1 Diabetes. 5th ed. American Diabetes Association, Alexandria, VA, 2008.
9. Weyer C, Bogardus C, Mott DM, Pratley RE. The natural history of insulin secretory dysfunction and insulin resistance in the pathogenesis of type 2 diabetes. J Clin Invest 1999; 104:787–794.
10. Feldstein AD, Nichols GA, Smith DH, et al. Weight change in diabetes and glycemic and blood pressure control. Diabetes Care 2008; 31:1960–1965.
11. Watts NB, Spanheimer RG, DiGirolamo M, et al. Prediction of glucose response to weight loss in patients with non-insulin-dependent diabetes mellitus. Arch Intern Med 1990; 150:803–806.
12. Franz MJ. The dilemma of weight loss in diabetes. Diabetes Spectrum 2007; 20: 133–136.
13. Riddle MC, Rosenstock J, Gerich J. Insulin Glargine 4002 Study Investigators. The Treat-to-Target Trial: randomized addition of glargine or human NPH insulin to oral therapy of type 2 diabetic patients. Diabetes Care 2003; 26:3080–3086.
14. Wei M, Gibbons LW, Kampert JG, et al. Low cardiorespiratory fitness and physical activity as predictors of mortality in men with type 2 diabetes. Ann Intern Med 2000; 132:605–611.
15. Church TS, Cheng YJ, Earnest CP, et al. Exercise capacity and body composition as predictors of mortality among men with diabetes. Diabetes Care 2004; 27:83–88.
16. Franz MJ. Facilitating lifestyle behavioral changes. Rev Endocrinol 2008; 2(8):44–48.
17. Wolever TMS, Gibbs Al, Mehling C, et al. The Canadian Trial of Carbohydrates in Diabetes (CCD), a 1 yr controlled trial of low-glycemic index carbohydrate in type 2 diabetes: no effect on glycated hemoglobin but reduction in C-reactive protein. Am J Clin Nutr 2008: 87:114–125.
18. Vega-López S, Ausman LM, Griffith JL, Lichtenstein AH. Interindividual variability and intra-individual reproducibility of glycemic index values for commercial white bread. Diabetes Care 2007; 30:1412–1417.
19. Gannon MC, Nuttall JA, Damberg G, et al. Effect of protein ingestion on the glucose appearance rate in people with type 2 diabetes. J Clin Endocrinol Metab 2001; 86: 1040–1047.
20. Howard AA, Arnsten JH, Gourevitch MN. Effect of alcohol consumption on diabetes mellitus: a systematic review. Ann Intern Med 2004; 140:211–219.

24 Lifestyle Interventions to Stem the Tide of Type 2 Diabetes

Marion J. Franz

Key Points

- Prevention of obesity is one of the most important steps for diabetes prevention.
- For persons with pre-diabetes, encourage a moderate and maintainable weight loss and provide individuals with support for behavioral changes.
- For persons with pre-diabetes, recommend a cardioprotective energy-restricted diet and 150 min/week of physical activity.
- Some support is available for reducing fat intake, especially saturated fats and increasing intake of whole grains and fiber; glycemic index/load and alcohol recommendations are less clear.
- For persons at very high risk for diabetes, in combination with lifestyle interventions, metformin and acarbose may be considered.

Key Words: Type 2 diabetes; prevention of diabetes; lifestyle interventions; glycemic index

1. INTRODUCTION

Worldwide, the number of persons with diabetes and those who are at risk for diabetes is increasing at an alarming rate, largely driven by the rising prevalence of obesity and inactivity. Of concern in the United States are the approximately 57 million people who have pre diabetes and the greater than 50 million with metabolic syndrome *(1)*. These individuals are at high risk for conversion to type 2 diabetes and for cardiovascular disease if lifestyle prevention strategies are not implemented.

Preventing obesity is a high priority for the prevention of type 2 diabetes as many individuals are overweight or obese at the onset. However, the disease can also be diagnosed in nonobese individuals, while many obese

From: *Nutrition and Health: Nutrition Guide for Physicians*
Edited by: T. Wilson et al. (eds.), DOI 10.1007/978-1-60327-431-9_24,
© Humana Press, a part of Springer Science+Business Media, LLC 2010

people never develop it. Therefore, it is likely that genetic predisposition is also an important factor in the development of type 2 diabetes.

Risk factors, both nonmodifiable (genetics and aging) and modifiable (central obesity, sedentary lifestyle, and high-fat diets), have been identified as contributing to insulin resistance, a common factor in the development of diabetes and cardiovascular disease. However, elevated plasma free fatty acids (lipotoxicity) may also be a common denominator and this is generally associated with obesity and in particular, intraabdominal obesity. Measurement of waist circumference may help identify individuals at risk.

Large clinical trials have demonstrated the role of nutrition therapy including both modest weight loss and increased physical activity in the prevention or delay of type 2 diabetes (2–5).

2. DIAGNOSIS OF PRE-DIABETES

Hyperglycemia that is not sufficient to meet the diagnostic criteria for diabetes is classified as either impaired fasting glucose (IFG) or impaired glucose tolerance (IGT). IFG and IGT have been officially termed "pre-diabetes" (6). The following are criteria used for diagnosis:

- IFG = fasting plasma glucose (FPG) 100 mg/dL (5.6 mmol/L) to 125 mg/dL (6.9 mmol/L)
- IGT = 2-h plasma glucose 140 mg/dL (7.8 mmol/L) to 199 mg/dL (11.0 mmol/L)

3. PREVENTION TRIALS

Based on evidence from earlier epidemiological and intervention studies suggesting the benefits of lifestyle interventions for the prevention of type 2 diabetes, four larger and well-designed trials were undertaken – the Finnish Diabetes Prevention Study (2), the Diabetes Prevention Program (DPP) (3), the Indian Diabetes Prevention Programme (4), and a Japanese diabetes prevention study (5).

In the Finnish study, subjects in the control group were given general information on diet and exercise, whereas each subject in the intervention group received detailed counseling by dietitians on how to reduce weight, as well as total intake of fat and saturated fat, and how to increase intake of fiber and physical activity. After 3.2 years of follow-up the lifestyle intervention was associated with a significant reduction in weight (–4.2 vs. –0.8 kg) and waist circumference (–4.4 vs. –1.3 cm) compared to the control group and a significant reduction in 2-h plasma glucose and serum insulin, triglycerides, and blood pressure. The risk of developing diabetes was reduced by 58% in the intervention group *(2)*. At 7-yr follow-up, participants in the intervention group still had a 43% lower diabetes risk *(7)*. This was the first study to report that an intensive lifestyle program in people with pre-diabetes results in continued lifestyle changes, which remained even after the individual lifestyle counseling had stopped.

In the DPP, conducted in 27 centers around the United States, subjects were randomly assigned to one of three groups: (1) an intensive lifestyle change emphasizing a 7% weight loss and 150 min/week of physical activity, (2) metformin (850 mg/day for 1 month, increasing to 850 mg bid), or (3) a placebo group. After 2.8 years of follow-up, average weight loss was 5.6, 2.1, and 0.1 kg in the lifestyle, metformin, and placebo groups, respectively, and 58% of the participants in the lifestyle arm were exercising 150 min/week. Compared with placebo, the incidence of diabetes was reduced by 58% by lifestyle and 31% by metformin *(3)*. The lifestyle intervention also resulted in improvements in hypertension, triglycerides, and HDL cholesterol.

Table 1
Diabetes Prevention Trials: Interventions and Effectiveness

Study	Total n Randomized	Population	Duration (yr)	Intervention (Daily Dose)	Relative Risk
Finnish Diabetes Prevention Study	522	IGT, BMI ≥ 25	3.2	Individual diet/exercise	0.42
Diabetes Prevention Program	2161	IGT, BMI ≥24, FPG >95 mg/dL (5.3 mmol/L)	3	Individual diet/exercise	0.42
Chinese Da Qing Study	577	IGT	6	Group diet/exercise	0.62
Japanese Trial	458	IGT (men), BMI = 24	4	Individual diet/exercise	0.33
Indian Diabetes Prevention Program	531	IGT	2.5	Individual diet/exercise	0.71
Diabetes Prevention Program	2161	IGT, BMI ≥24, FPG >95 mg/dL (5.3 mmol/L)	2.8	Metformin (1700 mg)	0.69

(Continued)

Table 1
(Continued)

Study	Total n Randomized	Population	Duration (yr)	Intervention (Daily Dose)	Relative Risk
Indian Diabetes Prevention Program	531	IGT	2.5	Metformin (500 mg)	0.74
STOP NIDDM: Study to Prevent Non-Insulin Dependent Diabetes	1429	IGT, FPG >100 mg/dL (5.6 mmol/L)	3.2	Acarbose (300 mg)	0.75
XENDOS: Xenical in the Prevention of Diabetes in Obese Subjects	3305	BMI >30	4	Orlistat (360 mg)	0.63
TRIPOD: Troglitazone in Prevention of Diabetes	266	Previous GDM	2.5	Troglitazone (400 mg)	0.45
DREAM	5269	IGT or IFG	3	Rosiglitazone (8 mg)	0.40

IGT, impaired glucose tolerance; FFG, fasting plasma glucose; BMI, body mass index; GDM, gestational diabetes mellitus
Source: Adapted from Ref. *(8)*.

Six randomized controlled trials have examined the effects of pharmacological agents on the prevention of type 2 diabetes *(8)*. Metformin, as noted above reduced the incidence of diabetes by 31%, acarbose by 25%, troglitazone by 55%, xenical by 37%, and rosiglitazone by 60%. The American Diabetes Association recommendations state that in addition to lifestyle counseling, metformin may be considered in those who are at very high risk (combined impaired fasting glucose and impaired glucose tolerance) and who are obese and under 60 years of age *(6)*. The American Association of Clinical Endocrinologists recommends that for persons with pre-diabetes at particularly high risk, pharmacologic glycemic treatment (metformin and acarbose) may be considered in addition to lifestyle strategies. They note that thiazolidinediones also reduce risk but safety concerns include congestive heart failure or fractures *(9)*. Table 1 summarizes therapies proven to be effective in diabetes prevention trials *(8)*.

4. LIFESTYLE INTERVENTION RECOMMENDATIONS

Three lifestyle interventions are consistently associated with decreased risk of type 2 diabetes in the prevention trials: moderate weight loss, regular physical activity, and frequent participant contact. Observational studies provide support for reduced dietary fat and an increase in whole grain and dietary fiber interventions. The role of the glycemic index/glycemic load and alcohol is unclear.

4.1. Encourage a Moderate and Maintainable Weight Loss and Provide Participant Support

In the past, achieving an ideal body mass index (BMI) was often recommended for participants in weight loss programs. But it has become clear that clinical improvements begin to appear with relatively small amounts of weight loss (approximately 5–7%), suggesting the importance of emphasizing weight loss for health benefits rather than for cosmetic reasons *(10)*.

To answer the question about expected weight loss from weight loss interventions, a systematic review of randomized clinical weight loss trials with a minimum duration of 1 yr was performed *(11)*. A mean weight loss of 5–8.5 kg (5–9%) was observed during the first 6 months from interventions involving a reduced-energy diet (and exercise) and/or weight loss medications, with weight plateaus at approximately 6 months. In studies extending to 48 months, a mean 3–6 kg (3–6%) of weight loss was maintained with none of the interventions experiencing weight regain to baseline *(11)*. In contrast, advice-only and exercise alone intervention groups experienced minimal weight loss at any time point. Study participants in the clinical trials appeared to benefit from the continued professional support they received.

Changes in body weight in the DPP were similar to the weight loss/maintenance outcomes reported above. Participants in the intensive lifestyle group experienced a mean weight loss of 7 kg at 6 months, experienced a weight plateau to 12 months, with a gradual weight regain; the average weight loss was 5.6 kg at study end *(3)*. Considerable support from well-trained staff was needed to achieve this weight loss outcome.

4.2. Recommend a Cardioprotective, Energy-Restricted Diet

The primary diet intervention in the diabetes prevention trials was a lower energy, lower fat diet. Basic behavioral strategies that are core and are used in nearly all weight loss interventions include self-monitoring, goal setting, stimulus control, reinforcement, and cognitive change. Other behavioral strategies shown to be beneficial are problem solving, relapse prevention, and stress management. Social support from partners, family, friends, or others, along with the support of health professionals, has also been shown to be helpful.

An area of controversy is the macronutrient content of the energy-reduced diet. Low-carbohydrate, high-protein/high-fat diets have been shown to achieve greater short-term (6 months) weight loss, but not long-term (12 months), than a low-fat diet *(12)*. Recently, a 2-yr weight loss trial reported a mean weight loss of 3.3, 4.6, and 5.5 kg in completers of a low-fat, Mediterranean, or low-carbohydrate diets, respectively *(13)*. Of interest was the more favorable effect on plasma glucose and insulin levels in subjects assigned to the Mediterranean diet. Providing support for a Mediterranean-style diet (use of unsaturated oils such as olive oil, fruits, nuts, legumes, and fish with relatively low consumption of meat and dairy) is a recent study that followed 13,380 adults for an average of 4.4 years *(14)*. Those with the highest adherence to a Mediterranean diet were 83% less likely to be among those who developed diabetes. Even more moderate adherence was associated with a 59% relative reduction in risk.

Table 2 summarizes nutrition recommendations from health organizations for the preventions of diabetes and cardiovascular disease *(4, 9, 10)*. It is unlikely that one diet is optimal for all overweight/obese persons.

Table 2
Food Recommendations for the Prevention of Diabetes

- Encourage a food pattern that includes carbohydrate from fruits, vegetables, whole grains, legumes, and low-fat/skim milk for good health.
- Limit saturated fat to <7% of total calories; *trans* unsaturated fatty acids to <1%, and food cholesterol to <200 mg/day; substitute unsaturated fat from vegetables, fish, nuts, and legumes.
- Emphasize a diet rich in fruits, vegetables, whole grain, high-fiber foods, nuts, and low-fat dairy products.
- Recommend two or more servings of fish per week (with the exception of commercially fried fish filets) for *n*–3 polyunsaturated fatty acids.
- Limit sodium intake to 2300 mg/day by choosing foods low in sodium and limiting the amount of salt added to food.
- Minimize intake of beverages and foods with added sugars.
- Limit alcohol to no more than 2 drinks/day (men) and 1 drink/day (women) in those who choose to drink alcohol.

Source: Adapted from Ref. *(10)*.

Recommendations should be individualized to allow for specific food preferences and individual approaches to reducing energy intake. Two important considerations are can the diet be followed long term and does it encourage healthful eating habits and regular physical activity?

4.3. Recommend 150 Min/Week of Physical Activity

Regular physical activity and aerobic fitness improve insulin sensitivity, independent of weight loss *(15)*, and reduce the risk of developing diabetes *(16)*. To assist with weight loss and maintenance and reduce risk of CVD, at least 150 min of moderate-intensity aerobic physical activity or at least 90 min of vigorous aerobic exercise per week is recommended. The physical activity should be divided over at least 3 days/week, with no more than 2 consecutive days without physical activity. For long-term maintenance of major weight loss, a larger amount of exercise (7 h/week of moderate or vigorous aerobic physical activity) may be helpful. In the absence of contraindications, individuals should be encouraged to perform resistance training three times per week *(6)*. Table 3 summarizes physical activity recommendations *(17)*.

Table 3
Physical Activity Recommendations

- For fitness and reduced risk of chronic health conditions: 30 min/day of moderate physical activity (e.g., walking 3–4 miles/h), above usual activity, on most days of the week.
- For prevention of weight gain: 60 min/day (increased energy expenditure by ~150–200 kcal) of moderate-to-vigorous activity on most days of the week while not exceeding caloric intake requirements.
- To avoid regain of weight loss: 60–90 min/day moderate-intensity physical activity while not exceeding caloric intake requirements.
- Vigorous intensity or longer duration physical activity provides greater benefits
- Cardiovascular conditioning, stretching exercises for flexibility, and resistance exercises for muscle strength and endurance are also recommended.

Source: Adapted from Ref. *(17)*.

In previously inactive patients, an initial exercise session should be of short duration (i.e., 10 min/day) of activity and gradually increase to 30 min/day of low-intensity activity. Intensity can be increased as the patient's strength and fitness improves *(10)*.

4.4. Other Nutrition-Related Factors

4.4.1. CARBOHYDRATE/FATS

There is no evidence that a high-carbohydrate diet contributes to insulin resistance; it may be beneficial for insulin sensitivity *(18, 19)*. This is a difficult issue to resolve because as carbohydrate in the diet increases, fat, especially saturated fats, decreases. High-fat intakes, especially of saturated and *trans* fats, are associated with a decline in insulin sensitivity *(20)*. Therefore, it is unclear if the improvement in insulin sensitivity is because of the increase in carbohydrate or the decrease in fat.

In a review of high-carbohydrate diets compared to low-carbohydrate diets, in subjects without diabetes, seven studies reported increased insulin sensitivity from the high-carbohydrate diets, whereas, four reported no differences. In subjects with diabetes, five studies reported increased insulin sensitivity from the high-carbohydrate diets, whereas, two studies reported no differences *(19)*.

Both the DPP and the Finnish Diabetes Prevention Study focused on reduced dietary fat as key component of the intervention. Reducing intake of fat, particularly saturated fat, may reduce risk for diabetes by producing an energy-independent improvement in insulin resistance. Six clinical trials, comparing high- and low-fat diets from 3 days to 4 weeks with weight kept constant, demonstrated that low-fat diets result in significant improvements in insulin sensitivity, whereas 3 other studies did not observe any difference between high- and low-fat diets on insulin sensitivity *(20)*. However, it should be remembered that excess energy intake, regardless of the energy source, and positive energy balance contribute to insulin resistance by way of obesity.

4.4.2. WHOLE GRAINS AND DIETARY FIBER

Increased intake of foods containing whole grains is associated with improved insulin sensitivity, independent of body weight *(21)*. Increased intake of dietary fiber is associated with improved insulin sensitivity as well as improved ability to secrete insulin adequately to overcome insulin resistance. Increased fiber intake was a recommendation in the Finnish Diabetes Study – participants were instructed to increase fiber intake to at least 15 g/1000 kcal. However, only 25% of the intervention group were able to achieve this goal *(2)*. Clearly, modest weight loss and regular physical activity remain the primary components of an intensive lifestyle intervention.

4.4.3. GLYCEMIC INDEX/GLYCEMIC LOAD

Two early epidemiologic studies from Harvard suggested that a low glycemic index (GI)/glycemic load (GL) may play a role in the prevention of diabetes; however, the Iowa Health Study did not find this association *(22)*. At this time, ten observational studies have reported on the effects of GI/GL and risk of diabetes. Three studies reported a positive association between GI/GL and diabetes risk or insulin resistance (Nurses Health Study 1997, Health Professional Study 1997, and Framingham Offspring Cohort 2004), whereas, seven do not (Iowa Women's Study 2000, Zutphen Elderly Study 2000, Atherosclerosis Risk in Communities (ARIC) 2002, Inter99 Study 2005, Insulin Resistance and Atherosclerosis Study (IRAS) 2005, Whitehall II 2007, and Health, Aging and Body Composition Study 2008). Interestingly, in three studies fiber was positively associated with insulin sensitivity whereas GI/GL was not (ARIC 2002, Inter99 Study 2008, and IRAS 2005).

Although many popular diet books promote the use of a low-GI diet for weight loss, there is minimal evidence to suggest that it contributes to weight loss. Studies supporting the role of a low-GI diet for weight loss are less than 6 months in duration and conducted primarily in adolescents. Longer term clinical trials in adults have not found a benefit for weight loss *(23)*.

Although it is often suggested there is no harm in recommending low-GI foods even if there is no evidence of benefit, this is not necessarily true. The GI may not be the best indicator of healthful food choices. Although many healthful foods have a moderate or low GI (e.g., whole grains, fruits, vegetables, legumes, diary products), many foods of questionable value also have low or moderate GIs. For example, Coke has a moderate GI of 58, Snickers Bar a GI of 55, premium ice cream a low GI of 37, and fructose a low GI of 19 *(24)*. If a food company wishes to produce a food with a low GI, they have only to sweeten it with more fructose or sucrose or add fat. Furthermore, whole wheat bread, brown rice, and brown spaghetti have the same GI value as their refined white versions. Fruits often have a low GI, but whole fruits and juice have the same GI.

4.4.4. ALCOHOL

Observational studies suggest a U- or J-shaped association between moderate consumption of alcohol (1–3 drinks/day [*15*–45 g alcohol]) and decreased risk of diabetes *(25, 26)*. A meta-analysis based on 32 studies found that compared to no alcohol use, for the general public, moderate amounts of alcohol were associated with a 33–56% lower incidence of diabetes. In contrast, a heavy/chronic amount of alcohol (greater than 3 drinks/day) was associated with a 43% increase in the incidence *(25)*. Small clinical trials and observational studies have shown light to moderate amounts of alcohol improve insulin sensitivity and raise HDL cholesterol levels. The type of alcoholic beverage does not make a difference.

5. SUMMARY

Well-designed randomized controlled trials clearly documented that diabetes can be prevented or delayed with moderate changes in weight and physical activity – a 5–7% weight loss and 150 min/week of activity. However, well-trained staff providing continued support was needed to achieve these results. Pharmacologic therapy also significantly lowers the incidence of diabetes.

In the American Diabetes Association *2008* nutrition recommendations and interventions for diabetes position statement *(27)*, the following lifestyle recommendations for the prevention of diabetes were made:

- Among individuals at high risk for developing type 2 diabetes, structured programs that emphasize lifestyle changes that include moderate weight loss (7% body weight) and regular physical activity (150 min/week), with dietary strategies including reduced calorie and reduced intake of dietary fat, can reduce the risk for developing diabetes and are therefore recommended.
- Individuals at high risk for type 2 diabetes should be encouraged to achieve the Dietary Reference Intakes recommendation for dietary fiber (14 g fiber/1000 kcal) and foods containing whole grains (one-half of grain intake).
- There is not sufficient, consistent information to conclude that low-glycemic load diets reduce the risk for diabetes.
- Observational studies report that moderate alcohol intake may reduce the risk for diabetes, but the data do not support recommending alcohol consumption to individuals at risk of diabetes.

SUGGESTED FURTHER READING

World Health Organization. Preventing Chronic Disease: A Vital Investment. WHO Press, Geneva, 2005.

Katzmarzyk PT, Janssen I, Ross R et al. The importance of waist circumference in the definition of metabolic syndrome. Diabetes Care 2006; 29:404–409.

America on the Move. Preventing Weight Gain. http://www.americaonthemove.org. Accessed August 18, 2008.

Klein S, Burke LE, Bray GA, et al. Clinical implications of obesity with specific focus on cardiovascular disease. A statement for professionals from the American Heart Association Council on Nutrition, Physical Activity, and Metabolism. Circulation 2004; 110: 2952–2967.

REFERENCES

1. Centers for Disease Control and Prevention. National Diabetes Fact Sheet, 2007. Atlanta, GA: Department of Health and Human Services, Centers for Disease Control and Prevention, 2007. Available at: www.cdc.gov/diabetes. Accessed October 21, 2008.
2. Tuomilehto J, Lindström J, Eriksson JG, et al. Prevention of type 2 diabetes mellitus by changes in lifestyle among subjects with impaired glucose tolerance. N Engl J Med 2001; 344:1343–1350.

3. Diabetes Prevention Research Group. Reduction in the incidence of type 2 diabetes with lifestyle intervention or metformin. N Engl J Med 2002; 346:393–403.

4. Ramachandran A, Snehalatha C, Mary S, et al. The Indian Diabetes Prevention Programme shows that lifestyle modification and metformin prevent type 2 diabetes in Asian Indian subjects with impaired glucose tolerance (IDPP-1). Diabetologia 2006; 49: 289–297.

5. Kosaka K, Noda M, Kuzuya T. Prevention of type 2 diabetes by lifestyle intervention: A Japanese Trial in IGT Males. Diabetes Res Clin Pract 2005; 67:152–162.

6. American Diabetes Association. Executive summary: Standards of Medical Care in Diabetes – 2008. Diabetes Care 2008; 31(Suppl 1):S5–S54.

7. Lindström J, Ilanne-Parikka P, Peltonen M, et al. Sustained reduction in the incidence of type 2 diabetes by lifestyle intervention: Follow-up of the Finnish Diabetes Prevention Study. Lancet 2006; 369:1673–1679.

8. Gerstein HC. Point: If it is important to prevent type 2 diabetes, it is important to consider all proven therapies within a comprehensive approach. Diabetes Care 2007; 30: 431–434.

9. American Association of Clinical Endocrinologists Consensus Statement of the AACE Task Force on Pre-diabetes. Released July 23, 2008.

10. Klein S, Sheard NF, Pi-Sunyer X, et al. Weight management through lifestyle modification for the prevention and management of type 2 diabetes: Rationale and Strategies. Diabetes Care 2004; 27:2067–2073.

11. Franz MJ, VanWormer JJ, Crain AL, et al. Weight-loss outcomes: A systematic review and meta-analysis of weight loss clinical trials with a minimum 1-year follow up. J Am Diet Assoc 2007; 107:1755–1767.

12. Foster GD, Wyatt HR, Hill JO, et al. A randomized trial of a low-carbohydrate diet for obesity. N Engl J Med 2003; 348:2082–2090.

13. Shai I, Schwarzfuchs D, Henkin Y, et al. Weight loss with a low-carbohydrate, Mediterranean, or low-fat diet. N Engl J Med 2008; 359:229–241.

14. Basterra-Gortari FJ, Martinez-González MA. Mediterranean diet in type 2 diabetes. Diabetolgia 2008; 10:1933–1934.

15. Duncan GE, Perri MG, Theriaque DW, et al. Exercise training without weight loss, increases insulin sensitivity and postheparin plasma lipase activity in previously sedentary adults. Diabetes Care 2003; 26:557–562.

16. Wei M, Gibbons LW, Mitchell TL, et al. The association between cardiorespiratory fitness and impaired fasting glucose and type 2 diabetes mellitus in men. Ann Intern Med 1999; 130:89–96.

17. Dietary Guidelines for Americans 2005. Physical Activity. Available at: http://health. gov/dietaryguidelines/dga2005. Accessed August 18, 2008.

18. Bessesen DH. The role of carbohydrate in insulin resistance. J Nutr 2001; 131: 2782S–2786S.

19. McClenaghan NH. Determining the relationship between dietary carbohydrate intake and insulin resistance. Nut Res Rev 2005; 18:222–240.

20. Lovejoy JC. The influence of dietary fat on insulin resistance. Curr Diab Rep 2002; 2:435–440.

21. Liese AD, Roach AK, Sparks KC, et al. Whole-grain intake and insulin sensitivity: The Insulin Resistance Atherosclerosis Study. Am J Clin Nutr 2003; 78: 965–971.

22. Franz MJ. The evidence is in: lifestyle interventions can prevent diabetes. Am J Lifestyle Medicine 2007; 1:113–121.

23. Das SK, Gilhooly CH, Golden JK, et al. Long-term effects of 2 energy-restricted diets differing in glycemic load on dietary adherence, body composition, and metabolism in CALERIE: A 1-y Randomized Controlled Trial. Am J Clin Nutr 2007; 85: 1023–1030.

24. Foster-Powell K, Holt SHA, Brand-Miller JC. International table of glycemic index and glycemic load values: 2002. Am J Clin Nutr 2002; 76:5–56.

25. Howard AA, Arnsten JH, Gourevitch MN. Effect of alcohol consumption on diabetes mellitus: A Systematic Review. Ann Intern Med 2004; 140:211–219.

26. Koppes LLJ, Dekker JM, Hendriks HFJ, et al. Moderate alcohol consumption lowers risk of type 2 diabetes. Diabetes Care 2005; 28:719–725.

27. American Diabetes Association. Nutrition recommendations and interventions for diabetes. A position statement of the American Diabetes Association. Diabetes Care 2008; 31(Suppl 1)31:S61–S78.

25 Coronary Heart Disease: Nutritional Interventions for Prevention and Therapy

Jayne V. Woodside, Claire McEvoy, and Norman J. Temple

Key Points

- Coronary heart disease (CHD) is a major cause of morbidity and mortality in the Western world.
- Diets low in saturated and trans fats can reduce CHD risk.
- Strong evidence suggests that increased consumption of fatty fish and of n–3 polyunsaturated fatty acids (n–3 PUFA) is likely to reduce CHD risk.
- While supplementation with antioxidants and B-group vitamins are unlikely to reduce CHD risk, diets rich in these micronutrients (e.g., diets rich in fruits, vegetables, and whole grain cereals) are associated with lower CHD risk.
- Maintaining a healthy weight and being physically active have each been shown to reduce CHD risk factors and CHD incidence.

Key Words: Cardiovascular risk factors; coronary heart disease; dietary fat; diet and prevention

1. INTRODUCTION

Coronary heart disease (CHD) is a major cause of morbidity and mortality in the Western world. Factors that are strongly associated with elevated risk of CHD are increasing age, male sex, smoking, lack of exercise, hypertension, and type 2 diabetes. In addition, blood lipid levels are strong predictors of CHD risk. A pattern of blood lipids that accelerates atherosclerosis is one where total cholesterol (TC) and low-density lipoprotein cholesterol (LDL-C) are elevated and high-density lipoprotein (HDL-C) is relatively low

From: *Nutrition and Health: Nutrition Guide for Physicians*
Edited by: T. Wilson et al. (eds.), DOI 10.1007/978-1-60327-431-9_25,
© Humana Press, a part of Springer Science+Business Media, LLC 2010

(1). A 1% reduction in circulating LDL-C is associated with a reduction in CHD risk of about 1% *(2)*.

A large body of evidence, collected over several decades from observational epidemiological studies and randomized controlled clinical trials (RCTs), strongly supports a major role for diet in the prevention and treatment of CHD. Dietary factors that have been proposed to affect the risk of CHD include saturated fatty acids (SFA), trans fatty acids (TFA), polyunsaturated fatty acids (both n–6 and n–3 PUFA), dietary fiber, B-vitamins, and antioxidant vitamins. This chapter examines how each of these food components, as well as whole dietary patterns, affect CHD risk. Obesity and exercise are also considered. Early studies focused on the effect of diet on blood lipids but it is now accepted that diet affects CHD etiology through multiple mechanisms, including insulin resistance, blood pressure, endothelial function, inflammation, and thrombosis.

2. DIETARY FAT AND CHD

2.1. Fat Intake

Much attention has been paid to the question of the total intake of dietary fat. A major reason for this is that increased intake of fat can lead to a positive energy balance and contribute to obesity. However, the relationship between the quantity of fat intake and the risk of CHD is much weaker. There is no strong evidence that low-fat diets reduce mortality rates from CHD. Low-fat diets (10–20% of total energy) reduce circulating LDL-C but this benefit can be cancelled out by the simultaneous reduction in HDL-C level and increase in triglyceride (TG) level, largely through the replacement of dietary fat by carbohydrate. Additionally, compliance with low-fat diets is often difficult.

The critical aspect of fat intake with regard to risk of CHD is the type of fat. Different fats have very different effects on blood lipid levels and this is the key mechanism that explains how fat affects risk of CHD *(3)*.

Public health strategies over the past two decades emphasized the reduction of total fat in the diet. The most common recommendation was that fat intake should be "less than 30%" of energy intake. In recent years, this recommendation has shifted to a more liberal 20–35%. Common dietary recommendations for fat intake are shown in Table 1.

2.2. Saturated Fat and Dietary Cholesterol

Many studies over the past 30 years have established that SFA is consistently positively correlated with TC and LDL-C levels. Dietary cholesterol also increases TC and LDL-C levels but to a much lesser degree than SFA.

Table 1
Dietary Fat Recommendations for Modification of Blood Lipids for the Prevention of CHD

Dietary Fat	Recommendation*	Major Dietary Sources
Total fat	20–35% total energy intake	As below
Saturated fatty acids (SFA)	<7% total energy intake	Animal products (fatty meat, processed meat, cheese, butter, cream, lard, shortening, full-fat milk, ice cream), cocoa butter, chocolate, coconut oil, palm oil, cakes, pastry products, cookies
Trans fatty acids (TFA)	<1% total energy intake	Stick margarine, cakes, pastry products, cookies, chips, many fast foods
Cholesterol	<200 mg/day	Liver, kidney, egg yolk, shellfish
Polunsaturated fatty acids (PUFA)	4% to 10% total energy intake	Soft margarines, vegetable oils (corn, safflower, soybean, sunflower)
Monounsaturated fatty acids (MUFA)	<20% total energy intake	Olive oil, canola oil, peanut oil, avocados, olives, almonds, cashews, peanuts
n–3 PUFA	2 or more servings fatty fish per week	Sardines, herring, pilchards, salmon, tuna, sardines. Walnuts, flaxseed oil, canola oil

*The recommendations shown are not necessarily ideal for minimizing risk of CHD but are the most common ones currently given.

RCTs have demonstrated that diets low in SFA (<7% of total energy intake) and cholesterol (<200 mg/day) bring about reductions in LDL-C levels of approximately 10%. This would be expected to have a clinically important protective impact on the risk of CHD. This dietary strategy was known for some years as a Step 2 diet and more recently as Therapeutic Lifestyle Change.

2.3. Trans Fatty Acids

Like SFA, TFA also raises TC and LDL-C levels. However, whereas SFA tends to increase HDL-C, TFA lowers it. A recent meta-analysis found that a 2% increase in energy from TFA is associated with a 23% increase in the incidence of CHD (4). These findings reinforce the importance of recent public health initiatives directed at minimizing dietary intake of TFA.

2.4. n–6 PUFA and MUFA

n–6 PUFA are usually referred to simply as PUFA as they represent the great majority of all PUFA. PUFA and MUFA are the major unsaturated fats. PUFA are found in abundance in vegetable oils, while olive oil and canola oil are rich sources of MUFA. PUFA lower TC and LDL-C levels whereas MUFA tend to have a neutral effect (3). A number of studies have suggested that MUFA may be preferable to carbohydrates as a replacement for SFA as they do not induce a fall in HDL-C or rise in TG. However, more research is required in this area.

We can summarize the above findings as follows: replacing SFA and TFA with PUFA and MUFA reduces TC and LDL-C and is likely to be protective against CHD. In general, diet change induces a greater fall in TC and LDL-C in persons with hypercholesterolemia.

2.5. n–3 PUFA

Eicosapentaenoic acid (EPA) and docosahexaenoic acid (DHA) are long-chain n–3 PUFA that are found in fatty fish (Table 1). Alpha linolenic acid (ALA) is an n–3 PUFA with a slightly shorter chain and is found in some oils, namely flaxseed (richest source), soybean, and canola oil (poorest source). Walnuts are another source. ALA can be converted to a limited extent in humans to EPA but almost not at all to DHA (3).

n–3 PUFA from fatty fish exert several different cardioprotective actions. They improve endothelial function and reduce the risk of thrombosis, inflammation, and arrhythmias. In addition, they lower TG levels, but tend to increase TC and LDL-C (3). The benefits of ALA are less clear.

Most prospective cohort studies have demonstrated inverse associations between fish consumption and risk of CHD. These studies indicate that eating fish between once and five times per week reduces risk of CHD (especially death) by around 40%. However, results are not completely consistent. The same story has emerged from the results of RCTs. In these the effects of fish or fish oil have been studied in patients with CHD. Most of those studies have reported impressive reductions in fatal MI and overall mortality in subjects given fish or fish oil (3). The protection afforded by n–3 PUFA against CHD appears to extend to ALA: several epidemiological studies have reported a strong inverse relationship between intake of ALA and risk of CHD (3). Support for this comes from the Lyon Diet Heart Study, a RCT on free-living subjects. While there were several dietary changes, the dominant one was an increase in ALA. Those in the intervention group had a 50-70% reduction of cardiac endpoints (5). Clearly, the very encouraging findings on n–3 PUFA, as discussed above, require further confirmation.

Current recommendations for n–3 PUFA are shown in Table 1.

3. PLANT STEROLS AND STANOLS

Phytosterols or plant sterols are structurally similar to cholesterol. Stanols are closely related substances. Plant sterols and stanols reduce the absorption of cholesterol (which comes from both the diet and from bile), and thereby lower the blood level of TC and LDL-C *(3)*. An intake of 2 g/day of plant sterols or stanols lowers LDL-C by around 10%. Consumption of sterols or stanols may result in reduced absorption of fat-soluble vitamins, such as vitamin E and β-carotene, but this should not be a problem provided a nutritious diet is consumed. Products containing added sterols or stanols include certain brands of orange juice, cereal bars, salad dressings, and Benecol and Take Control spreads. Such products can be classed as functional foods.

4. THCY AND B-VITAMINS

Homocysteine (tHcy) is an amino acid which is an intermediate product in methionine metabolism. Its metabolism requires folate and vitamins B_{12} and B_6. Epidemiological evidence indicates that elevated blood levels of tHcy are associated with an increase in CHD risk. tHcy can be lowered by supplementation with folate and vitamins B_{12} and B_6. These findings suggest that supplementation might be an effective prevention strategy against CHD. However, RCTs have failed to produce the hoped-for results *(3)*. The results of more RCTs are expected over the next few years.

5. ALCOHOL

Consistent evidence from cohort studies suggest an inverse relationship between daily consumption of alcohol and risk of CHD *(6)*. Moderate consumption (1–2 drinks/day) reduces risk by 10–40%. The major mechanism by which alcohol achieves this effect is by increasing HDL-C. In addition, alcohol has an antithrombotic action *(6)*.

There has been much speculation that wine, especially red wine, is more potent than other forms of alcoholic beverages. The origin of this belief is the low rates of CHD in France compared to certain other countries, such as Britain. This has been referred to as the "French paradox." These differences cannot be easily explained by looking at the "usual suspects," particularly smoking and intake of SFA. Many people found it attractive to assume that red wine deserved the credit. However, when the epidemiological evidence is looked at as a whole, especially cohort studies, then a different story emerges: all forms of alcoholic beverages – beer, spirits, and wine, both red and white – are similarly protective *(6)*. This saga serves as a valuable reminder of the golden rule in this type of research: epidemiology shows association, not causation.

Recommendations for the general public regarding intake of alcoholic beverages are discussed in chapters (Chapters 9 and 11).

6. ANTIOXIDANTS

Many observational studies have demonstrated an association between intake of antioxidant vitamins and risk of CHD. The association is strongest for vitamin E but less consistent for vitamin C *(3, 7)*. We see the same lessons here as we saw above with red wine. Many researchers were quick to jump to the conclusion that the epidemiological evidence means that supplements of vitamins C and E will prevent CHD. In the case of vitamin E a plausible biochemical explanation was available, namely that vitamin E prevents the oxidation of LDL particles and thereby slows the progression of atherosclerosis. A similar biochemical explanation had been proposed to help explain why red wine prevents CHD, namely that it is a rich source of resveratrol, a phytochemical with antioxidant properties.

Based on the above reasoning several large RCTs have been conducted. In most cases the trials were conducted on patients with existing CHD (i.e., they were secondary prevention trials). In addition to clinical trials on vitamins C and E, RCTs have also been conducted using supplements of β-carotene, another antioxidant vitamin. However, the primary goal of the RCTs using β-carotene was the prevention of cancer rather than CHD. Looked at as a whole, the results of the RCTs on antioxidant vitamins have been mostly negative with regard to reducing the risk of CHD.

The most important finding from these RCTs is the effect of antioxidant vitamins on all-cause mortality. After all, what use is it to save a person from CHD or cancer if the price is premature death from some other cause? A recent Cochrane review and meta-analysis was carried out on 67 RCTs that had included 233,000 participants. Of these, 164,000 were healthy at the start of the trial while 68,000 already had an existing disease. The key finding was that supplementing with antioxidant nutrients (β-carotene or vitamin C or E) led to an increase of about 5–6% in all-cause mortality *(8, 9)*. These results compel the conclusion that these vitamin supplements should not be recommended in any class of patient.

The story of red wine, antioxidants, and the prevention of CHD holds a valuable lesson for many people with an interest in diet and disease. While epidemiology is a tremendously valuable research tool, it is prone to generating spurious associations. This can lead to people making claims that particular dietary components are either causative or preventive of particular diseases. Such claims should be viewed cautiously until such time as they are verified by well-conducted RCTs.

7. DIETARY FIBER

Dietary fiber was discussed in Chapter 3. Fiber represents a diverse group of substances which can be divided into two main groups: soluble fiber (or viscous fiber) and insoluble fiber. Major food sources of soluble fiber are fruit, oats, and beans. This type of fiber brings about modest, albeit useful, lowering of the TC and LDL-C *(3)*. Sources of soluble fiber that can be added to the diet as a supplement include oat bran and psyllium. An appropriate dose is around 10–15 g/day. Insoluble fiber, present in abundance in most types of whole grain cereals, has little effect on blood lipids.

8. WHOLE DIET APPROACHES TO CHD RISK REDUCTION

A number of studies have moved beyond food components and have investigated whether whole foods are protective against CHD. Some studies have explored the efficacy of a whole diet approach for CHD prevention and therapy *(10)*.

8.1. Fruit, Vegetable, and Whole Grain Cereals

Fruits and vegetables are complex foods and contain many bioactive components, including folate, potassium, hundreds of phytochemicals, and dietary fiber, while also having a negligible amount of fat. Epidemiological studies have repeatedly shown that consumption of fruit and vegetables has a strong protective association with risk of CHD *(11)*. This is not surprising when we consider the various healthful effects of these foods. By virtue of their high content of fiber, combined with a negligible content of fat, a generous intake of fruit and vegetables helps counter the development of obesity. These foods have also been used as part of the DASH diet, a dietary strategy to lower blood pressure (Chapter 26).

Epidemiological studies have also generated strong evidence that intake of cereal fiber is strongly and negatively associated with risk of CHD *(12)*. The most plausible explanation of this finding is that cereal fiber is a proxy indicator of consumption of whole grain cereals. These foods are likely to be protective against CHD for much the same reasons as fruit and vegetables.

8.2. Nuts

Nuts are rich in unsaturated fat. Their consumption tends to displace SFA from the diet. Not surprisingly, therefore, they tend to lower the TC and LDL-C while some epidemiological studies have suggested that they may help lower the risk of CHD. Any recommendation to eat nuts should specifically mention unsalted brands.

8.3. The Portfolio Diet

The portfolio diet is a plant-based diet that includes <7% SFA, <200 mg/day cholesterol, viscous fiber 10 g/day, plus phytosterols/stanols, almonds, and soy protein. The diet is designed to maximize the reduction in serum LDL-C levels. Among subjects who adhered to the dietary advice, LDL-C levels fell by 30% after 1 year *(13)*, which is comparable to the results achieved using statins. It is important to bear in mind that while changes in LDL-C are predictive of changes in CHD risk over the next several years, diet affects risk of CHD in multiple ways and LDL-C may be a crude predictor. Large-scale studies with clinical end points are therefore required.

9. OBESITY

Obesity is strongly associated with risk of CHD. However this association becomes weak after age 65. Much of the association between obesity and CHD, possibly all of it, can be accounted for by the frequent presence of established CHD risk factors in obese people, notably hypertension, hyperlipidemia, and insulin resistance (including glucose intolerance and diabetes) *(3)*.

BMI is the most widely used index of obesity. However, waist circumference, a measures of abdominal adiposity, appears to have a stronger association with CHD risk than does BMI *(3)*. For the practicing physician, waist circumference offers a quick and useful tool to assess the degree to which a patient is carrying excess abdominal fat and its threat to cardiac health. While cut-points for BMI for overweight and obesity are well-established and accepted, further research is required to determine analogous cut-points for waist circumference in different sex, age, and ethnic groups. However, commonly used cut-points are waist circumferences of >102 cm (>40 in) for men and of >88 cm (>35 in) for women.

10. PHYSICAL ACTIVITY

Physical activity, by which we mean aerobic exercise, has consistently been associated with a reduction in CHD events in both primary and secondary prevention. This has been shown in both prospective cohort studies and in RCTs *(3)*. Indeed, a sedentary lifestyle is now recognized as one of the big four risk factors, alongside elevated LDL-C, smoking, and hypertension (five, if we include diabetes). Much of this benefit of physical activity can be explained in terms of its favorable effects on several factors associated with CHD, namely body weight, blood pressure, the blood lipid profile (including a rise in HDL-C), insulin resistance, and glucose tolerance *(3)*.

There is widespread agreement among medical organizations that everyone should be encouraged to engage in an exercise program. Typical recommendations are for at least 30 min of moderate intensity physical activity, such as walking at a speed that induces mild exertion, at least 5 days per week. As the benefits are cumulative, the exercise can be done as several short activities every day or as one or two long activities at the weekend. However, there is some uncertainty regarding the exact relationship between the quantity and the intensity of exercise and the degree of risk reduction. In general, our best evidence suggests that the majority of the risk reduction comes from following the recommendations just stated while significant additional benefit comes from doubling the time spent in exercise and from engaging in vigorous intensity exercise, such as jogging.

A major challenge in this area is to determine what behavioral strategies will motivate individuals to engage in a long-term program of physical activity.

11. CONCLUSION

Compelling evidence exists that diet and lifestyle changes can substantially reduce the risk of CHD. Based on the strongest evidence presently available, we can state, with a high degree of confidence, that diets low in SFA and TFA, and with generous amounts of fruit, vegetables, whole grains, and foods that supply n–3 PUFA, are highly protective against CHD. This dietary pattern has much in common with that found in the traditional Mediterranean diet. The diet should also be low in refined grains (so as to make room for whole grains).

It has been demonstrated that simply lowering the percentage of energy from total fat will be unlikely to reduce TC and LDL-C or reduce CHD incidence. Different fats have very different effects on blood lipid levels and this is the key mechanism that explains how fat affects risk of CHD.

Maintaining a healthy body weight and engaging in a regular program of exercise will also reduce CHD risk. Therefore, public health policies encouraging consumption of a healthy diet (as outlined above), maintenance of a healthy weight, physical activity, and smoking avoidance have the potential to substantially reduce the burden of CHD.

The focus of this chapter has been CHD. We can conclude with some comments on other cardiovascular diseases, most notably stroke. While the relative importance of different risk factors varies from one form of cardiovascular disease to the next, the general recommendations made here will go far to achieving the prevention of all cardiovascular disease.

SUGGESTED FURTHER READING

Van Horn L, McCoin M, Kris-Etherton PM, et al. The evidence for dietary prevention and treatment of cardiovascular disease. J Am Diet Assoc 2008; 108:287–331.

REFERENCES

1. Brunner EJ, Rees K,Ward K, Burke M, Thorogood M. Dietary advice for reducing cardiovascular risk. Cochrane Database of Systematic Reviews 2007, Issue 4. Art. No.: CD002128. DOI: 10.1002/14651858.CD002128.pub3.
2. Grundy SM, Cleeman JL, Merz CN. Implications of recent clinical trials for the National Cholesterol Education Program Adult Treatment Panel III Guidelines. J Am Coll Cardiol 2004; 44:720–732.
3. Van Horn L, McCoin M, Kris-Etherton PM, et al. The evidence for dietary prevention and treatment of cardiovascular disease. J Am Diet Assoc 2008; 108:287–331.
4. Mozaffarian D, Katan MB, Ascherio A, Stampfer MJ, Willett WC. Trans fatty acids and cardiovascular disease. N Engl J Med 2006; 354:1601–1613.
5. De Lorgeril M, Salen P, Martin J-L, Monjaud I, Delaye J, Mamelle N. Mediterranean diet, traditional risk factors, and the rate of cardiovascular complications after myocardial infarction. Final report of the Lyon Diet Heart Study. Circulation 1999; 99:779–785.
6. Rimm E, Temple NJ. What are the health implications of alcohol consumption? In: Wilson T, Temple N, eds. Nutritional Health. Humana Press, Totowa, NJ, 2001, pp. 211–221.
7. Moats C, Rimm EB. Vitamin intake and risk of coronary disease: observation versus intervention. Curr Atheroscler Rep 2007; 9:508–514.
8. Bjelakovic G, Nikolova D, Gluud LL, Simonetti RG, Gluud C. Antioxidant supplements for prevention of mortality in healthy participants and patients with various diseases. Cochrane Database Syst Rev 2008: CD007176.
9. Bjelakovic G, Nikolova D, Gluud LL, Simonetti RG, Gluud C. Mortality in randomized trials of antioxidant supplements for primary and secondary prevention: systematic review and meta-analysis. JAMA 2007; 297:842–857.
10. Woodside JV, McCall D, McGartland C, Young IS. Micronutrients: dietary intake v. supplement use. Proc Nutr Soc 2005; 64:543–553.
11. He FJ, Nowson CA, Lucas M, MacGregor GA. Increased consumption of fruit and vegetables is related to a reduced risk of coronary heart disease: meta-analysis of cohort studies. J Hum Hypertens 2007; 21:717–728.
12. Pereira MA, O'Reilly E, Augusston K, et al. Dietary fiber and risk of coronary heart disease: A pooled analysis of cohort studies. Arch Intern Med 2004; 164:370–376.
13. Jenkins DJ, Kendall CW, Faulkner DA, et al. Assessment of the longer-term effects of a dietary portfolio of cholesterol-lowering foods in hypercholesterolemia. Am J Clin Nutr 2006; 83:582–591.

26 Diet and Blood Pressure: The High and Low of It

David W. Harsha and George A. Bray

Key Points

- Hypertension poses significant risks for stroke and heart disease.
- Weight gain and obesity increase blood pressure (BP); weight loss can reverse it.
- Diets high in fruits and vegetables and low-fat dairy products and low in red meat and sugar-containing foods (DASH Diet) can significantly lower BP.
- Dietary sodium has an important impact on BP in some people, and lowering sodium intake can lower BP.
- Alcohol intake increases BP.

Key Words: Hypertension; stroke; sodium; blood pressure; antihypertensive therapy

1. INTRODUCTION

Hypertension is a global public health problem. Roughly 1 billion people worldwide are estimated to have clinically significant elevations in blood pressure (BP) with about 50 million of them in the United States *(1)*. Hypertension, in turn, is associated with increased risk for coronary heart disease (CHD), stroke, renal disease, and all-cause mortality *(1)*. BP is significantly affected by nutrition which is the subject of this chapter.

The public health burden of hypertension is clearly enormous. Although perhaps impossible to tease out due to associations with other risk factors, including overweight, hypertension is a major contributor to most categories of chronic disease *(2)*. Diseases of the heart and cerebrovascular diseases are the first and third leading causes of mortality in the United States, accounting for more than one-third of all deaths. Hypertension is a major risk factor for both of these diseases *(1)*. Therefore, reduction in hypertension

From: *Nutrition and Health: Nutrition Guide for Physicians*
Edited by: T. Wilson et al. (eds.), DOI 10.1007/978-1-60327-431-9_26,
© Humana Press, a part of Springer Science+Business Media, LLC 2010

constitutes a major health goal. The federal government, through the Healthy People 2010 initiative, proposes to increase to 50% the proportion of the adult hypertensive population whose BP is under control. This contrasts with the current estimated figure of 34% (1).

In clinical trials antihypertensive therapy can result in reductions of incidence of stroke, myocardial infarction, and heart failure of between 20 and 50% (3). Ogden et al. (4) estimate that a 12 mmHg decline in systolic BP maintained over a period of 10 years in a population with initial stage 1 hypertension will reduce incident mortality by between 9 and 11%. A population-wide reduction of 5.5 mmHg systolic or 3.0 mmHg diastolic will lower incident CHD by 15% and stroke by 27%.

2. DEFINITIONS OF HYPERTENSION

The JNC VII report divides BP into several categories (Table 1). Normal BP is defined as a level of less than 120/80 (systolic/diastolic in mmHg). Hypertension is a sustained elevated BP above 140/90 mmHg. Stage 1 hypertension is defined as a BP of 140–159 mmHg systolic and 90–99 mmHg diastolic; stage 2 is >160/100 mmHg. This report also establishes a category of prehypertension (systolic BP of 120–140 mmHg or diastolic of 80–89 mmHg). Prehypertension and stage 1 hypertension are deemed to be appropriate primary targets for lifestyle interventions, including weight loss. Higher levels of BP should be addressed primarily with medications or other appropriate treatments.

Table 1
JNC-VIII Classification of Blood Pressure Levels

Blood Pressure Categories from JNC VII	
Normal	< 120/80
Prehypertension	120–139/80–89
Hypertension	> 140/90
Stage 1	140–159/90–99
Stage 2	> 160/100

3. BLOOD PRESSURE AND BODY WEIGHT

Overweight is an increasingly prevalent condition throughout the world. In the United States, recent data indicate that as much as 66% of the adult population is overweight or obese (4).

There is a positive relationship between overweight or obesity, on the one hand, and BP and risk for hypertension, on the other. The Framingham Study found that in both sexes hypertension is about twice as prevalent in the obese as the nonobese. Stamler and colleagues *(5)* noted an odds ratio for hypertension of obese relative to nonobese (BMI of <25) of 2.4 for younger adults and 1.5 for older ones. The Nurses' Health Study compared women with BMIs of <22 with those >29 and found a two- to sixfold greater prevalence of hypertension among the obese. More recent data from the Framingham Study add further support to this relationship. Divided into BMI quintiles, Framingham participants of both sexes demonstrated increasing BPs with increased overweight. In this instance those in the highest BMI quintile exhibited 16 mmHg higher systolic and 9 mmHg higher diastolic BPs than those in the lowest BMI quintile. For systolic BP this translated into an increase of 4 mmHg for each 4.5 kg of increased weight. In younger Canadian adults there is a fivefold greater prevalence of hypertension in individuals of both sexes with BMIs of >30 relative to those <20.

Consistent with the above findings numerous clinical interventions have reported that weight loss is associated with a decrease in BP. In a meta-analysis of 25 studies Neter et al. *(6)* concluded that a 1 kg loss of body weight is associated with an approximate 1 mmHg drop in BP. This was achieved without the necessity of also attaining normal weight status. The Trial of Hypertension Prevention, one of the largest of these studies, included a weight loss intervention arm. In this trial, a 2 kg loss in weight over a 6-month period resulted in a decline of 3.7 mmHg in systolic and 2.7 mmHg in diastolic BP. There was also a 42% decline in the prevalence of hypertension *(7)*.

Another analysis examined eight trials for the effects of weight gain and loss on BP. The findings revealed that weight gain was associated with increased BP while, conversely, weight loss resulted in reduced BP. BP reductions were approximately 5.2 mmHg for both systolic and diastolic pressures for varying degrees of weight reduction.

4. DIET AND BP

4.1. Dietary Sodium

The jury of scientific opinion is still out on the degree to which weight loss or sodium restriction make independent contributions to BP reduction. An early study found that sodium restriction in low-calorie diets was thought to be the primary cause of BP reduction. Several more recent studies have sided with weight loss as having an independent effect on BP reduction *(8)*.

Chief among perceived dietary influences on BP is sodium consumption. A large literature supports the notion that decreasing sodium consumption below that typical in Western society will result in a decline in BP. Numerous epidemiological studies have demonstrated this relationship *(9)*. Reductions in sodium intake of around 75 mmol/day are associated with a decline in BP of about 1.9 mmHg systolic and 1.1 mmHg diastolic. The previously mentioned Trial of Hypertension Prevention (TOHP) found that a decrease of 44 mmol/day of sodium leads to a 38% reduction in the prevalence of hypertension in one of its treatment arms.

The Dietary Alterations to Stop Hypertension Study (DASH-Na) observed in persons with elevated BP who were eating a typical American diet that an approximate 100 mmol/day reduction in sodium intake leads to a maximum reduction in systolic and diastolic BP of about 6.7 and 3.5 mmHg, respectively. When the reduction in sodium consumption was only half as much (approximately 50 mmol/day), there was much less decline in systolic and diastolic BP (2.1 and 1.1 mmHg, respectively) *(10)*. These findings were produced in the absence of weight loss.

The TOHP examined 181 participants for the effect of either weight loss or sodium reduction on BP *(11)*. The subjects were randomly assigned to a nontreated control, a sodium-reduction, or a weight-loss arm. The active component of the intervention lasted 18 months but individuals were further monitored for BP, weight, and dietary status for 7 years. Incident hypertension was the outcome variable of interest. This was 32.9% in the control group. The weight-loss group (in the absence of sodium restriction) had an average reduction of 5 kg in weight at 18 months; they demonstrated an incidence of hypertension of 18.9% after 7 year. This contrasts with the sodium-reduction group (in the absence of weight loss) which had a prevalence of hypertension of 22.4% over the same period. These results were found in spite of the fact that much of the weight in the weight-loss group had been regained at year 7. The odds of hypertension was reduced by 77% in the weight-loss group and by 35% in the sodium-reduction group compared with their control groups.

The results of the various studies looked at above support the recommendations of the Dietary Guidelines for Americans and the American Heart Association for a heart-healthy diet. Both recommend that people choose and prepare foods with little salt (less than 2300 mg of sodium per day or approximately one teaspoon of salt).

4.2. Potassium and BP

The contention that increased potassium intake is associated with decreased BP levels has received somewhat mixed support in the scientific literature. The INTERSALT study *(12)* found a negative correlation between urinary potassium excretion and BP. In contrast, the TOHP 1 trial found little maintained impact on BP accompanying a 44 mmol/day supplementation of potassium chloride. A meta-analysis conducted by Whelton et al. *(13)* concluded that most instances of oral potassium supplementation were associated with decreases in systolic and diastolic BP of approximately 3.1 and 2.0 mmHg, respectively. However, most of these findings occurred in groups consuming high sodium intakes *(14)* thereby making interpretation somewhat more complicated. Moreover, physicians view potassium supplementation with a cautious eye due to its potential for damage from acute hyperkalemia and instead prefer to recommend increased potassium intake.

4.3. Dietary Patterns and BP

Other studies have investigated the effect of manipulations of dietary patterns on BP *(15)*. The motivation for this line of research was the recognition of the inconsistent effects of micronutrient supplementation.

Vegetarian diets are widely associated with lower BP levels. The DASH Trial demonstrated that a diet high in fruit, vegetables, and low-fat dairy servings could reduce systolic and diastolic BP by 5.3 and 3.0 mmHg, respectively, in the absence of either weight loss or sodium restriction *(15)*. Raben et al. *(16)* found that significantly increased sucrose consumption leads to noteworthy increases in both weight and fat mass as well as increases in BP by about 4 mmHg.

4.4. Dietary Fat

Dietary fat intake is variably associated with BP. This is likely due to the different kinds of fat consumed. The Multiple Risk Factor Intervention Trial (MRFIT) found that a diet high in cholesterol and saturated fat is positively associated with both systolic and diastolic BP. Concurrently, the study found an inverse relationship between diastolic blood pressure and polyunsaturated fat intake. In other studies, *n*–3 fatty acids typically show a negative association with BP in those with elevated BP. Monounsaturated fat consumption is inconsistently associated with BP *(14)*.

4.5. Dietary Protein

The relationship between dietary protein and BP may vary with the type of protein. Studies examining this association have produced variable results. The previously cited INTERSALT study found an inverse relationship between protein consumption and BP with higher consumption of protein associated with a 3.0 mmHg lower systolic BP relative to lower consumption *(12)*. The MRFIT also found a very modest negative association between protein intake and BP. In contrast, some observational studies indicate that cultures with high protein consumptions typically have higher average BPs *(17)* and high-protein diets are contraindicated in individuals with high BP and accompanying renal deficit *(14)*. One possibility is that vegetable sources of protein may promote BP reduction *(17)*.

4.6. Alcohol Intake

Alcohol intake is positively associated with BP in most studies. The MRFIT program noted a positive relationship with amount of alcohol consumed and both systolic and diastolic BP. Subsequent decrease in alcohol intake was also associated with a decrease in BP. The INTERSALT study also noted this relationship, at least in those who routinely consumed larger amounts of alcohol. Viewing the data in the larger perspective, JNC VII recommendations are to limit alcohol consumption to two drinks per day for men and one drink per day for women *(1)*.

5. SUMMARY

Numerous dietary manipulations have a significant impact on BP. The array of dietary patterns, macro- and micronutrients implicated in control of BP and hypertension is impressive and growing over time. Much further research is still necessary, particularly in the areas of micronutrient interactions and in elucidating the roles of dietary fat and protein in BP management. Findings resulting from such investigations will ultimately help fine-tune dietary approaches to the management of BP and the control hypertension.

SUGGESTED FURTHER READING

www.nhlbi.nih.gov/hbp The National Heart Lung and Blood Institute provides information for preventing and controlling high blood pressure.

www.nhlbi.nih.gov/health/public/heart/hbp/dash Access the DASH Eating Plan – "Lowering Your Blood Pressure with DASH." Click on the brochure for the full report.

REFERENCES

1. JNC VII Express. The Seventh Report of the Joint National Committee on Prevention, Detection, Evaluation, and Treatment of High Blood Pressure. National Institutes of Health, Bethesda, MD. Publication No. 03-5233; 2003.
2. Havas S, Roccella EJ, Lenfant C. Reducing the public health burden from elevated blood pressure levels in the United States by lowering intake of dietary sodium. Am J Public Health 2004; 94:19–22.
3. Neal B, MacMahon S, Chapman N. Effects of ACE inhibitors, calcium antagonists, and other blood-pressure-lowering drugs: results of prospectively designed overviews of randomised trials. Blood Pressure Lowering Treatment Trialists' Collaboration. Lancet 2000; 356:1955–1964.

4. Ogden CL, Carroll MD, Curtin LR, McDowell MA, Tabak CJ, Flegal KM. Prevalence of overweight and obesity in the United States. 1999–2004. JAMA 2006; 295:1549–1555.

5. Stamler R, Stamler J, Riedlinger WF, Algera G, Roberts R. Weight and blood pressure: findings in hypertension screening of 1 million Americans. JAMA 1978; 240:1607–1609.

6. Neter JE, Stam BE, Kok FJ, Grobbee DE, Gelseijnse JM. Influence of weight reduction on blood pressure: a meta-analysis of randomized controlled trials. Hypertension 2003; 42:878–884.

7. Stevens VJ, Obarzanek E, Cook NR, et al. Trials of hypertension prevention, phase II. Ann Intern Med 2001; 134:1–11.

8. Maxwell MH, Kushiro T, Dornfeld LP, Tuck ML, Waks AU. BP changes in obese hypertensive subjects during rapid weight loss. Comparison of restricted v unchanged salt intake. Arch Intern Med 1984; 144:1581–1584.

9. Cutler JA, Follman D, Allender PS. Randomized trials of sodium reduction: an overview. Am J Clin Nutr 1997; 65:643S–651S.

10. Sacks FM, Svetkey LP, Vollmer WM, et al. DASH-Sodium Collaborative Research Group. Effects on blood pressure of reduced dietary sodium and the Dietary Approaches to Stop Hypertension (DASH) Diet. N Engl J Med 2001; 344:3–10.

11. He J, Whelton PK, Appel LJ, Charleston J, Klag MJ. Long-term effects of weight loss and dietary sodium reduction on incidence of hypertension. Hypertension 2000; 35: 544–549.

12. Intersalt Cooperative Research Group. Intersalt: an international study of electrolyte excretion and blood pressure. Results for 24 hour sodium and potassium excretion. BMJ 1988; 297: 319–328.

13. Whelton PK, He J, Cutler JA, Brancatti FL, Appel LJ, Follmann D, Klag MJ. Effects of oral potassium on blood pressure. Meta-analysis of randomized controlled clinical trials. JAMA 1997; 297:1624–1632.

14. Hermansen K. Diet, blood pressure and hypertension. Br J Nutr 2000; 83(suppl 1): S113–S119.

15. Appel LJ, Moore TJ, Obarzanek E, et al. DASH Collaborative Research Group. N Engl J Med 1997; 336:1117–1124.

16. Raben A, Vasilaras TH, Møller AC, Astrup A. Sucrose compared with artificial sweeteners: different effects on ad libitum food intake and body weight after 10 wk of supplementation in overweight subjects. Am J Clin Nutr 2002; 76:721–729.

17. Elliot P, Stamler J, Dyer AR, et al. Association between protein intake and blood pressure, the Intermap study. Arch Intern Med 2006; 166:79–87.

27 Gastrointestinal Disorders: Does Nutrition Control the Disease?

Alice N. Brako

Key Points

- Nutrition has a role in the etiology and management of gastrointestinal (GI) diseases.
- Overnutrition leading to overweight and obesity is a risk factor for gastroesophageal reflux disease.
- Nutritional requirements greatly increase with severe malabsorptive diseases such as celiac disease and Crohn's disease.
- To prevent weight loss associated with malabsorptive GI diseases, a variety of feeding methods, with emphasis on a high-calorie, high-protein diet that also includes micronutrient supplementation, should be the key.

Key Words: Gastroesophageal reflux disease (GERD); constipation; peptic ulcers; diverticulosis; inflammatory bowel disease; colon cancer

1. INTRODUCTION

"Nutrition" is the term used in this chapter to characterize a relatively new scientific discipline that examines how food nourishes the body and influences health. Nutrition encompasses how food is consumed, digested, absorbed, and, also, how the waste products of digestion are eliminated. The gastrointestinal system receives food and, through complex mechanical and chemical processes involving several organs, extracts nutrients. Nutrients are substances in foods that are necessary for providing the body with energy and building blocks to support its structure and for regulating metabolism. Gastrointestinal disorders occur when there is malfunction of one or more of the digestive organs, or when there is disruption of the mechanical or

From: *Nutrition and Health: Nutrition Guide for Physicians*
Edited by: T. Wilson et al. (eds.), DOI 10.1007/978-1-60327-431-9_27,
© Humana Press, a part of Springer Science+Business Media, LLC 2010

chemical processes of digestion. GI diseases are common in primary care, and the prevalence of some is increasing. Additionally, of the top 10 high-cost physical health conditions affecting people in the United States, GI disorders rank second *(1)*.

Gastroesophageal reflux disease and peptic ulcers are common problems that affect the upper GI tract. They are serious conditions characterized by excessive acid production that causes frequent discomfort and tissue damage. Disorders of the lower GI tract include constipation, diarrhea, diverticulosis and diverticulitis, celiac disease, inflammatory bowel disease, and colorectal cancer. Constipation is characterized by infrequent bowel movements, altered stool consistency or straining, that is difficulty with passage of bowel movements. Diarrhea is associated with passage of frequent stools of watery to loose consistency. Diverticulosis refers to the presence of pouches in the intestinal wall; it can lead to diverticulitis if the pouches are inflamed. Celiac disease is a genetic problem characterized by an abnormal immune response to proteins (e.g., gluten) in wheat, barley, and rye. Inflammatory bowel diseases are chronic conditions associated with extensive damage to intestinal tissue which causes serious complications to the GI tract. They include Crohn's disease and ulcerative colitis. Colorectal cancer is the third most diagnosed malignant neoplasm in the United States. A food allergy is a hypersensitivity reaction of the immune system to a particular food substance, usually a protein *(2)*.

Because of the intricate relationship between nutrition and the GI tract, diet has an impact on the development and subsequent medical management of GI disorders, and the diseases discussed subsequently may benefit from dietary adjustments.

2. CONSTIPATION

Constipation is a common problem of the lower gastrointestinal tract and is associated with stools that are hard to pass and infrequent bowel movements. The prevalence of constipation ($\sim$15–20%) is higher in women than men and appears to increase with age over 65 yr. A low-fiber diet often contributes to constipation. The lack of bulk that comes with fiber causes slow colonic transit, resulting in excessive absorption of water from the colon. This leaves dry hard stools that are hard to pass. Other nutritional-related causes of constipation include use of aluminum-containing antacids and iron and calcium supplements *(2)*. Paradoxically, these substances are often used to treat other GI disorders or are a part of standard vitamin/mineral supplementation regimens.

3. DIARRHEA

Diarrhea is characterized by frequent (more than three) watery to loose stools in a 24-h period. Diarrhea can be classified as acute or chronic. Acute diarrhea is usually caused by an infection from a bacteria, virus, or parasite, which may be present in animal and human fecal matter or contaminated food, milk, and water. Symptoms may persist for 1–2 days with or without serious consequences; however, persistent diarrhea lasting more than 3 days often leads to dehydration and electrolyte imbalance and can be fatal, particularly in children and the elderly. Other symptoms of diarrhea may include cramping, abdominal pain, bloating, nausea, fever, and bloody stools. Prolonged diarrhea that lasts for a month or longer is chronic; it may be caused by a large number of diseases, some of which are related to nutrients, such as allergies to cow's milk, lactose intolerance, and celiac disease.

Nutritional therapy for diarrhea is aimed at replacing fluids and electrolytes through consumption of water, juices, and sports drinks; and eliminating the cause of diarrhea (contaminated foods). Juices should be diluted down since they are often hyperosmolar and would otherwise aggravate the diarrhea. The optimal fluid replacement therapy has an osmolality at or below that of plasma ($\sim$280 mOsm/kg). If solid foods are tolerated, restricting insoluble fiber can assist in slowing gut transit time; yogurt intake may be helpful in replacing commensal gut flora; and increasing soluble dietary fiber intake may be helpful with chronic diarrhea; however, these suggestions are based more on belief than evidence (3).

4. IRRITABLE BOWEL SYNDROME

In addition to the symptoms of chronic constipation or diarrhea, the association of altered bowel function and abdominal pain is commonly recognized as irritable bowel syndrome (IBS). This is sometimes associated with abdominal bloating and passage of gas. These symptoms are reduced by dietary supplementation with single probiotics like *Bifidobacterium infantis* or combination probiotics, as with VSL#3. Probiotics are discussed below under inflammatory bowel diseases.

5. FOOD ALLERGY

A food allergy is characterized by an abnormal immune reaction to a particular component in food, usually a protein. Food allergies are far less common than most other GI disorders, but their prevalence has increased markedly over the last 50 yr. Approximately 30,000 Americans require emergency room treatment and 150 people die each year because of allergic reactions to food, however, these are predominantly generalized anaphylactic reactions, as may occur with peanut allergy, rather than allergies with GI symptoms. Food allergy usually manifests in early childhood as part of the so-called atopic march and most commonly involves one or more of the following foods: cow's milk, hen's egg, soy, peanuts and tree nuts, wheat, sesame seed, kiwi fruit, and seafood *(4)*.

The diagnostic approach to adverse reactions to food is based on accurate clinical history and objective examination, and further execution of specific tests when allergy or intolerance is suspected. Symptoms may be localized or systemic, and the latter may lead to anaphylactic shock. The therapy for food allergies is the elimination of the food to which hypersensitivity has been found; this strategy can lead, especially in pediatric age, to tolerance. If elimination diets cannot be completely performed, or if it is not possible to identify the food to eliminate, some drugs (e.g., antihistaminics, steroids) can be administered. Specific allergen immunotherapy has been recently introduced. It is fundamental to prevent food allergy, especially in high-risk subjects *(5)*.

6. DIVERTICULOSIS AND DIVERTICULITIS

Diverticulosis refers to a disorder in which pouches develop in weakened areas of the intestinal wall, typically at the site where arteries normally penetrate from the outside of the wall toward the internal lining or mucosa. Most people with diverticulosis are asymptomatic. However, some people may develop inflammation (diverticulitis) typically when the pouch is blocked; this can manifest as persistent abdominal pain, and alternating constipation and diarrhea, with possible loss of fluids and electrolytes. Patients have tenderness on examination over the inflamed area of colon.

About 10% of Americans older than age 40 and about 50% of people over 60 yr have colonic diverticulosis *(6)*. A major risk factor for developing this includes a low-fiber diet. Such a diet facilitates development of increased intraluminal pressure that induces tubular sacs to form and protrude on the serosal side, away from the intestinal lumen of the colon.

Nutrition may play a role in treatment of diverticulosis and diverticulitis. When diverticulitis occurs, a low-fiber diet is recommended to facilitate smooth passage of stools through the inflamed area. Once healing is restored, the approach is to encourage an increase in fluids and the insoluble fiber content of the diet to prevent future diverticuli. Previous recommendations for patients with diverticular disease to avoid nuts and seeds are no longer indicated since there is no firm evidence that these foods trigger inflammation.

7. GASTROESOPHAGEAL REFLUX DISEASE

Gastroesophageal reflux disease (GERD) is a painful condition of the upper gastrointestinal tract characterized by heartburn that occurs more than twice a week. About 19 million people in the United States experience GERD each year, making it one of the most prevalent GI disorders (7). The main cause of GERD is a transient relaxation or weakening of the lower esophageal sphincter (LES) which allows regurgitation of gastric acid and other gastric contents, including bile, back into the esophagus, thereby causing substernal discomfort and heartburn. The esophageal lining is susceptible to irritation by acid because it does not have the thick mucous protection of the stomach, attributable to the mucin-secreting gastric epithelial cells. Some people with GERD do not experience heartburn, but may have difficulty swallowing, burning sensation in the mouth, a feeling that food is stuck at any level of the esophagus, or hoarseness in the morning (7).

There are a number of predisposing factors associated with GERD, including a hiatal hernia, cigarette smoking, alcohol use, being overweight or obese, and pregnancy. Foods such as citrus fruits, chocolate, caffeinated drinks, fried foods, garlic, onions, spicy foods, and tomato-based foods, such as chili, pizza, and spaghetti sauce are associated with heartburn symptoms. Consumption of large high-fat meals requires prolonged gastric passage times and the increased stomach pressure may lead to movement of hydrochloric acid from the stomach into the esophagus. Additionally, lying prone after a meal promotes backflow of stomach contents and the development of symptoms (8). GERD may result in persistent irritation of the esophageal lining; the resulting esophagitis may lead to malnutrition due to development of a stricture leading to dysphagia and a loss of appetite. Bleeding related to chronic inflammation or surface epithelial erosive change causes loss of iron as well as other blood nutrients (minerals, vitamins, amino acids, glucose, fatty acids).

Effective treatments for GERD include identifying and avoiding foods that trigger increased acid production. People can reduce symptoms by eating smaller meals, waiting at least 3 h after a meal before lying down, and elevating the head of the bed by four to six inches to allow gravity to keep stomach contents down. Diet therapy may also require replacing lost nutrients with the use of vitamin and mineral supplements. Patient compliance may be low but these lifestyle modifications are the first step in management, before prescription of a proton pump inhibitor.

8. PEPTIC ULCERS

Ulcers are erosions or sores of the mucosal lining of the stomach and duodenum. The majority of ulcers occur in the duodenum which lacks the thick, protective mucosal lining of the stomach and is therefore more susceptible to damage by the acidic chyme before it is neutralized by bicarbonate secreted from the pancreas. One in 10 Americans develops a peptic ulcer at some time in his or her life *(8)*.

The primary cause of peptic and duodenal ulcers is now widely accepted to be due to an infection with *Helicobacter pylori* (*H. pylori*); prolonged use of nonsteroidal anti-inflammatory drugs (NSAIDs) remains an additional cause. For many years, the cause of ulcers was thought to be stress, alcohol, and spicy foods but this focus on lifestyle and diet has changed since the discovery of *H. pylori* as the chief causative agent. However, stress is still thought to play a role because of its effects on behavioral changes such as increased use of alcohol which is a potential risk factor *(8)*.

Upper abdominal pain occurring 1–3 h after eating remains a primary symptom. Duodenal ulcer discomfort may be relieved by eating, while the discomfort due to gastric ulcers may also be paradoxically aggravated by food and cause loss of appetite and subsequent weight loss. Peptic ulcers can also be accompanied by hemorrhaging, resulting in iron deficiency anemia, and vomiting, leading to electrolyte losses.

The goals for peptic ulcer treatment include relief of symptoms, promotion of mucosal repair, and prevention of recurrence. This is achieved with a combination of medications including antibiotics to eradicate *H. pylori*, mucosal protectants, antacids, and proton pump inhibitors, and stopping NSAID use. Dietary recommendations are adapted to individual food tolerances. Foods that trigger acid secretion such as alcohol, caffeine and caffeine-containing beverages, and spicy foods should be avoided. Patient compliance is generally poor and this is less important with the highly effective treatments with antibiotics and proton pump inhibitors. A bland diet has not been shown to increase the rate of healing *(9)*.

9. INFLAMMATORY BOWEL DISEASES

Inflammatory bowel diseases (IBDs) are characterized by chronic inflammation and diarrhea of the lower gastrointestinal tract and include Crohn's disease and ulcerative colitis. Crohn's disease usually affects the small and large intestines, and less frequently the mouth, esophagus, and stomach, and causes damage that may extend through all layers of the gut wall. In contrast, ulcerative colitis involves the colon and the very end of the small intestine with tissue damage limited to the surface layers. IBDs usually present between 15 and 30 yr of age and are now generally classified as autoimmune diseases with a genetic basis *(9)*.

The pattern of ulcerations in Crohn's disease is patchy, with normal tissue separated by diseased regions. Patients with Crohn's disease may require surgical resection to remove affected areas, but new regions often become ulcerated.

The main consequence of Crohn's disease is malnutrition resulting from intestinal resections as well as from impaired digestion and absorption. Reduced nutrient intake and eventual weight loss are common due to poor absorption of bile salts as a result of the interruption of the enterohepatic circulation. Thus, if the ileum is involved, bile acids may become depleted because of the loss of the active transport site for bile acids; this may cause malabsorption of fat, fat-soluble vitamins, calcium, magnesium, and zinc. Additionally, vitamin B12 deficiency can occur with ileal involvement, resulting in anemia.

The rectum is always involved in ulcerative colitis and lesions may extend into the colon. In mild cases, patients experience diarrhea and there may be weight loss, fever, and weakness, but in more severe forms, the disease is characterized by anemia, dehydration, electrolyte imbalance, and protein losses.

Dietary treatment for both Crohn's disease and ulcerative colitis should aim at preventing symptoms associated with the diseases, correcting malnutrition, promoting healing of affected tissue, and enhancing normal growth and development in children. Approaches to nutritional therapy are variable and are based on individual symptoms, complications, and documented nutritional deficiencies. A high-calorie, high-protein diet is generally indicated, and adults with advanced disease may require 40 kcal/kg/d, or approximately 2.2 times the basal metabolic energy needs *(10)*. Nutritional supplements may be recommended, especially for children whose growth has been retarded. Special high-calorie liquid formulas are sometimes used for this purpose. A small number of patients may require periods of parenteral feeding to provide extra nutrition, allow the intestines to rest and hopefully heal, or to bypass the intestines for individuals whose guts cannot absorb enough nutrition from ingested food. Because of fat malabsorption, limiting fat intake may help, and medium-chain triglycerides may be better tolerated as they can be absorbed without the participation of bile salts. In some patients, a low-fiber diet may be indicated if there is a partial narrowing of the small intestine, while in others lactose restriction is to be recommended if the patient has proven lactose intolerance *(10)*.

Prebiotics are nondigestible dietary oligosaccharides that affect the host by selectively stimulating growth, activity, or both of selective intestinal (probiotic) commensal bacteria. These bacteria may provide protection, stimulate local immune responses to combat infectious organisms, or suppress inflammation caused by antigens *(11)*. Although more clinical studies need to be done, preliminary results from animal models and humans indicate that prebiotics and probiotics may provide effective treatments for people with IBD *(12)*. There is convincing evidence to support the use of probiotics in the treatment of pouchitis, a common problem among those who have had ileal pouch-anal anastomosis surgery for ulcerative colitis.

Currently, there is an explosion of these products in the market. They are added to dairy products, such as yogurt drinks, and are also sold in the form of capsules. The role of *n*–3 fatty acids in the management of IBD is not clear. Results from some studies show they may have the potential to alleviate intestinal inflammation *(13)*, but findings from other investigations do not support this anti-inflammatory role *(14)*.

10. COLORECTAL CANCER

People with either ulcerative colitis or Crohn's disease are at an increased risk of colon cancer. Approximately 48 cases of colorectal cancer were diagnosed per 100,000 people in the United States in 2004, making it the third most commonly diagnosed cancer *(15)*.

Although a high-fat diet was thought to contribute to an increased risk of colon cancer, recent studies reveal factors found in red meat, other than fat, that are correlated with a higher risk *(16)*. Some epidemiological data indicate that a high-fiber diet is protective against colorectal cancer, however, short-term human clinical trials have not produced supportive findings. Other population studies show that people who consume higher amounts of raw and cooked garlic lower their risk for colorectal cancer *(15)*. A recent study on the adherence to the USDA Food Guide, Dietary Approaches to Stop Hypertension (DASH) Eating Plan, and Mediterranean Dietary Pattern concluded that people who follow these dietary recommendations have a reduced risk of colorectal cancer, and the risk reduction is higher for men *(17)*. It is possible that these diets are protective against colorectal cancer because they emphasize consumption of generous amounts of fruits and vegetables – foods rich in antioxidants and fiber – though their causative links remain unconfirmed. Intriguingly, colorectal cancer mortality was found to be inversely proportional to serum vitamin D levels *(18)*. Further investigation of vitamin D's effects is needed and will hopefully clarify this apparent correlation. Similarly, further long-term studies are needed to clarify the role of nutrients, including folic acid and fat, as well as fiber.

11. CELIAC DISEASE

Celiac disease or Sprue is a genetic disorder characterized by intolerance to gluten, the primary protein found in wheat, rye, and barley. Approximately one in 133 people in the United States is affected by this disease, a proportion higher than previously estimated *(19)*. More than 95% of celiac patients share the major histocompatibility complex II class human leukocyte antigen (HLA) DQ2 or DQ8 haplotype; patients negative for both haplotypes are unlikely to suffer from the disease *(20)*. Some cases of Sprue develop in infancy or childhood, and others occur later in life.

In susceptible individuals, the cells of the small intestine mount an immune response against gluten, with subsequent damage and erosion of the intestinal villi. The damage to the brush border, which normally absorbs nutrients, can lead to malabsorption and, over time, malnutrition can occur. Deficiencies of fat-soluble vitamins (A, D, E, and K), iron, folic acid, and calcium are common in people afflicted with celiac disease. There is increased risk of osteoporosis, from poor calcium absorption, diminished growth because of overall nutrient malabsorption, and seizures as a result of inadequate folate absorption *(21)*. The only effective treatment for celiac disease is a gluten-free diet *(22)*. There are many gluten-free foods, such as meats, milk, eggs, fruit, and vegetables. Rice, potatoes, corn, and beans are also gluten free. Specialty food stores and many supermarkets now provide specially formulated gluten-free breads, pasta, and cereal products.

12. CONCLUSION

The digestive system serves as the gateway into the body for nutrients that are derived from mechanical and chemical digestion of food. Foods and nutrients, such as caffeine and caffeine-containing beverages, alcohol, spicy foods, onions, garlic, and fried foods, affect the secretory function of the stomach, possibly aggravating GERD and peptic ulcers. Inadequate fiber and fluids in the diet can cause hypomotility of the intestinal wall, leading to constipation.

The absorptive function of the gut is impaired by diseases of the small and large intestines, including celiac disease, IBDs, diverticulitis, and colorectal cancer. In severe cases, these malabsorptive diseases can result in serious energy and nutritional deficiencies. Nutritional care is important in the prevention and management of GI diseases and should adapt food intake to the symptoms and complications of the disease and at the same time consider individual food tolerances. Current dietary recommendations, such as the USDA's Food Guide and the DASH diet, provide useful dietary practices for reducing risk of some diseases, such as colorectal cancer. Additionally, prebiotics and probiotics have potential as treatments for Crohn's disease, ulcerative colitis, and irritable bowel syndrome and warrant further investigation.

SUGGESTED FURTHER READING

Hark L, Morrison G. Medical Nutrition and Disease: A Case-based Approach (3rd ed.). Blackwell, Malden, MA, 2003.

Feagan BG, Sandborn WJ, Mittman U, et al. Omega-3 free fatty acids for the maintenance of remission in Crohn disease: the EPIC randomized controlled trials. JAMA 2008; 299:1690–1697.

Mitsuyama K, Sata M. Gut microflora: a new target for therapeutic approaches in inflammatory bowel disease. Expert Opin Ther Targets 2008; 12:301–312.

Freedman DM, Looker AC, Chang SC, Graubard BI. Prospective study of serum vitamin D and cancer mortality in the United States. J Natl Cancer Inst 2007; 99:1594–1602.

Westerberg DP, Gill JM, Dave B, et al. New strategies for diagnosis and management of celiac disease. J Am Osteopath Assoc 2006; 106:145–151.

REFERENCES

1. Goetzel RZ, Ozminkowski RJ, Meneades L, Stewart M, Schutt DC. Top 10 high cost physical health conditions. J Occup Environ Med 2000; 42:338–351.

2. Whitney E, DeBruyne LK, Pinna K, Rolfes SR. Nutrition for Health and Health Care (3rd ed.). Thomson Wadsworth, Belmont, CA, 2007.

3. Hark L, Morrison G. Medical Nutrition and Disease: A Case-Based Approach (3rd ed.). Blackwell, Malden, MA, 2003.

4. Meyer R. New guidelines for managing cow's milk allergy in infants. J Fam Health Care 2008; 18:27–30.

5. Montalto M, Santoro L, D'Onofrio F, et al. Adverse reactions to food: allergies and intolerances. Dig Disease 2008; 26:96–103.

6. Diverticulosis and Diverticulitis. Available at www.digestive.niddk.nih.gov/ddiseases/pubs/diverticulosis/index.htm#1. Last accessed April 29, 2008.

7. Thompson J, Manore M. Nutrition: An Applied Approach (2nd ed.). Pearson Benjamin Cummings, New York, 2008.

8. Whitney E, DeBruyne LK, Pinna K, Rolfes SR. Nutrition for Health and Health Care (3rd ed.). Thomson Wadsworth, Belmont, CA, 2007.

9. McGuire M, Beerman KA. Nutritional Sciences: From Fundamentals to Food. Thomson Wadsworth, Belmont, CA, 2007.

10. Hark L, Morrison G. Medical Nutrition and Disease: A Case-Based Approach (3rd ed.). Blackwell, Malden, MA, 2003.

11. Leenen CHM, Dieleman LA. Inulin and oligofructose in chronic inflammatory bowel disease. J Nutr 2007; 137:2572S–2575S.

12. Mitsuyama K, Sata M. Gut microflora: a new target for therapeutic approaches in inflammatory bowel disease. Expert Opin Ther Targets 2008; 12:301–312.

13. Innis SM, Jacobson K. Dietary lipids in early development and intestinal inflammatory disease. Nutr Rev 2007; 65:S188–193.

14. Feagan BG, Sandborn WJ, Mittman U, et al. Omega-3 free fatty acids for the maintenance of remission in Crohn disease: the EPIC randomized controlled trials. JAMA 2008; 299:1690–1697.

15. Garlic and cancer: questions and answers. Available at www.cancer.gov/cancertopics/factsheet/Prevention/garlic-and-cancer-prevention. Last accessed April 29, 2008.
16. Martinez ME, Jacobs ET, Ashbeck EL, et al. Meat intake, preparation methods, mutagens and colorectal adenoma recurrence. Carcinogenesis 2007; 28:2019–2027.
17. Dixon B, Subar AF, Peters U, et al. Adherence to the USDA food guide, DASH eating plan, and Mediterranean dietary pattern reduces risk of colorectal adenoma. J Nutr 2007; 137:2443–2450.
18. Freedman DM, Looker AC, Chang SC, Graubard BI. Prospective study of serum vitamin D and cancer mortality in the United States. J Natl Cancer Inst 2007; 99:1594–1602.
19. Blake JS. Nutrition and You. Pearson Benjamin Cummings, New York, 2008.
20. Kaukinen K, Partanen J, Maki M, Collin P. HLA-DQ typing in the diagnosis of celiac disease. Am J Gastroenterol 2002; 97:695–699.
21. Presutti RJ, Cangemi JR, Cassidy HD, Hill DA. Celiac disease. Am Fam Physician 2007; 76:1795–1802.
22. Westerberg DP, Gill JM, Dave B, et al. New strategies for diagnosis and management of celiac disease. J Am Osteopath Assoc 2006; 106:145–151.

28 Nutrition in Patients with Diseases of the Liver and Pancreas

Roman E. Perri

Key Points

- Protein-calorie malnutrition (PCM) is common in patients with cirrhosis and screening should be performed to detect its presence.
- Dietary protein intake of 1.2–1.5 g/kg/d is safe for patients with advanced liver disease. Significant protein restriction should be avoided in cirrhotics, even those with hepatic encephalopathy.
- Chronic overnutrition and resultant obesity/insulin insensitivity is associated with the development of chronic liver disease; nutritional counseling should be provided to patients with obesity and liver disease. Gradual weight loss through diet and exercise is warranted in this group of patients.
- Severe acute pancreatitis can result in marked malnutrition and mortality is high. Nutritional support through enteral nutrition is the preferred method of maintaining adequate nutrition in this setting.
- Chronic pancreatitis is associated with exocrine insufficiency that may require supplemental pancreatic enzymes and dietary adjustments to control symptoms and maintain adequate nutrition.

Key Words: Protein-calorie malnutrition

1. PATIENTS WITH LIVER DISEASE

Patients with the end-stage liver disease of cirrhosis frequently exhibit significant malnutrition, and the proper medical management of the cirrhotic patient focuses, in large part, on nutritional aspects of therapy. The liver is a fundamental organ for maintenance of metabolic homeostasis and therefore,

From: *Nutrition and Health: Nutrition Guide for Physicians*
Edited by: T. Wilson et al. (eds.), DOI 10.1007/978-1-60327-431-9_28,
© Humana Press, a part of Springer Science+Business Media, LLC 2010

when the liver's ability to maintain homeostasis is compromised, it can be expected that significant metabolic abnormalities will result. The prevalence of protein-calorie malnutrition (PCM) has been found to be up to 80% in patients with alcoholic liver disease. Other etiologies of cirrhosis, including viral liver disease and biliary cirrhosis, are also associated with high prevalence of malnutrition (1). In addition to PCM, patients with cirrhosis often have significant abnormalities in the homeostasis of fluids and electrolytes. The nutritional management of patients with cirrhosis is complex, but as the presence of malnutrition has been shown to independently predict poor survival, it is imperative that close attention be paid to the nutritional and metabolic complications of liver disease.

Patients at the highest risk of nutritional compromise are those with advanced liver disease; this is characterized by decreased liver synthetic function and complications such as the development of hepatic encephalopathy or ascites. Those patients who have well-compensated cirrhosis without these complicating developments may also be at risk of nutritional deficits (2). The process by which PCM develops in the cirrhotic patient is complex and is likely secondary to anorexia, nausea, poor dietary intake, and hypermetabolism, all of which are prevalent in patients with cirrhosis. It is therefore of utmost importance to assess all patients with chronic liver disease for evidence of PCM.

Patients with cirrhosis require sufficient protein intake; an intake of 1.2–1.5 g/kg/d is considered appropriate (3). Administration of a late-night snack was found to augment the typical dietary intake of patients and to result in improved serum albumin and markers of energy metabolism (4). The use of enteral supplementation for cirrhotic patients found to be undernourished has been demonstrated to be clinically beneficial in those with alcoholic liver disease.

The administration of moderate amounts (1.2–1.5 g/kg/d) of dietary protein to patients with advanced liver disease is a somewhat controversial topic as it is recognized that a significant dietary protein load can be a precipitant for hepatic encephalopathy. Therefore, the traditional instruction for patients who have decompensated cirrhosis is to avoid excessive quantities of protein at meals. In patients who are hospitalized for hepatic encephalopathy, this has been extrapolated to include the placement of patients on a protein-restricted diet while in the hospital. While the abrupt though temporary withdrawal of dietary protein during the search for an etiology of hepatic encephalopathy is reasonable, a prolonged limitation of dietary protein is not warranted. A recent study has demonstrated that protein intake of 1.2 g/kg/d can be safely administered to patients hospitalized with hepatic encephalopathy throughout the course of their hospitalization (5). Liver disease is characterized by amino acid metabolism that results in low levels of branched-chain amino acids, a finding that likely results from many potential sources *(6)*. It is theorized that the altered ratios of amino acids in the cirrhotic patient may contribute to the development of hepatic encephalopathy. In rare patients who are unable to clear changes of hepatic encephalopathy while receiving standard amounts of dietary protein, the use of branched-chain amino acid supplements has been shown to be useful in allowing clinical improvement while permitting adequate protein administration *(7)*.

Overnutrition and obesity are recognized risk factors for the development of nonalcoholic steatohepatitis. It is paradoxical that PCM can even be present in this group together with obesity *(1)*. Nonalcoholic fatty liver disease (NAFLD), the hepatic manifestation of insulin resistance, is increasing in prevalence and is an important cause of cryptogenic cirrhosis. Despite numerous trials of medical therapy to improve inflammation and fibrosis associated with hepatic steatosis, gradual weight loss achieved through lifestyle remains the preferred NAFLD treatment protocol and has been demonstrated to result in improvement of markers of liver inflammation and hepatic steatosis *(8)*. Gradual weight loss through use of low-calorie diets as well as ketogenic low-carbohydrate diets have both been studied as treatment of NAFLD; the optimal diet with which to treat nonalcoholic steatohepatitis is unknown. Rapid weight loss through very low-calorie diets, however, has been associated with worsened hepatic inflammation and fibrosis and should therefore be avoided.

Ascites is the most common of the major complications of cirrhosis and heralds a 2-year mortality of 50%. The presence of ascites can result in decreased gastric accommodation and resultant early satiety leading to malnutrition. The etiology of ascites is retention of sodium, not water. The fluid that accumulates in ascites and edema is passively associated with retained sodium. The initial therapy of ascites, therefore, is to decrease dietary sodium intake thereby inducing a negative sodium balance. Dietary sodium restriction to 2000 mg/d allows retained palatability of diet with a likely negative sodium balance. When dietary interventions fail, diuretic therapy with spironolactone +/– furosemide may be required to increase urinary sodium loss *(9)*.

2. LIVER DISEASE ASSOCIATED WITH NUTRITIONAL SUPPORT

Nutritional support for patients who cannot utilize their intestines, either temporarily due to medical or surgical need or permanently due to gut failure, is by total parenteral nutrition (TPN). While this intervention has been helpful in the maintenance of the patient's nutrition, well-defined hepatic complications of TPN include the development of end-stage liver disease in 15% of those receiving long-term TPN *(10)*. Elevation in hepatic transaminases and alkaline phosphatase is seen in patients treated with TPN, while hepatic steatosis is associated with excessive amounts of infused dextrose *(10)* and possibly choline deficiency. Administration of supplemental choline during TPN administration was demonstrated, in a small trial, to ameliorate hepatic steatosis *(11)*. In addition to hepatic abnormalities, patients on TPN have an increased risk of biliary disease as both calculous and acalculous cholecystitis *(10)*.

Patients are typically inundated with information from various sources expounding on the benefits of various herbal or homeopathic dietary supplements for the treatment of chronic liver disease. These supplements are frequently misconstrued by vague labeling as being a part of "good nutrition." The general problem of dishonest and unscientific marketing of supplements is further discussed in   Chapter 13   on dietary supplements by Temple and Anwar. The most common herbal supplement taken is silymarin, or milk thistle extract. While silymarin has been evaluated for up to 2 years in patients with chronic liver disease and has been found to be safe, there have been no convincing objective data found that indicate a protective effect on morbidity or mortality in patients with chronic liver disease. Other herbal preparations advocated include phyllanthus, glycyrrhizin, and Liv 52; claims have been made that they improve various aspects of chronic liver disease though there are no placebo-controlled studies that demonstrate their usefulness. In the absence of adequate evidence, the use of herbal dietary supplements for the treatment of chronic liver disease is not recommended *(12)*. Ironically, there are reports of hepatotoxicity that have been developed after the use of herbal supplements taken specifically to treat liver disease *(13)*.

3. PATIENTS WITH PANCREATIC DISEASE

Acute pancreatitis is characterized by abdominal pain and characteristic biochemical abnormalities. Eating is commonly associated with exacerbations of abdominal pain early in the course of the disease and has been attributed to stimulation of the pancreas that typically occurs during the digestion process. Acute pancreatitis can be characterized as mild, in which edema of the pancreas is noted on abdominal imaging, and abdominal pain typically abates over a few days. The patient is almost always able to resume eating within a few days of the onset of symptoms. The standard management of these patients is initiation of eating when pain has subsided and signs of bowel function, such as bowel sounds and flatus, have returned. Because oral intake can typically be started within a few days of symptom onset, it is not felt that bouts of mild acute pancreatitis pose significant nutritional risks to patients *(14)*.

In contrast, the management of severe acute pancreatitis has proven to be more complicated. Without adequate nutritional support, this class of patients has a tenfold increased mortality *(15)*. Nutritional support during bouts of severe acute pancreatitis is important as this condition has been demonstrated to be characterized by marked negative nitrogen balance, hypermetabolism, and catabolism.

The classical management of patients with bouts of severe acute pancreatitis was to place them on prolonged bowel rest and provide TPN. Stimulation of the pancreas is avoided so as to not worsen pancreatic inflammation or prolong the disease duration. Unfortunately, the use of TPN is complicated by high costs, risk of catheter-related infections, and metabolic complications such as hyperglycemia. Recently, it has found that enteral nutrition early in the course of severe acute pancreatitis is superior to the use of TPN in that it is well tolerated, less expensive, and associated with fewer infectious complications *(16)*. Enteral feeding is therefore the accepted practice in severe acute pancreatitis as the preferred route of nutrition *(17)*. The benefits of enteral nutrition are primarily seen in the avoidance of TPN-related complications as well as in the enhanced maintenance of the enteric immune and barrier functions. The trophic effects of enteral nutrition lead to decreased gut-derived infections of pancreatic fluid collections.

Even with the use of enteral nutrition, avoidance of pancreatic stimulation is still felt to be of importance. The delivery of nutrition to distal sites of the intestine has been shown to result in minimal pancreatic stimulation *(18)*, therefore the jejunal placement of feeding tubes in patients with severe acute pancreatitis is the preferred mode of nutrition administration. Recent studies have now challenged the prevailing belief that avoidance of pancreatic stimulation is of paramount importance by demonstrating that intragastric nutrition is tolerated even in patients with severe acute pancreatitis *(19)*. While the results of these studies may eventually change the current paradigm of nutritional support in patients with severe acute pancreatitis, larger studies will be required before intra-gastric nutrition is recommended as initial management for such patients.

Chronic pancreatitis is the condition where progressive inflammatory changes in the pancreas result in structural changes. These consist of fibrosis and calcification of the interstitium of the pancreas as well as ductular abnormalities. With time, both endocrine and exocrine functions of the pancreas can be impaired. The most common cause of chronic pancreatitis is long-standing alcohol abuse. Alcoholic patients may have significant nutritional deficits of their own, irrespective of associated diseases of the liver and pancreas. Chronic pancreatitis is a cause of chronic pain that in turn can result in anorexia and consequent undernutrition. When pancreatic exocrine function declines significantly, maldigestion of food can occur. The lack of pancreatic enzymes such as lipase and trypsin manifests as steatorrhea due to inability to digest fats. This may cause deficiencies in vitamins, particularly the fat-soluble vitamins A, D, E, and K.

With respect to the nutrition of patients with chronic pancreatitis the treatment goal is to maintain adequate caloric intake. Abstinence from alcohol may help in the control of maldigestion due to exocrine dysfunction. In addition, adequate control of abdominal pain with the use of analgesics or surgical/endoscopic therapy may diminish pain-associated anorexia *(14)*.

The two available approaches to management of steatorrhea are dietary fat restriction and the use of supplemental pancreatic enzymes. Restriction of dietary fat to 20 g daily allows for adequate digestion with limited endogenous lipase production; it ameliorates steatorrhea in many patients with pancreatic exocrine insufficiency. If this intervention is not tolerated by the patient, does not result in improvement of steatorrhea, or results in insufficient caloric intake, then administration of supplemental pancreatic enzymes (SPE) with a normal fat diet is required *(14)*. Typically, the administration of around 30,000 IU of pancreatic lipase ingested with each meal allows for proper digestion of dietary fat. As the effect is greatest if the enzymes properly mix with ingested food, it is therefore important that the SPE be taken during the meal and not before or after it. SPE should be taken with all ingested foods, though the amount taken can be reduced for snacks. Some types of SPE are susceptible to inactivation by gastric acid; medical control of gastric acidity may therefore be required for full effectiveness. Fat-soluble vitamin supplementation (A, D, E, and K) should be offered to all patients with chronic pancreatitis in whom maldigestion or steatorrhea is seen.

In the rare patient in whom weight loss and steatorrhea persist despite the use of SPE, medium-chain triglycerides can be used as a dietary supplement *(20)*. They are absorbed by the intestine in a lipase-independent manner and can therefore result in absorbed fat-derived calories despite the lack of sufficient pancreatic function. The use of TPN is generally not required in patients with chronic pancreatitis, though rare indications may be discovered.

4. CONCLUSION

Patients with chronic liver disease and those with severe acute pancreatitis or chronic pancreatitis have significant nutritional needs. All are characterized as significantly catabolic states. Patients with chronic liver disease are commonly protein-calorie malnourished and the clinician should be aware of the need for close nutritional assessment. It is important to maintain adequate dietary protein intake and significant protein restriction should be avoided, even in patients with hepatic encephalopathy. If a patient is unable to tolerate adequate dietary protein intake, supplementation with branched-chain amino acids may be beneficial.

Chronic overnutrition and obesity can result in significant liver disease; gradual weight loss through the use of diet and exercise should therefore be encouraged, with the goal of approaching an ideal body weight. The use of herbal dietary supplements should not be encouraged in patients with chronic liver disease due to lack of evidence of benefit and potential hepato-toxicity.

Patients with mild acute pancreatitis are not typically at risk for significant nutritional deficits. In contrast, patients with severe acute pancreatitis require significant nutritional support. The early use of enteral nutrition has supplanted the use of parenteral nutrition in this population, as clinical outcomes are improved, and the significant risks of parenteral nutrition are avoided. In patients with chronic pancreatitis, pancreatic exocrine insufficiency is commonly seen. Treatment with supplemental pancreatic enzymes results in improved digestion of oral nutrition. Fat-soluble vitamin deficiency is common in patients with steatorrhea and supplemental vitamins A, D, E, and K are warranted.

SUGGESTED FURTHER READING

Plauth M, Cabre E, Riggio O, et al. ESPEN guidelines on enteral nutrition: Liver disease. Clin Nutr 2006; 25:285–294.
Matos C, Porayko M, Francisco-Ziller N, et al. Nutrition and chronic liver disease J Clin Gastroenterol 2002; 35:391–397.
Meier R, Ockenga J, Pertkiewicz M, et al. ESPEN guidelines on enteral nutrition: pancreas. Clin Nutr 2006; 25:275–284.
O'Keefe S, Sharma S. Nutrition support in severe acute pancreatitis. Gastroenterol Clin N Am 2007; 36:297–312.

REFERENCES

1. Matos C, Porayko MK, Francisco-Ziller N, DiCecco S. Nutrition and chronic liver disease. J Clin Gastroenterol 2002; 35:391–397.
2. Carvalho L, Parise ER. Evaluation of nutritional status of nonhospitalized patients with liver cirrhosis. Arq Gastroenterol 2006; 43:269–274.
3. Plauth M, Cabre E, Riggio O, et al. ESPEN guidelines on enteral nutrition: Liver disease. Clin Nutr 2006; 25:285–294.
4. Nakaya Y, Okita K, Suzuki K, et al. BCAA-enriched snack improves nutritional state of cirrhosis. Nutrition 2007; 23:113–120.
5. Cordoba J, Lopez-Hellin J, Planas M, et al. Normal protein diet for episodic hepatic encephalopathy: results of a randomized study. J Hepatol 2004; 41:38–43.
6. Blonde-Cynober F, Aussel C, Cynober L. Abnormalities in branched-chain amino acid metabolism in cirrhosis: influence of hormonal and nutritional factors and directions for future research. Clin Nutr 1999; 18:5–13.

7. Charlton M. Branched-chain amino acid enriched supplements as therapy for liver disease. J Nutr 2006; 136:295S–298S.
8. Ueno T, Sugawara H, Sujaku K, et al. Therapeutic effects of restricted diet and exercise in obese patients with fatty liver. J Hepatol 1997; 27:103–107.
9. Runyon BA. Management of adult patients with ascites due to cirrhosis. Hepatology 2004; 39:841–856.
10. Montalvo-Jave EE, Zarraga JL, Sarr MG. Specific topics and complications of parenteral nutrition. Langenbecks Arch Surg 2007; 392:119–126.
11. Buchman AL, Dubin MD, Moukarzel AA, et al. Choline deficiency: a cause of hepatic steatosis during parenteral nutrition that can be reversed with intravenous choline supplementation. Hepatology 1995; 22:1399–1403.
12. Dhiman RK, Chawla YK. Herbal medicines for liver diseases. Dig Dis Sci 2005; 50:1807–1812.
13. Seeff LB. Herbal hepatotoxicity. Clin Liver Dis 2007; 11:577–596, vii.
14. Meier R, Ockenga J, Pertkiewicz M, et al. ESPEN guidelines on enteral nutrition: pancreas. Clin Nutr 2006; 25:275–284.
15. Sitzmann JV, Steinborn PA, Zinner MJ, Cameron JL. Total parenteral nutrition and alternate energy substrates in treatment of severe acute pancreatitis. Surg Gynecol Obstet 1989; 168:311–317.
16. Kalfarentzos F, Kehagias J, Mead N, Kokkinis K, Gogos CA. Enteral nutrition is superior to parenteral nutrition in severe acute pancreatitis: results of a randomized prospective trial. Br J Surg 1997; 84:1665–1669.
17. Marik PE, Zaloga GP. Meta-analysis of parenteral nutrition versus enteral nutrition in patients with acute pancreatitis. BMJ 2004; 328:1407.
18. Vu MK, van der Veek PP, Frolich M, et al. Does jejunal feeding activate exocrine pancreatic secretion? Eur J Clin Invest 1999; 29:1053–1059.
19. Eatock FC, Chong P, Menezes N, et al. A randomized study of early nasogastric versus nasojejunal feeding in severe acute pancreatitis. Am J Gastroenterol 2005; 100:432–439.
20. Scolapio JS, Malhi-Chowla N, Ukleja A. Nutrition supplementation in patients with acute and chronic pancreatitis. Gastroenterol Clin North Am 1999; 28:695–707.

29 Medical Nutrition Therapy in Chronic Kidney Disease and Other Disorders

Luanne DiGuglielmo

Key Points

- Chronic kidney disease (CKD) often coexists with cardiovascular disease and diabetes and requires medical nutrition therapy for optimal outcomes.
- Effective nutritional management should be correlated to the stage of CKD as dietary restriction will vary according to stage.
- Prevention of malnutrition is an important goal of medical nutrition therapy.
- Management of blood pressure and diabetes will have the greatest impact on delaying the progression of chronic kidney disease.
- Diabetes is the leading cause of end-stage renal disease (ESRD).
- Nutritional requirements in acute renal failure encompass both the catabolic state and the needs of the patient in renal failure.

Key Words: Chronic kidney disease; acute renal failure; nutritional management; medical nutrition therapy; hemodialysis; peritoneal dialysis; urinary tract infections

1. INTRODUCTION

The prevalence of chronic kidney disease (CKD) is rising in the United States with a rise in the aging population as well as from an increase in the prevalence of comorbidities associated with CKD (1, 2). One in nine Americans suffers from kidney disease with estimates approaching 20 million people (1). Diabetes, hypertension, and primary kidney diseases account for most of the kidney failure seen in this country. Diabetes is the leading cause of end-stage renal disease (ESRD).

Medical nutrition therapy is a vital part of the management for the CKD patient population. Nutrition therapy is correlated to the stage of CKD as

From: *Nutrition and Health: Nutrition Guide for Physicians*
Edited by: T. Wilson et al. (eds.), DOI 10.1007/978-1-60327-431-9_29,
© Humana Press, a part of Springer Science+Business Media, LLC 2010

nutrient needs change as CKD progresses to ESRD. Nutritional status is a strong predictor of patient outcomes, including morbidity and mortality. Patients who begin renal replacement therapy (either dialysis or transplantation) with compromised nutritional status have a higher morbidity and mortality than those who are adequately nourished. Because of this, particular attention to nutrition in the earlier stages of CKD is crucial *(3)*.

Primary nutritional goals for the management of the early stages of CKD include

1. Prevent protein–energy malnutrition
2. Minimize the buildup of uremic toxins and associated symptoms
3. Delay the progression of the disease
4. Prevent secondary hyperparathyroidism and control acidosis
5. Treat any complications resulting from lifestyle issues

2. STAGES OF CHRONIC KIDNEY DISEASE

The National Kidney Foundation (NKF) Kidney Disease Outcome Quality Initiatives (K/DOQI) has defined CKD as described in Table 1. Clinical practice guidelines classify CKD into five stages based on kidney function indicated by glomerular filtration rate (GFR) and evidence of kidney damage. Table 2 outlines the five stages with corresponding medical nutrition therapy *(4)*.

Table 1
Definition of Chronic Kidney Disease Criteria

---

1. Kidney Damage for > or equal to 3 mo, as defined by structural or functional abnormalities of the kidney, with or without decreased GFR, manifest by *either*:
   *Pathological abnormalities; or
   *Markers of kidney damage, including abnormalities in the composition of the blood or urine, or abnormalities in imaging tests
2. GFR < 60 ml/min/1.73 m^2 for > or equal to 3 mo, with or without kidney damage

---

Reprinted with permission from the National Kidney Foundation. National Kidney Foundation. K/DOQI clinical practice guidelines for chronic kidney disease: Evaluation, classification and stratification. Am J Kidney Dis 2002; 39 (2 suppl 1):S1–S266.

3. OVERVIEW OF NUTRITIONAL MANAGEMENT OF CKD FOR STAGES 1–4

Medical and nutritional management in CKD stages 1–4 can impact overall patient health and potentially delay progression to stage 5 or ESRD. Studies in animals and humans have suggested that controlling protein intake

Table 2

Stages of Chronic Kidney Disease and Corresponding Nutrition Recommendations

Stage	Description	GFR(ml/min/1.73 m^2)	Protein (g/kg/day)	Calories	Sodium (g/day)	Potassium (g/day)	Phosphorous (g/day)	Calcium (g/day)	Vitamins
1	Kidney damage with normal or increasing GFR	= 90	0.75	Based on energy expenditure	Varies from 1–4 to no added salt, depending on comorbidities	Usually no restriction unless serum level is high	Monitor and restrict if serum levels >4.6	1.2–1.5, maintain serum Ca on lower end	DRI
2	Kidney damage with mild decreasing GFR	60–89	0.75	Based on energy expenditure	Same a stage 1	Same as stage 1	Same as stage1	Same as stage 1	DRI
3	Moderate decreasing GFR	30–59	0.75	Based on energy expenditure	Same as stage 1	Same as stage 1	8–12 mg/g protein or 800–1000 mg/day	Same as stage 1	B complex and C: DRI. Individualize vitamin D, zinc, and iron

(Continued)

Table 2
(Continued)

Stage	Description	GFR(ml/ min/ 1.73 m^2)	Protein (g/kg/day)	Calories	Sodium (g/day)	Potassium (g/day)	Phosphorous (g/day)	Calcium (g/day)	Vitamins
4	Severe decreasing GFR	15–29	0.6	30–35 kcal/kg/ day	Same as stage 1	Same as stage 1	Same as stage 3	Same as stage 1 but not to exceed 2000 mg/day	Same as stage 3
5	Kidney failure	<15 or dialy-sis	0.6–0.75	30–35 kcal/kg/ day	Same as stage 1	Same as stage 1	Same as stage 3	Same as stage 4	Same as stage 3

Abbreviations: DRI, dietary reference intake; GFR, glomerular filtration rate.
Copyright 2004 American Dietetic Association. Reprinted with permission.

may delay disease progression as well as minimize uremic toxicity. Blood pressure and glycemic control will have the greatest impact on delaying the progression of chronic kidney disease *(5)*. The Modification of Diet in Renal Disease study demonstrated that good blood pressure control could slow the progression of renal disease and that patients could be maintained on a low-protein diet without adverse effects on nutritional status *(6)*. Another large clinical trial, the Diabetes Control and Complications Trial, showed that microalbuminuria, a significant marker for diabetic nephropathy, was reduced in patients with very tight blood glucose control. Although research has not definitively demonstrated that dietary protein restriction will stop or slow the progression of renal disease, it continues to be part of the dietary treatment of CKD patients.

CKD patients are at high risk for cardiovascular disease, Therefore, overall lifestyle management for the patient with impaired renal function is critical. Since CKD shares common risk factors with cardiovascular disease and diabetes, lifestyle changes directed at modifiable risk factors such as smoking, obesity, alcohol consumption, physical activity, and diet are important *(5)*. Modification of these risk factors can promote organ blood flow, can potentially reduce kidney damage, and can slow the progression of CKD *(2)*.

4. DIET PRESCRIPTION IN CKD STAGES 1–4

Protein. Recommendation for protein intake in CKD stages 1–3 is 0.75 g/kg/day which is close to the 0.8 g/kg/day necessary for the non-CKD population *(7)*. Because typical consumption is much higher, this constitutes a significant reduction for the average individual. Of the 0.75 g/kg/day, at least 50% should be of high biological value (HBV) providing all of the essential amino acids needed for protein synthesis.

Foods of animal origin are HBV proteins. As the individual progresses to stages 4 and 5 protein restriction becomes more stringent leveling out at 0.6 g/kg/day *(2)*. Because this is below the RDA for protein (0.8 g/kg/day), patient utilization of a registered dietitian is critical for patient education, follow-up coaching for dietary adherence, and prevention of malnutrition.

Energy. In general, calorie needs are similar to the general population and should be correlated to energy expenditure to maintain a healthy weight. However, it has been shown that CKD patients tend to consume less than the 30–35 kcal/kg recommended in stages 4 and 5 *(8)*. Inadequate energy intakes not only lead to malnutrition but will decrease any positive benefit afforded by a low-protein diet.

Minerals and Water. Recommendations for sodium, potassium, phosphorous, calcium, and fluid in CKD stages 1–4 depend on the presence of comorbidities and serum levels. Sodium intake can range from 1 to 4 g/day depending on blood pressure, fluid balance, and the presence of congestive heart failure and other diseases. Fluid intake is closely linked with urine output and is not restricted unless oliguria is present *(4)*. Potassium restriction in CKD stages 1–4 is generally not necessary unless urine output decreases to less than 1000 ml/day or serum level is high *(4)*. Preserving bone health and preventing vascular and soft tissue calcification is the focus of phosphorous and calcium control in CKD. Control of serum phosphorous is key in the management of the complications of secondary hyperparathyroidism. In the earlier stages (1–3) of CKD, dietary restriction of phosphorous is effective in controlling serum levels. As kidney function declines further, phosphate-binding medications are needed along with diet therapy to maintain recommended serum levels. In the earlier stages of CKD, calcium levels should be maintained within normal lab value ranges with a calcium intake not to exceed 2000 mg/day due to the risk of vascular calcification and bone disease *(4)*.

5. MEDICAL NUTRITION THERAPY FOR HEMODIALYSIS

Nutrient needs change when a patient reaches ESRD (end-stage renal disease) and begins regular hemodialysis treatment, and malnutrition becomes a significant concern. The prevalence of malnutrition in this population ranges from 10 to 75%. It has been documented that hemodialysis patients often consume less than the recommended amounts of calories and protein *(9)*. Reasons for poor appetite and oral intake are many. The presence of comorbid conditions such as diabetes, chronic inflammation, and cardiovascular disease affect oral intake and contribute to declining nutritional status *(9)*. Hemodialysis patients show evidence of chronic inflammation with elevated levels of C-reactive protein *(10)*. Chronic inflammation has been found to be associated with decreased oral intake *(11)*. Additionally, depression and social and economic issues factor into a patient's overall well-being and nutritional status. Although serum albumin is used as a marker for chronic inflammation, it is also used as an important marker of protein intake and nutritional status in the dialysis patient along with body weight *(12)*. Patients with serum albumins of less than 3.5 g/dL have a mortality rate 1.38 times higher than those above 3.5 g/dL *(13)*. The goal is for albumin to reach 4.0 g/dL *(12)*. Liberalization of diet, oral supplements, and nasogastric or PEG feedings can all be used to increase energy and protein intake.

Potassium, Sodium, and Fluid. Most hemodialysis patients who are anuric or oliguric with a urine output of less than 1000 ml/day will become hyperkalemic without potassium restriction. A reduced daily intake of 2500 mg potassium is usually sufficient to prevent hyperkalemia in most hemodialysis patients *(11)*. As kidney function declines, the gut compensates and becomes more efficient at removing potassium through the stool contributing to potassium balance *(2)*. Nevertheless, individual differences will exist, therefore 40 mg/kg of ideal body weight or standard body weight is recommended. Along with dietary excess and constipation, hyperkalemia may also result from inadequate dialysis, metabolic acidosis, and certain medications *(10)*. As outlined in Table 3, sodium and fluid requirements depend on urine output.

Phosphorous, Calcium, PTH, and Vitamin D. Controlling the balance between phosphorous, calcium, PTH, and vitamin D is crucial in the

Table 3
Daily Recommended Nutrient Intakes for Adults on Hemodialysis

Nutrient	Daily Recommendation for Adults on Hemodialysis
Protein	1.2 g/kg average weight (50% high biological value)
Energy	Energy
Adults <60 yr	35 kcal/kg
Adults >60 yr or obese	30–35 kcal/kg
Sodium and fluid	Sodium and fluid
▶or equal to 1 L fluid output	2–4 g Na and 2 L fluid
< or equal to 1 L fluid output	2 g Na and 1–1.5 L fluid
Anuria	2 g Na and 1 L fluid
Potassium	40 mg/kg IBW or SBW
Phosphorous	800–1000 mg or <17 mg/kg IBW or SBW
Calcium	Individualized
Magnesium	0.2–0.3 g
Iron	Individualized
Zinc	8–11 mg
Vitamin A	700–900 μg
Vitamin D	5–15 μg
Vitamin E	15 mg
Vitamin K	90–120 mg
Thiamin	1.1–1.2 mg
Riboflavin	1.1–1.3 mg
Biotin	Unknown
Pantothenic acid	Unknown
Niacin	Unknown
Folic Acid	800–1000 μg
Vitamin B$_6$	1.3–1.7 mg
Vitamin B$_{12}$	2.4 μg
Vitamin C	75–90 mg

Abbreviations: IBW, ideal body weight; SBW, standard body weight.
Copyright 2004 American Dietetic Association. Reprinted with permission *(10)*.

prevention of secondary hyperparathyroidism. This complication of kidney disease affects about 300,000 ESRD patients as well as more than 3 million patients with CKD *(14)*. Excessive dietary intake of phosphorous contributes to hyperphosphatemia, elevated calcium phosphate product, and high circulating levels of PTH, which in turn can lead to renal osteodystrophy and soft tissue and vascular calcification *(11)*.

Decreasing phosphorous intake, preventing absorption with phosphate binding medications and along with the administration of vitamin D analogs has been shown to effectively suppress PTH secretion and prevent complications. Newer drugs, like calcimimetics, also work to suppress PTH by increasing the sensitivity of calcium-sensing receptors sites to *extracellular* calcium *(14)*. In addition to protein foods, other examples of high phosphorous foods include dairy products, dried beans, beer, nuts, chocolate, and colas.

Intake of calcium is individualized as indicated in Table 3. Given the risk of vascular calcification, in persons undergoing hemodialysis, calcium intake should not exceed 2000 mg/day. This includes dietary intake, calcium-containing phosphate binders, and dialysate calcium. For this reason, binders that do not contain calcium are usually the ones of choice. Patients with an intact PTH of greater than 300 pg/ml should be evaluated for vitamin D therapy *(11)*. Vitamin D analogs not only suppress the secretion of PTH but also seem to have beneficial effects on bone as well as improving survival of ESRD patients on dialysis *(14)*.

Vitamins and Other Minerals. Table 3 outlines vitamin and mineral requirements. Because vitamins A and E accumulate in kidney failure, these are not supplemented over usual requirements. Losses of vitamins B_6, B_{12}, and folate occur with dialysis so they are supplemented. Vitamin C is not supplemented above the RDA, as excessive levels are associated with the formation of oxalate kidney stones. Low zinc levels have been associated with decreased taste acuity so zinc is often supplemented. Lastly iron deficiency is common in dialysis patients due to the use of synthetic erythropoietin and chronic blood loss. IV iron is more effective than oral iron in replacement. Transferrin saturation less than 20% and ferritin less than 100 ng/ml indicate the need for IV iron. Recommendations are individualized based on the patient's response to iron and need for erythropoietin therapy *(11)*.

6. MEDICAL NUTRITION THERAPY IN PERITONEAL DIALYSIS

Energy and Protein. Energy requirements in peritoneal dialysis (PD) are similar to hemodialysis. Energy needs should be individualized to achieve or maintain desirable body weight, including the calories from dextrose in the dialysate solution. PD patients can absorb up to a third of their total energy requirement from the dialysate *(15)*. Protein intake must compensate for the loss of protein in PD effluent. Typically, between 5 and 15 g are lost daily, mostly as albumin *(15)*. During an episode of peritonitis, the peritoneal membrane becomes hyperpermeable resulting in greater protein losses *(3)*. Therefore, recommendations for protein intake are 1.2–1.3 g/kg of standard or adjusted body weight, 50% of which should be of high biological value *(2)*. This amount may need to be individualized on a case-by-case basis with some patients having higher protein needs due to low albumins and the presence of malnutrition. In these cases, protein supplementation may be necessary.

Potassium and Sodium. Potassium is usually unrestricted in PD patients as it is very easily cleared by PD *(15)*. In some cases, potassium supplementation is required. Most patients will remain in potassium balance with 3–4 g of potassium daily, which is consistent with an unrestricted diet. Very few patients will require further restriction but in those that do a 2 g potassium diet is usually sufficient *(15)*. Sodium is also easily cleared on PD. Patients consuming excess sodium will need to use higher dextrose dialysate exchanges to remove excess fluid retained as a result of increased sodium intake. Frequent use of high dextrose exchanges can damage the peritoneal membrane affecting its ultrafiltration capabilities. This practice can also aggravate existing diabetes, hypertriglyceridemia, and hypercholesterolemia and contribute to overweight and obesity from the absorption of dextrose calories. Sodium intake should be individualized but remain between 2 and 4 g/day to maintain adequate fluid balance *(15)*.

Cholesterol and Triglycerides. PD patients are at risk for hyperlipidemia due to weight gain and absorption of dextrose from the dialysate. Patients should be taught how to limit sugars, saturated fats, and cholesterol but without compromising protein intake *(15)*.

7. ACUTE RENAL FAILURE

Acute renal failure (ARF) is associated with alterations in protein, carbohydrate, and lipid metabolism as well as disturbances in fluid and electrolyte and acid–base balance *(16)*. These metabolic changes, while associated with the uremic state, are also the result of the catabolism of critical illness, a complication of sepsis, trauma, or multiple organ failure *(10)*. Therefore, nutritional requirements in ARF encompass both the catabolic state and the needs of the patient in renal failure. Muscle protein catabolism is accelerated in ARF resulting in large reductions in lean body mass *(16)*. Protein recommendations will differ based on whether the patient is receiving dialysis. For those not treated with dialysis, no less than 0.8 g/kg/day is recommended with an upper limit of 1.2 g/kg/day *(16)*. More often than not patients are treated with dialysis. The recommendation of 1.2–1.5 g/kg/day is similar to that of the critically ill patient *(10)*. The hypercatabolism of critical illness and ARF cannot be overcome by increasing protein intake. Intakes greater than 1.5 g/kg/day show no benefit and may actually aggravate the uremia *(16)*. Protein provided should be a mixture of essential and nonessential amino acids. Energy requirements should be based on critical illness as there is minimal increase in energy expenditure due to ARF *(17)*. The goal is to provide adequate calories to minimize protein catabolism without overfeeding; 25–35 kcal/kg/day can be used to estimate energy needs *(17)*. Fluid needs are dependent on level of renal function and the patient's fluid status. In general, urine output plus 500 ml for insensible losses (e.g., through skin, sweat, stool) is a good guideline. Electrolytes are individualized based on lab values and the mode of nutrition support *(17)*. Patients can be fed orally, enterally, or parenterally based on the severity of illness.

8. OTHER KIDNEY-RELATED CONDITIONS

The discussion of urinary tract infections (UTIs) is adapted from Ref. *(18)*. UTIs represent a major health problem and occur when bacteria (primarily *Escherichia coli* or *E. coli*) adhere to the uroepithelial cells that line the bladder, kidney, or urethra and then multiply. Bacterial adhesion to uroepithelial cells requires the production of a set of structures called p-fimbriae on the cell walls of the colonizing bacteria. P-fimbria are fibers that form adhesions to carbohydrates on the surface of uroepithelial cells, thereby allowing the bacteria to adhere. Adhesion leads to colonization of the urinary tract epithelium and destruction of the lining of the bladder, as well as inflammation and rupturing of the underlying blood vessels, causing blood in the urine in some cases. The resultant inflammation promotes a painful burning sensation; persistent, untreated UTI can lead to cystitis and pyelonephritis *(19)*, which can ultimately lead to the loss of one or both kidneys.

UTIs are most typically found in women, with 60% of American women being affected over a lifetime, but can also occur in men *(20)*. Persons at very high UTI risk include the elderly, paraplegics, and quadriplegics. Cranberry juice has been used in folk medicine for millenia. There has been much speculation as to the mechanism by which cranberry products protect against UTIs. In 1984 Sabota used *E. coli* isolates from UTI-afflicted humans to determine that cranberry juice contains a nondialyzable material that specifically inhibits the expression of the p-fimbria of bacteria, hence preventing their attachment to and colonization of the urinary tract *(21)*. The first double-blind human clinical trial confirming the effect of cranberry juice was not published until 1994 *(22)*. In this trial, elderly women were randomized to 300 ml/day of a saccharine-sweetened 27% cranberry beverage or a synthetic placebo drink. Cranberry juice consumption leads to significant reductions in the numbers of both bacteria and white blood cells in the urine over the 6-mo-study period. Recent clinical studies have confirmed its usefulness for the prevention of UTI. The active agents are proanthocyanidins which prevent bacterial adhesion to the urinary tract. While other fruits and vegetables contain proanthocyanins, only the cranberry, and its close relative the blueberry, have the ability to prevent p-fimbriae expression and bacterial adhesion to uroepithelial cells *(23)*. However, consumer and researcher understanding of how cranberries affect human health remains difficult to determine in part because of the large range of product formulations and the differences in the amount of cranberry juice actually present in these beverages.

9. SUMMARY

Medical nutrition therapy plays a vital role in all stages of kidney disease. Ongoing monitoring and evaluation is necessary to maintain optimal nutritional status and quality of life. The role of the registered dietitian is vital in the achievement of these goals

SUGGESTED FURTHER READING

National Kidney Foundation, http://www.kidney.org/professionals/KDOQI/
McCann L. Pocket Guide to Nutrition Assessment of the Patient with Chronic Kidney Disease. 3rd ed. Council on Renal Nutrition, National Kidney Foundation, NY, 2002.
Beto JA, Bansal VK. Medical nutrition therapy in chronic kidney failure: integrating clinical practice guidelines. J Am Diet Assoc 2004; 104:404–409.

REFERENCES

1. Compton, A. Chronic kidney disease. Clinician Rev 2007; 9:37–53.
2. Beto JA, Bansal VK. Medical nutrition therapy in chronic kidney failure: integrating clinical practice guidelines. J Am Diet Assoc 2004; 104:404–409.
3. Wells C. Optimizing nutrition in patients with chronic kidney disease. Nephrology Nursing J 2003; 12:637–657.
4. National Kidney Foundation Kidney Disease Outcome Quality Initiatives (K/DOQI). 2002. Available at www.kidney.org/professionals/KDOQI/guidelines_ckd/toc.htm. Last accessed May 6, 2008.
5. Levin A, Hemmelgarn B, Culleton B, et al. Guidelines for the management of chronic kidney disease. Canadian Medical Association Journal 2008: 179:1154–1162.
6. Fedje L, Maralis M. Nutrition management in early stages of chronic kidney disease. In: Byham-Gray L, Wiesen K, eds. A Clinical Guide to Nutrition Care in Kidney Disease. American Dietetic Association, Chicago, IL, 2004, pp. 21–28.

7. National Kidney Foundation Kidney Disease Outcome Quality Initiatives (K/DOQI), 2000. Available at www.kidney.org/professionals/KDOQI/guidelines_updates/nut_a24. html.

8. Cuppari L, Avesani CM. Energy requirements in patients with chronic kidney disease. J Renal Nutr 2004; 14:121–126.

9. Burrowes JD, Dalton S, Backstrand J, Levin NW. Patients receiving maintenance hemodialysis with low vs high levels of nutritional risk have decreased morbidity. J Am Diet Assoc 2005; 105:563–572.

10. Mitch E, Klahr S. Handbook of Nutrition and the Kidney. Lippincott Williams and Wilkins, Philadelphia, 2002.

11. Biesecker R, Stuart N. Nutrition management of the adult hemodialysis patient. In: Byham-Gray L, Wiesen K, eds. A Clinical Guide to Nutrition Care in Kidney Disease. American Dietetic Association, Chicago, IL, 2004, pp. 43–55.

12. National Kidney Foundation Kidney Disease Outcome Quality Initiatives (K/DOQI), 2000. Available at www.kidney.org/professionals/KDOQI/guidelines_updates/nut_a03. html. Last accessed on May 7, 2008.

13. Combe C, McCullough KP, Asano Y, Ginsberg N, Maroni BJ, Pifer TB. Kidney Disease Outcomes Quality Initiative (K/DOQI) and the Dialysis Outcomes and Practice Patterns Study (DOPPS): Nutrition guidelines, indicators, and practices. Am J Kidney Dis 2004; 44:39–44.

14. Torres PU, Prie D, Beck L, Friedlander G. New therapies for uremic secondary hyper-parathyroidism. J Renal Nutr 2006; 16:87–99.

15. McCann L. Nutritional management of the adult peritoneal dialysis patient. In: Byham-Gray L, Wiesen K, eds. A Clinical Guide to Nutrition Care in Kidney Disease. American Dietetic Association, Chicago, IL, 2004, pp. 57–69.

16. Bickford A, Schatz SR. Nutrition management in acute renal failure. In: Byham-Gray L, Wiesen K, eds. A Clinical Guide to Nutrition Care in Kidney Disease. American Dietetic Association, Chicago, IL, 2004, pp. 29–41.

17. Kalista-Richards M, Pursell R, Gayner R. Nutritional management of the patient with acute renal failure. Renal Nutr Forum 2005; 24:1–12.

18. Wilson T. Cranberry juice effects on health. In: Wilson T, Temple NJ, eds. Beverage Impacts on Health and Nutrition. Humana Press, Totowa, NJ, 2003, pp. 51–62.

19. Dowling KJ, Roberts JA, Kaack MB. P-fimbriated Escherichia coli urinary tract infection: a clinical correlation. South Med J 1987; 80:1533–1536.

20. Foxman B, Barlow R, D'Arcy H, Gillespie B, Sobel JD. Urinary tract infection: self-reported incidence and associated costs. Ann Epidemiol 2000; 10:509–515.

21. Sobota AE. Inhibition of bacterial adherence by cranberry juice: potential use for the treatment of urinary tract infections. J Urology 1984; 131:1013–1016.

22. Avorn J, Monane M, Gurwitz JH, Glynn RJ, Choodnovskiy I, Lipsitz LA. Reduction of bacteriuria and pyuria after ingestion of cranberry juice. JAMA 1994; 271:751–754.

23. Ofek I, Goldhar J, Sharon N. Anti-Escherichia coli adhesion activity of cranberry and blueberry juices. Adv Exp Med Biol 1996; 408:179–183.

30 Bone Health: Sound Suggestions for Stronger Bones

Laura A.G. Armas, Karen A. Rafferty, and Robert P. Heaney

Key Points

- Bone requires calcium, vitamin D, protein, and phosphorus for optimal growth and maintenance.
- Food is the best source for most of the nutrients required by bone.
- Many in the population are consuming diets with inadequate calcium
- Most adults require additional vitamin D supplementation, especially if they have little sun exposure.
- Improvements in nutrition can make a significant difference to bone health, even if started later in life.

Key Words: Bone health; calcium; vitamin D; phosphorus; magnesium

1. INTRODUCTION

Bone is a complicated organ made of collagen, proteins, calcium, phosphate, and cells that remodel and maintain bone. It requires many nutrients obtained from the diet for remodeling and maintaining the bony structure. Nutrition science has identified a select few of these nutrients as particularly important for bone health. We will highlight those here. But remember that in food, these nutrients do not occur in isolation; they are present in nature packaged in various combinations of fat, protein, minerals, etc. Only in the past few decades has it been possible to consume these nutrients in isolation in the form of supplements. As in many cases the whole seems to be greater than the sum of its parts; in making recommendations for bone health

From: *Nutrition and Health: Nutrition Guide for Physicians*
Edited by: T. Wilson et al. (eds.), DOI 10.1007/978-1-60327-431-9_30,
© Humana Press, a part of Springer Science+Business Media, LLC 2010

we will emphasize obtaining these nutrients from food sources whenever possible.

If a patient is being treated with medication for osteoporosis, we emphasize that these nutrients are the building blocks that the medication uses to form bone. This seems a simplistic explanation, but many patients think that the medications themselves contain these nutrients. All bone-active pharmacologic agents have been tested with additional supplemental calcium and most with vitamin D as well. Presumably, the effects of the pharmacologic agents depend to some extent on these supplemental nutrients.

2. CALCIUM

For over 100 years we have been aware of calcium's effects on bone health. Of the nearly 100 clinical trials using calcium supplements or dairy foods, all but four have shown positive outcomes, i.e., greater bone mass during growth, reduced bone loss with age, and reduced fractures. Despite this knowledge, about 85% of the female population fails to get the recommended intake of calcium.

The body's calcium requirements have to come from dietary sources. The *blood* level of calcium is tightly maintained despite fluctuations in dietary intake. This constancy is ensured in the face of poor dietary intake by decreasing urinary calcium output, by improving gastrointestinal calcium absorption, and, more importantly, by increasing resorption of bone tissue, thereby releasing its calcium. In brief, *blood* levels of calcium are maintained during long-term dietary calcium deprivation at the expense of the skeleton.

The body systems do not act in isolation: calcium intake and regulation of the calcium economy have effects on other body systems and diseases including hypertension, colon cancer, renolithiasis, obesity, premenstrual syndrome, and polycystic ovary syndrome. However, this review will confine itself to the skeletal effects of calcium (and of nutrition, generally).

2.1. Dietary Calcium Requirements

The gut absorbs about 30% of dietary calcium, but the mineral is also lost through gastrointestinal secretions. As a result net intestinal absorption is only 10–15%. Additionally, calcium is lost in urine and sweat *(1, 2)*. These so-called "obligatory losses" amount to about 200 mg/day in adults. Hence, net absorption must be at least that much to maintain zero balance. That much net absorption requires a daily total intake of 1000–1500 mg (the equivalent of 3–5 dairy servings). *See* Table 1.

During growth, net absorption is more efficient and bones will accumulate mass (and calcium), although when persons consume a low-calcium diet the

Table 1
Dietary Reference Intakes for Calcium

Childhood	500–800 mg
Adolescence	1300 mg
Adult	1000 mg
Elderly	1200 mg

bones cannot reach their full potential. Later in life, absorption and retention are less efficient and the bones are unable to maintain their mass. Calcium retention rises in proportion to the intake up to a certain threshold level, above which excess calcium is excreted. There is no storage mechanism for extra calcium except what is needed by the skeleton.

Because blood levels of calcium are so tightly regulated, a serum measurement tells one little about the body's calcium intake or reserve. The reserve must be severely depleted for hypocalcemia to occur.

Dietary sodium needs a brief mention here. Sodium chloride increases urinary calcium excretion (i.e., it contributes to the obligatory loss), and this could theoretically lead to bone loss on a low-calcium diet. This sodium-induced urinary calcium loss can generally be offset by consuming more calcium in the diet.

2.2. Calcium Sources

Important sources of calcium are natural foods (principally dairy, a few greens and nuts, and a few crustaceans) and calcium-fortified foods (some cereals, breads, and fruit juices). Dairy products are the richest dietary sources of calcium. In fact, it is difficult to get enough calcium on a dairy-free diet. One serving of dairy has approximately 300 mg of calcium in addition to protein, phosphorus, vitamins, and trace minerals. Even patients with lactose intolerance can "wean" themselves onto dairy foods if done slowly and milk is taken with other foods (3).

Not all food sources of calcium are equally bioavailable. For example, spinach contains 122 mg of calcium per 90 g serving, but very little (about 5%) is absorbed because the oxalate in the spinach interferes with calcium absorption. This can be source of clinical confusion to patients who are depending on the calcium content of certain foods but are still deficient with respect to calcium stores and bone mineral density.

Calcium supplements may be needed in order to reach the recommended daily intake. Most calcium salts (citrate, carbonate, phosphate) exhibit similar bioavailability. Brand name or chewable products have been shown to be the most reliable. Even relatively less soluble salts, such as carbonate, absorb well if taken with food. All calcium sources should be taken with meals and in small amounts throughout the day to ensure optimal absorption.

3. VITAMIN D

A second nutrient that has been closely linked to bone health is vitamin D. Deficiency of this vitamin is classically associated with unmineralized bone matrix, expressed as rickets in the growing skeleton and osteomalacia in the fully formed skeleton. Vitamin D is not truly a nutrient, at least in humans, because the body makes the vitamin for itself when a precursor in the skin is exposed to ultraviolet B light. This reaction forms pre-vitamin D, which is then spontaneously converted to vitamin D. At prevalent levels of sun exposure, vitamin D is converted almost entirely to 25-hydroxyvitamin D (25OHD) by the liver. 25OHD is the form of vitamin D that correlates best with calcium absorption in adults and is converted by the kidney and other cells to the active form of vitamin D, 1,25-dihydroxyvitamin D ($1,25OH_2D$). Like calcium, $1,25OH_2D$ is physiologically regulated and serum measurements do not reflect vitamin D status. The mechanism by which vitamin D has been implicated in cancer prevention, immune response, and cell cycle regulation has been elucidated in recent years *(4)*.

Vitamin D is essential for active absorption of calcium. From multiple calcium absorption studies it has been established that absorption plateaus at about 32 ng/ml *(5)*. Population-based studies demonstrate that bone mineral density increases in relation to 25OHD status *(6)*. Reduction in risk of fracture has been reported in clinical trials of vitamin D supplements *(7)*. The decrease in fractures appears to be the result of at least two mechanisms: first, vitamin D increases calcium absorption, which in turn increases bone mineral density; and, second, vitamin D has an effect on muscle strength and balance. Even short-term studies show a reduction in falls *(8, 9)*.

3.1. Vitamin D Requirements

Vitamin D recommendations have been a moving target in recent years. In 1997, the Food & Nutrition Board (Institute of Medicine) recommended 200–600 IU daily, but that figure has been challenged in recent years as being too low for optimal health. Heaney *(10)* showed that about 4000 IU/d from all sources are needed to maintain optimal vitamin D levels (32 ng/ml). Unlike calcium and other nutrients, vitamin D is made in the skin. The total input is difficult to quantify and is dependent on many environmental factors; these are discussed below. Those of us who live away from the equator and work indoors are at greater risk of deficiency. The simplest way to assess vitamin D status is by checking 25OHD levels. If the level is less than

32 ng/ml, supplementation with an oral vitamin D product is the simplest way for a person to get an adequate amount (*see* below).

3.2. Sources of Vitamin D

3.2.1. FOOD

Few foods are sources of vitamin D. The best food source is oily fish such as salmon, but there are large differences in vitamin D content between farm-raised and wild salmon. Farm-raised salmon has approximately 188 IU/3.5 oz serving whereas wild salmon has much more, approximately 1090 IU/3.5 oz serving *(11)*. Milk in the United States and Canada is routinely fortified with some vitamin D, typically 100 IU per cup. Some cheeses, yogurt, and cereals are fortified with a small amount of the vitamin.

3.2.2. SUN

Many variables affect the skin's ability to produce vitamin D, including weather, season, latitude, altitude, pollution, clothing, age, and sunscreen. Skin pigmentation also interferes with vitamin D production as melanin acts as a natural sunscreen.

Season of the year plays a large part in determining the production of vitamin D. Those with light skin require an exposure to summer midday sun of about 15 min to allow adequate synthesis of vitamin D. This is with a relatively high proportion of the skin exposed and before sunscreen is applied. It is not necessary to burn or redden the skin. Those with darker skin require at least twice as much time in the sun. In the winter, UVB rays do not penetrate the atmosphere, except close to the equator. During that season, therefore, no vitamin D can be produced and most patients will need to use supplements.

The light source used in tanning booths may be able to produce UVB rays and this can therefore be a source of vitamin D. However, tanning booths are not regulated by the FDA and it is difficult to know how much, if any, UVB rays are produced. Moreover, the light source may also generate UVA rays which can cause skin aging.

3.2.3. SUPPLEMENTS

Nutritional supplements for vitamin D come in two forms. Vitamin D_2 is produced by irradiating yeast, while vitamin D_3 is the animal form produced by the skin. Several studies have shown that vitamin D_3 is between three and nine times more potent at maintaining 25OHD levels *(12)*. The question always arises as to how much to give. Rather than rely on a "one size fits all" recommendation, which does not account for differences in skin pigmentation, sun exposure, age, or weight, the simplest method is to measure the patient's 25OHD level. In calculating supplement dose, a good rule of thumb is 100–150 IU daily will raise 25OHD levels by ~1 ng/ml. In practice, this translates to between 1000 and 2000 IU daily for most patients. Occasionally, patients with malabsorption or gastrointestinal surgery may require substantially more vitamin D.

These recommendations are based on several clinical studies of different doses of vitamin D and also on clinical experience. This approach treats patients with lower vitamin D levels with higher amounts of vitamin D. Of course, empiric treatment regimens can be used and again, 1000–2000 IU daily seems to be adequate for many patients and is a good place to start without risk of toxicity.

3.2.4. SAFETY

Vitamin D is a fat-soluble vitamin and there is a valid concern that toxicity may occur at high intakes. The good news is there is a wide gap between the amounts of vitamin D that we typically recommend to patients and potentially toxic amounts. A review of toxicity reports and clinical trials found that doses <30,000 IU daily or achieved 25OHD levels <200 ng/ml were not associated with toxicity and concluded that the tolerable upper limit should be 10,000 IU daily (13). We find in practice that we rarely need to give 10,000 IU to a patient with malabsorption.

4. PROTEIN

Bone is one of the most protein-dense tissues. When bone is remodeled and new bone is laid down, it requires fresh dietary protein. Dietary protein is known to increase urine calcium excretion but this effect is offset by higher calcium intakes. Studies of protein intake show that, overall, it is good for bone both as a source of building materials and through effects of insulin-like growth factor. In the Framingham Study, age-related bone loss was inversely related to protein intake (14). In a calcium intervention trial, only subjects with the highest protein intake gained bone (15). In patients with hip fractures, mortality and recovery is improved if the patients have adequate protein intake ($\approx$1 g protein/kg body weight/day) (16).

The general population of the United States has adequate protein intake, but the population at most risk for fracture are the ones most likely to consume a diet deficient in protein. The recommended dietary allowances (RDA) for protein for adults is 0.8 g of protein per kg body weight per day. Animal protein foods include meat, poultry, fish, dairy products, and eggs. Plant foods include beans, nuts, and seeds.

5. PHOSPHORUS

Bone mineral consists of calcium phosphate. Adequate dietary phosphorus is therefore as important as calcium for building bone. Without it, the patient will develop a form of osteomalacia; they will not mineralize the skeleton. Fortunately, phosphorus is plentiful in many plant and animal tissues and if one has a diet with adequate protein, it likely also contains adequate phosphorus. Dairy products, meat, and fish are good sources of phosphorus.

Absorption of phosphorus is highly efficient. Net absorption is about 55–80%. Phosphorus is also efficiently retained by the body by reducing urinary phosphorus excretion. However, calcium supplements may interfere with phosphorus by acting as a binder and reducing its absorption from the GI tract. This is a good example of the general rule that food sources of nutrients are superior to a nutrient ingested in isolation. In this case, a serving of dairy food will supply phosphorus in addition to the calcium and protein needed for bone health.

The RDA for phosphorus for adults is 700 mg/day and most of the US population obtains enough of the mineral from their diet. However, some groups may have an inadequate intake such as people eating a weight-reduction diet. Another problem group is older women, eating poorly: 10% of women >60 years and 15% of women >80 years consume <70% of the RDA for phosphorus. This group is also likely to have a diet deficient in other nutrients, including calcium and protein. Also of concern are those easting very strict vegetarian diets as these do not contain enough phosphorus in a usable form.

6. MAGNESIUM

About 50% of the body's magnesium resides in the skeleton. It may serve as a reservoir for maintaining the extracellular magnesium concentration. Unprocessed foods are good sources of magnesium. Rich sources include fresh leafy vegetables, whole grains, and nuts. The body is efficient at absorbing magnesium from the diet and about 40–60% is absorbed. The kidney is also efficient at retaining magnesium unless the patient has diabetes or alcoholism that leads to urinary magnesium loss. Measuring magnesium status can be difficult clinically because serum measurements correlate poorly with intracellular levels.

Currently, the role of magnesium in maintaining bone density and preventing osteoporosis is unclear. Cross-sectional studies have not revealed any relationship between magnesium intake and bone density. Controlled studies of magnesium supplementation show a possible increase in bone mineral density. With the paucity of evidence for bone health, we would recommend that patients increase fruit and vegetable intake for general health, but would not make specific recommendations for magnesium supplementation.

SUGGESTED FURTHER READING

Heaney RP. Calcium intake and the prevention of chronic disease. In: Wilson T, Temple NJ, eds. Nutritional Health: Strategies for Disease Prevention. Humana Press, Totowa, NJ, 2001, pp. 31–50.
Heaney RP. Bone health. Am J Clin Nutr 2007; 85:300S–303S.
Holick MF. Sunlight and vitamin D for bone health and prevention of autoimmune diseases, cancers, and cardiovascular disease. Am J Clin Nutr 2004; 80(6 Suppl):1678S–1688S.

REFERENCES

1. Heaney RP, Recker RR, Stegman MR, Moy AJ. Calcium absorption in women: relationships to calcium intake, estrogen status, and age. J Bone Miner Res 1989; 4:469–475.
2. Nordin BEC, Polley KJ, Need AG, Morris HA, Marshall D. The problem of calcium requirement. Am J Clin Nutr 1987; 45:1295–1304.
3. Pribila BA, Hertzler SR, Martin BR, Weaver CM. Savaiano DA. Improved lactose digestion and intolerance among African-American adolescent girls fed a dairy-rich diet. J Am Diet Assoc 2000; 100:524–528.
4. Holick MF. Sunlight and vitamin D for bone health and prevention of autoimmune diseases, cancers, and cardiovascular disease. Am J Clin Nutr 2004; 80(6 Suppl): 1678S–1688S.
5. Heaney RP, Dowell MS, Hale CA, Bendich A. Calcium absorption varies within the reference range for serum 25-hydroxyvitamin D. J Am Coll Nutr 2003; 22:142–146
6. Bischoff-Ferrari HA, Dietrich T, Orav EJ, Dawson Hughes B. Positive association between 25-hydroxy vitamin D levels and bone mineral density: A population-based study of younger and older adults. Am J Med 2004; 116:634–639.
7. Trivedi DP, Doll R, Khaw KT. Effect of four monthly oral vitamin D3 (cholecalciferol) supplementation on fractures and mortality in men and women living in the community: Randomised double blind controlled trial. BMJ 2003; 326:469.
8. Bischoff HA, Stahelin HB, Dick W, et al. Effects of vitamin D and calcium supplementation on falls: A randomized controlled trial. J Bone Miner Res 2003; 18: 343–351.
9. Bischoff Ferrari HA, Dawson Hughes B, Willett WC, Staehelin HB, Bazemore MG, Zee RY, Wong JB. Effect of vitamin D on falls: A meta-analysis. JAMA 2004; 291: 1999–2006.
10. Heaney RP, Davies KM, Chen TC, Holick MF, Barger Lux MJ . Human serum 25-hydroxycholecalciferol response to extended oral dosing with cholecalciferol. Am J Clin Nutr 2003; 77:204–210.
11. Lu Z, Chen TC, Persons KS, et al. Vitamin D content in fish is highly variable: farm salmon is not a good source. J Bone Miner Res 2006; 21(S1):S326.
12. Armas LA, Hollis BW, Heaney RP. Vitamin D2 is much less effective than vitamin D3 in humans. J Clin Endocrinol Metab 2004; 89:5387–5391
13. Hathcock JN, Shao A, Vieth R, Heaney R. Risk assessment for vitamin D. Am J Clin Nutr 2007; 85:6–18.

14. Hannan MT, Tucker KL, Dawson-Hughes B, Cupples LA, Felson DT, Kiel DP. Effect of dietary protein on bone loss in elderly men and women: The Framingham Osteoporosis Study. J Bone Miner Res 2000; 15:2504–2512.
15. Dawson-Hughes B, Harris SS. Calcium intake influences the association of protein intake with rates of bone loss in elderly men and women. Am J Clin Nutr 2002; 75:773–779.
16. Delmi M, Rapin CH, Bengoa JM, Delmas PD, Vasey H, Bonjour JP. Dietary supplementation in elderly patients with fractured neck of the femur. Lancet 1990; 335:1013–1016.

31 Inherited Metabolic Disorders and Nutritional Genomics: Choosing the Wrong Parents

Asima R. Anwar and Scott P. Segal

Key Points

- We describe the categorization of inherited metabolic disorders to better aid in diagnosis.
- Inherited metabolic disorders can be classified into three categories for diagnostic purposes: disorders presenting as intoxication or encephalopathy; disorders of energy metabolism; and disorders involving complex molecules.
- General guiding principles for the nutritional management of inherited metabolic disorders are given.
- Specific approaches to nutritional therapy are discussed for the most common diseases in this group, such as medium-chain *acyl*-CoA dehydrogenase deficiency, maple syrup urine disease (MSUD), phenylketonuria (PKU), homocystinuria, and galactosemia.

Key Words: Inherited metabolic disorders; nutritional management; medium-chain acyl-CoA dehydrogenase deficiency; maple syrup urine disease; phenylketonuria; homocystinuria; galactosemia

1. INTRODUCTION

Many countries, including the United States and Canada, have screening services in place for the detection of inherited metabolic disorders in newborns. This is due to the fact that they are relatively common in the population, and are a significant cause of morbidity in infants, with one out of 1,000 newborns affected. Many inherited metabolic disorders (IMD) have severe symptoms which may lead to significant morbidity and mortality. Interestingly, these disorders are difficult to diagnose as symptoms

From: *Nutrition and Health: Nutrition Guide for Physicians*
Edited by: T. Wilson et al. (eds.), DOI 10.1007/978-1-60327-431-9_31,
© Humana Press, a part of Springer Science+Business Media, LLC 2010

may be easily mistaken for other similar metabolic conditions. IMD have been reported in relation to deficiencies, overproduction, and/or toxic accumulation of precursors or end products of metabolism, respectively.

Tandem mass electroscopy, a recent technological advance, allows a complete acylcarnitine and amino acid profile on a blood specimen. It is being used in an increasing number of states and countries to screen for organic acid and fatty acid oxidation and amino acid disorders, including maple syrup urine disease (MSUD), homocystinuria, phenylketonuria (PKU), and hereditary tyrosinemia (1). Most of these diseases respond well to dietary manipulations, but unfortunately a large number of patients suffer irreversible damage before any warning symptoms appear.

2. IMD DIAGNOSTIC CLASSIFICATIONS

IMD can be divided into three categories according to their clinical presentation (2).

2.1. Disorders Presenting as Intoxication or Encephalopathy

Syndromes of intoxication or encephalopathy may be caused by an accumulation of toxic metabolites due to a metabolic block deficiency of an essential product or a defective transport process. This group includes inborn errors of intermediary metabolism, such as aminoacidopathies, organic acidurias, urea cycle disorders, sugar intolerances, metal disorders, and porphyrias. Clinically, infants with these disorders appear normal at birth and are symptom free for hours or days. Lethargy, poor feeding, vomiting, increased muscle tone, seizures, liver failure, and coma ensue, often quite rapidly. Some newborns have respiratory symptoms, such as apnea or hyperventilation, the latter being more likely if the disorder causes metabolic acidosis. Neurologic findings, such as hyper- or hypotonia, opisthotonus, pedaling, coarse tremors, and myoclonic jerking, are typical of the disorders presenting as intoxication or encephalopathy.

2.2. Disorders of Energy Metabolism

Hypoglycemia is a consistent symptom of disorders of energy metabolism including fatty acid oxidation disorders. Other clinical features are lactic acidosis, hypotonia, and cardiac involvement (cardiomyopathy, arrhythmias, conduction disturbances, and congestive heart failure), but lethargy and coma rarely occur.

2.3. Disorders Involving Complex Molecules

These disorders affect either the synthesis or catabolism of complex molecules. These disorders involve cellular organelles, such as the lysosomes and peroxisomes. Symptoms of these disorders are generally present immediately after birth, and include facial dysmorphia (facial deformities) and severe neurologic dysfunction.

3. NUTRITIONAL MANAGEMENT OF INHERITED METABOLIC DISORDERS – THE GENERAL APPROACH

One common goal that is central to nutritional management of all inherited metabolic disorders is to provide sufficient energy, amino acids, and nitrogen to support and maintain normal growth and development. Shils et al. *(3)* have suggested 12 general approaches to therapy for this group of diseases which may be used sequentially or simultaneously:

1. Enhancing anabolism and depressing catabolism
2. Correcting the primary metabolic imbalance by using both the dietary restrictions to reduce substrate accumulation as well as provision of products that may be deficient
3. Enhancing excretion of accumulated substrate. The kidney may aid as a dialysis organ while maintaining the equilibrium between diuresis and hydration
4. Providing alternative metabolic pathways to decrease accumulated toxic precursors in blocked reaction sequences
5. Using metabolic inhibitors to lower overproduced products
6. Supplying products of blocked secondary pathways
7. Stabilizing altered enzyme proteins
8. Replacing deficient coenzymes
9. Artificially inducing enzyme production
10. Replacing enzymes
11. Transplanting organs
12. Correcting the underlying defects in DNA so that the body can manufacture its own functionally normal enzymes

4. NUTRITIONAL MANAGEMENT OF INHERITED METABOLIC DISORDERS – DISEASE-SPECIFIC APPROACH

Although more than 300 genetic disorders have been reported, only the primary examples of the more debilitating or common IMD are considered in this chapter. Until improved methods of providing patient gene therapy are developed, treatment must generally focus on nutritional management and palliative therapy.

4.1. Medium-Chain Acyl-CoA Dehydrogenase Deficiency (MCAD Deficiency)

The autosomal recessive disorder, medium-chain acyl-CoA dehydrogenase deficiency, is the most common form of fatty acid metabolism abnormalities seen in the population. Caucasians of Northern European descent exhibit the highest frequency of this disorder (4), with an incidence of one in 15,000. Common symptoms of MCAD disorder include recurrent hypoglycemia (when fasting for more than 10–12 h), vomiting, lethargy, encephalopathy, respiratory arrest, hepatomegaly, seizures, apnea, cardiac arrest, coma, and sudden death. Long-term outcomes may include developmental and behavioral disability, chronic muscle weakness, failure to thrive, cerebral palsy, and attention deficit disorder. Mutations in MCAD gene result in the autosomal recessive MCAD deficiency, which results in production of an abnormal MCAD enzyme.

Nutritional management focuses mainly on restricting dietary fat intake to 20% (5) or 30% or less (6) of total caloric intake. Due to decreased fat intake, caloric intake from carbohydrates as well as from night feeding (or extra snack before bed) should be increased to prevent lipolysis and hypoglycemia. For instance, children at 8 months of age (when pancreatic enzymes become fully functional) should be started on a diet of uncooked corn starch (7), with dosing initially at 1.0–1.5 g/kg and gradually increased to 1.75 g/kg by the second year of age (8). This will allow for the necessary sustained release of glucose. Carnitine supplementations may also be used during prolonged unavoidable fasting, such as for surgery as well as other medical testing. Medium-chain triglyceride oils, flaxseed, canola, walnut, or safflower oils are used for alternate fat form and to avoid essential fatty acid deficiency (9). Daily multi-vitamin and mineral supplements that include all fat soluble vitamins are also recommended.

Although no specific commercial dietary formulas are available to meet the complex needs of patients with fatty acid oxidation disorders, a combination of different formulas to provide a diet high in complex carbohydrate, low in fat, and adequate in vitamins and minerals (6) are usually prescribed.

4.2. Maple Syrup Urine Disease (MSUD)

This is a rare IMD in which the patient has a deficiency of the 2-keto acid dehydrogenase enzyme. This results in the inability to effectively metabolize branched-chain amino acids, such as isoleucine and leucine. Internationally, it has an incidence of one in 185,000 newborns; however, it has a significantly higher incidence of one in 176 in Mennonite populations. The excess buildup of branched-chain amino acids in these patients will cause the urine to have a sweet smell similar to maple syrup. Clinical symptoms of

MSUD include neurotoxicity, including opisthotonos, seizures, blindness, mental retardation, and coma, which are due to elevated plasma levels of branched-chain amino acids *(10)*. Without proper treatment, individuals with this disorder will die at a very early age.

Dietary therapy for MSUD requires lifelong restriction of branched-chain amino acid intake, to control the plasma levels of branched-chain amino acids, in particular levels of leucine. It is important to control the levels of branched-chain amino acids without impairing growth and intellectual development of the patient. Recommendations include the measurement of plasma amino acid levels at appropriate intervals for the first 6–12 months of life. In addition to dietary therapy, thiamine (10–1,000 mg/day) should be administered, irrespective of clinical phenotype *(11)*. This high dose has become common practice by pediatricians due to the fact that excess thiamine poses no harm and is excreted in the urine *(11)*.

4.3. Phenylketonuria (PKU)

PKU is caused by amino acid substitutions in the phenylalanine hydroxylase enzyme, which impair its ability to sufficiently metabolize the amino acid phenylalanine. One in 14,000 Caucasian newborns and one in 132,000 African-American newborns are affected by this disorder. Symptoms of PKU include mental retardation, seizures, hyperactivity, and muscular hypertonicity. Untreated maternal PKU during pregnancy has extremely harmful effects on fetal development, including mental retardation, microcephaly, maternal phenylketonuric syndrome, congenital heart disease, and intrauterine growth retardation *(1, 3, 12–14)*.

Therapy for PKU consists of a diet with a low content of phenylalanine. This includes a diet of fruits, vegetables, regular/special low-protein breads, pastas, and cereals, which are low in phenylalanine. Foods that contain large amounts of phenylalanine, such as milk, dairy products, meat, fish, chicken, eggs, beans, and nuts, must be eliminated. Since these foods are also high in protein, adequate protein intake is achieved by adding special phenylalanine-free formulas, and therefore, most of the patient's nutrient intake will be through phenylalanine-free formulas. Although phenylalanine intake should be restricted in individuals with PKU, it should not be outright eliminated, especially during the critical period of brain development early in infancy. Plasma phenylalanine levels maintained above 1–2 mg/100 mL were consistent with better growth and levels up to 7 mg/100 mL allowed for good mental development *(15)*.

Individuals with PKU should also show caution with respect their use of artificial sweeteners. Aspartame (Equol®) contains phenylalanine and is a common ingredient in many reduced- or low calorie foods and beverages. Suggested alternative phenylalanine-free artificial sweeteners such as sucralose (Splendra®) or saccharin (Sweet'n Low®) may be suggested.

4.4. Homocystinuria

Homocystinuria is an autosomal recessive disorder caused by deficiency of the enzyme cystathionine beta-synthase. This renders the patient unable to properly metabolize homocysteine, which is an intermediate in the metabolism of the amino acid methionine. Newborn screening in 13 countries found only one case in 334,000 infants but the frequency is much higher in infants of Irish descent: one in 58,000 (16). Common symptoms of include dislocated lenses, intravascular thrombosis, skeletal changes, osteoporosis, and mental retardation.

Patients with homocystinuria should be given a methionine-restricted diet, which is supplemented with betaine and l-cysteine (3). Some examples of commercially available methionine-free medical foods are HCY Powder, Hominex-1, Hominex-2, XMET Analog, XMET Maxamaid, and XMET Maxamum. Additionally, some patients may respond well to supplements of vitamin B_6 and folic acid (3). Nutritional support should be followed throughout adulthood, as termination of nutrition support in adulthood may increase the risk to thromboembolisms and lens dislocation (17, 18).

4.5. Galactosemia

Galactosemia is an autosomal recessive disorder caused by a deficiency of the galactose-1-phosphate uridyltransferase enzyme. This enzyme is necessary for the breakdown of the monosaccharide galactose and thus deficiencies of galactose-1-phosphate will manifest as hyperglycemia. The incidence of galactosemia, in the general population, is one in 8,000 births. Symptoms of galactosemia include acute hepatotoxicity. Prolonged jaundice may appear with the start of human milk or infant formulas containing lactose (a disaccharide that is digested to galactose and glucose). Other complications include delayed speech development, severe mental retardation, irregular menstrual cycles, and decreased ovarian function and ovarian failure. The condition is irreversible and requires abstinence from milk, milk products, and galactose-containing foods for life.

Generally, patients with galactosemia should have a diet of foods that contain neither galactose nor lactose (which when broken down will result in galactose and glucose). A few patients with a residual 5–10% of normal galactose-1-phosphate uridyltransferase. These individuals may be able to tolerate small amounts of galactose found in muscle meat, fruit, and vegetables (3). Due to the dairy restrictions these patients must endure, calcium supplements are recommended to offset the lack of dietary calcium intake. Infants with this disorder also should not be fed milk, instead they can be fed with soy formula, meat-based formula, Nutramigen (a protein hydrolysate formula), or other lactose-free formula *(19)*.

5. CONCLUSIONS

Many of the inherited metabolic disorders are now included in routine neonatal screening. Diagnosis of these disorders may facilitate early intervention based solely off data collected from the initial tests, prior to further confirmation from follow-up tests. Nutritional management prevents severe pathologic complications by reducing the overproduction and accumulation of toxic metabolites, and providing the necessary nutritional constituents that are deficient, while attempting to support and maintain sufficient growth and development throughout the lifespan.

SUGGESTED FURTHER READING

Shils M, Shike M, Ross A, Caballero B, Cousines, R. eds. Modern Nutrition in Health and Disease, 10th ed. Lippincott Williams and Wilkins, Philadelphia, PA, 2006.
Children living with inherited metabolic diseases. The National Information Centre For Metabolic Diseases. Crewe, UK. Available at http://www.climb.org.uk. Last accessed January 19, 2009. Website offers support to parents and family members with children suffering from inherited metabolic disorders.

REFERENCES

1. Burton B. Inherited metabolic disorders. In: Avery's Neonatology: Pathophysiology and Management of the Newborn, 6th ed. MacDonald M, Mullet M, Seshia M, eds. Lippincott Williams & Wilkins, Philadelphia, 2005.
2. Stokowski LA. The Unusual Suspects: Genetic Metabolic Disorders in the Newborn. Highlights of the National Association of Neonatal Nurses 23rd Annual Conference September 26–29, 2007, San Diego, California.
3. Elsas L, Acosta P. Amino acids, organic acids, and galactose. Shils ME, Olson JA, Shike M, Ross A, eds. In: Modern Nutrition in Health and Disease, 10th ed. Lippincott Williams & Wilkins, Philadelphia, 2006.
4. MCAD Deficiency Medium-chain acyl-CoA dehydrogenase. Available at www.cdc.gov/genomics/hugenet/factsheets/fs_mcad. Last accessed July 18, 2008.
5. Online support organization for Fatty Oxidation Disorder. Available at http://www.fodsupport.org. Last accessed January 19, 2009.
6. Solis J, Singh R. Management of fatty acid oxidation disorders: a survey of current treatment strategies. J Am Diet Assoc 2002; 102:1800–1806.
7. Hayde M, Widhalm K. Effects of cornstarch treatment in very young children with type I glycogen storage disease. Eur J Pediatr 1990; 149:630–633.
8. Vici C, Burlina AB, Bertini E, et al. Progressive neuropathy and recurrent myoglobinuria in a child with long-chain 3-hydroxyacyl-coenzyme a dehydrogenase deficiency. J Pediatr 1991; 118:744–746.

9. Vockley J, Renaud D. Inherited metabolic disorders: defects of *B*-oxidation. In: Shils M, Olson J, Shike M, Ross A, eds. Modern Nutrition in Health and Disease, 10th ed. Lippincott Williams & Wilkins, Philadelphia, 2006, pp. 960–978.

10. Korein J, Sansaricq C, Kalmijn M, Honig J, Lange B. Maple syrup urine disease: clinical, EEG, and plasma amino acid correlations with a theoretical mechanism of acute neurotoxicity. Int J Neurosci 1994; 79:21–45.

11. Chuang D, Chuang J, Wynn R. Branched-chain amino acids: metabolism, physiological function and application. J Nutr 2006; 136:243S–249S.

12. Rouse B, Azen C, Koch R, Matalon R, et al. Maternal Phenylketonuria Collaborative Study (MPKUCS) offspring: facial anomalies, malformations, and early neurological sequelae. Am J Med Genet 1997; 69:89–95.

13. Wilcken B, Wiley V, Hammond J, et al. Screening newborns for inborn errors of metabolism by tandem mass spectrometry. N Engl J Med 2003; 348:2304–2312.

14. Lenke R, Levy H. Maternal phenylketonuria and hyperphenylalaninemia. An international survey of untreated and treated pregnancies. N Engl J Med 1980; 303:1202–1208.

15. Wardlaw, G, Hampl J, DiSilvestro, R. Metabolism. In: Perspectives in Nutrition. McGraw-Hill, New York, NY, 2004.

16. Mudd S, Levy H, Kraus J. Disorders of transsulfuration. In: Scriver C, Beaudet A, Sly W, et al., eds. The Metabolic and Molecular Bases of Inherited Disease. 8th ed. McGraw-Hill, NY, 2001, pp. 2007–2056.

17. Marcus A. Editorial perspective: aspirin as an antithrombotic medication. N Engl J Med 1983; 309:1515–1517.

18. Davi G, Di Minno G, Coppola A, et al. Oxidative stress and platelet activation in homozygous homocystinuria. Circulation 2001; 104:1124–1128.

19. Pasternak J. Counseling, diagnostic testing and management of genetic disorders. In: An Introduction to Human Molecular Genetics. John Wiley and Sons, Hoboken, NJ, 2005.

32 Nutritional Challenges of Girls and Women

Margaret A. Maher
and Kate Fireovid

Key Points

- Physical demands of females with regard to reproductive function and child-bearing affect nutrition, appetite, and weight regulation. Nutrition and reproductive interactions may have both acute and long-lasting affects on female health that are distinct from that of men.
- Cultural and social factors emphasizing gender-specific roles, body shape, and weight in females increase risk of disordered eating, eating disorders, and likelihood that women will seek medical and nonmedical management of weight.
- Neural and hormonal regulation of appetite varies between males and females and within females at different stages in the lifespan; it may affect success of nutritional and medical management of weight and appetite.
- The female "athlete" triad, a condition involving amenorrhea, disordered eating (usually restrictive), and osteoporosis, is most often recognized in female athletes due to activity-associated pain and stress fractures, but also occurs in more sedentary girls and women.
- Polycystic ovary syndrome (PCOS) is a condition often associated with overweight and obesity, insulin resistance and resulting glucose intolerance, carbohydrate craving, and eating disorders. This condition may benefit from nutrition-related lifestyle changes along with drug treatment (sibutramine, metformin, etc.).
- Women may seek advice regarding nutritional supplements for relief of peri- and postmenopausal symptoms in addition to or as surrogate for hormone replacement therapy.

Key Words: Women; nutrition; appetite; weight regulation; amenorrhea; disordered eating; osteoporosis

From: *Nutrition and Health: Nutrition Guide for Physicians*
Edited by: T. Wilson et al. (eds.), DOI 10.1007/978-1-60327-431-9_32,
© Humana Press, a part of Springer Science+Business Media, LLC 2010

1. FEMALE REPRODUCTION AND NUTRITION

Demeter, the Greek goddess of grain and fertility, reflects the long-recognized ancient associations among females, fertility, and food. Nutrients may impact, and be impacted by, gender roles, menstrual cycling, fertility, pregnancy, labor and delivery, lactation, and peri- and postmenopausal adaptations. In addition, reproductive status in women may have long-lasting effects on other body systems, such as bone health. It follows, therefore, that clinicians need a solid understanding of nutritional issues that are specific to females. This chapter focuses on unique nutrition-related challenges for girls and women to complement the lifecycle chapters on nutrition during pregnancy by Francis (Chapter 15) and breast milk by Rorabaugh and Friel (Chapter 16).

Weight issues should be addressed with those women who are underweight or overweight. Very high or low body mass index (BMI >35 or BMI<20, respectively) is associated with reduced probability of conceiving *(1)*, complications during pregnancy, labor and delivery, and increased risk to the health of prospective children. However, careful assessment for presence or risk of development of disordered eating should be undertaken before weight gain or loss is encouraged. History of dieting and dietary restraint has been associated with increased weight gain during pregnancy in all but underweight women *(2)*. The health benefits of ideal weight range for both mother and prospective children should be emphasized.

Adequate calcium is recommended for women of all ages, but especially during adolescence and in young women; this is because peak bone mass is developed during the growing years, up to age 30 *(1)*, as is more thoroughly discussed in Chapter 30. Females 18–30-yr-old who consumed dairy calcium intake of 1,200–1,300 mg/day showed greater total hip bone mass density (BMD) at the end of the 1-yr intervention as compared to those who consumed less than 800 mg/day *(3)*. Although somewhat controversial, in some studies calcium supplementation and low-fat dairy products have also been associated with reduced postmenopausal weight gain or increased weight loss in overweight women *(1)*. Because of common preoccupation of girls and women with weight they may purposefully consume low levels of foods that are typically rich in calcium, for instance replacing milk with diet drinks. Promotion of three servings of low-fat dairy products that provide both calcium and vitamin D is recommended. If a vegetarian lifestyle or lactose intolerance are considerations, other calcium-fortified beverages or foods, such as orange juice, or a calcium and vitamin D supplement may be warranted. The daily recommendations for calcium, vitamin D, and other nutrients are listed in Appendix C. Use of certain hormonal contraceptives may increase osteoporosis risk in women who would otherwise be menstruating naturally *(3)*, but may reduce amenorrhea-associated osteoporosis risk in anorexia nervosa *(4)* or the female athlete triad reviewed below.

Women of reproductive age are at greater risk of anemia due to iron loss (15–20 mg) during menstruation and reduced dietary iron intake. Added concerns include especially heavy or frequent menses and athletic-induced hemolysis and anemia *(5)*. Iron supplementation is recommended as well as education on the difference between heme- and non-heme iron sources with regard to bioavailability. Non-heme iron is better absorbed in the presence of meat protein and should be consumed in the same meal with foods rich in vitamin C so as to enhance absorption *(1)*.

Adequate periconceptional and pregnancy intake of folate is well known to decrease the risk of neural tube defects but may also be linked to reduction of other complications of pregnancy including preeclampsia and miscarriage *(6)*. Repeated miscarriages and infertility have been linked to insufficient amounts of vitamin B_{12} and folate. Unlike iron, folic acid in supplement form has a higher bioavailability (85%) than food folate (50%) *(7)*.

A few nutrients have been linked to management of premenstrual symptoms. Some studies have shown calcium supplementation (1,000–1,300 mg/day) to alleviate some symptoms, including irritability and cramping. Vitamin B_6 in doses up to 100 mg/day may help reduce premenstrual symptoms and premenstrual depression *(1)*. The overall efficacy of nutritionally related measures for improved premenstrual symptoms is an area of growing interest and in need of further clinical study.

2. FEMALES, BODY DISSATISFACTION, AND NUTRITION

Girls and women of all ages, many ethnicities, and environments report struggling with body dissatisfaction that may affect nutrition *(8, 9)*. This dissatisfaction may lead females or their loved ones to express concern about their bodies and seek healthy or unhealthy ways to change their bodies *(9)*. While girls and women of all ages evaluate and report dissatisfaction with their bodies; as women age, the self-reported "importance" of their body shape and size declines. *(8)*. While both boys and girls undergo great body changes during adolescence, and sometimes into early adulthood, that can impact body image *(9)*, females have monthly body changes associated with menstrual cycling, enormous changes in physical size and shape associated with pregnancy and postpartum, as well as changes in body composition and fat deposition associated with midlife hormonal changes. Referral of girls and women (as well as boys and men) for counseling to explore and resolve body image as well as aging issues may improve nutrition outcomes and mental and physical health. The passage of mental health parity legislation should improve treatment options for individuals and families struggling with eating and body image disturbances.

3. WEIGHT MANAGEMENT IN FEMALES

Both obesity and eating disorders (as a group) are more common in females than males in developed countries. Although there is a well-known difference in body fat distribution among most women vs. most males, the interaction of factors dictating gender-specific fat storage and mobilization are not clear. Multiple appetite regulating hormones are currently under investigation for their roles in energy balance and inappropriate imbalance *(10)*. Weight management and appetite regulation in girls and women are complicated by gender-specific roles as family meal preparers, menstrual cycle fluctuations, major changes in sex hormone levels at the onset and end of the reproductive years, and body weight and shape changes associated with pregnancy and lactation *(10)*. For example, carbohydrate (vs. placebo) beverage consumption has been associated with reduction in premenstrual symptoms; an effect linked to carbohydrate craving and attributed to promotion of tryptophan and the serotonin system *(11)*.

Success rates for weight loss maintenance in overweight women and recovery from eating disorders are not encouraging. It is important for clinicians to recognize that a one-size-fits-all approach to treatment of disordered eating issues and weight management, in both males and females, may be less effective than individualized nutrition assessment and management approaches. Evidence is mixed with regard to whether reasonable calorie restriction is effective in the long-term or if it predisposes to eating disorders; however, any dieting should be done with caution, supervision, and with adequate dietary carbohydrate and protein to preserve lean body mass. There is also evidence that a size acceptance (health at all sizes) approach that emphasizes attention to internal hunger, satiety, and appetite cues may improve health and self-esteem more than dieting *(12)*.

4. THE FEMALE ATHLETE TRIAD

The female athlete triad (TRIAD) involves three interrelated conditions that may profoundly affect the skeletal and reproductive health of girls and women: amenorrhea, disordered eating (usually restrictive), and osteoporosis *(13)*. Eating disorders are covered in more detail in Chapter 22, by Allison. The prevalence of the TRIAD has been reported to range from 12 to 27% from elite athletes to regularly active females *(14)*. Screening for the TRIAD should occur at regular and athlete physical examinations. Detected presence of any one of the TRIAD components with screening or patient presentation of amenorrhea, stress fractures, or low body weight indicates assessment of the other two components. Diagnosis of the TRIAD should be followed by comprehensive evaluation and management by a physician, behavioral health professional, and registered dietitian *(13)*. More information about the underlying causes of the TRIAD may be provided by the following means: careful assessment of nutritional intake, social history, and body image; administration of a screening tool, such as EAT-26 *(15)*; measurement of bone mineral density (BMD) and body composition; and laboratory assessments to rule out other causes of amenorrhea. Restoration of normal eating patterns, energy balance, menses, and BMD are the goals of treatment. Adequate calcium and vitamin D consumption should also be monitored. Failure of the patient to comply with treatment plan and/or resume menses may indicate the need for medical treatment with hormonal replacement therapy (usually oral contraceptives), activity restrictions, and/or more intensive family or even inpatient supervision *(13)*.

5. POLYCYSTIC OVARIAN SYNDROME

Polycystic ovarian syndrome (PCOS), also known as Stein–Leventhol syndrome, is associated with an array of five clinical features: hyperandrogenism, small ovarian cysts, menstrual dysfunction, android-pattern overweight or obesity, and insulin resistance (with accompanying glucose intolerance and hyperinsulinemia). The prevalence of the condition is estimated to be 5–10% of women of reproductive age and there is often family history of PCOS or its signs. Indications of hyperandrogenism in women include hirsutism, acne, dysmenorrhea, and alopecia. The presence of insulin resistance and hyperinsulinemia are suggested by episodic hypoglycemia and related carbohydrate craving, acanthosis nigricans (dark patches on the skin), and unexplained weight gain. Other symptoms that may also be present include significant mood disorder, body image disturbance, and disordered eating, secondary to attempts to control weight gain. Results of sex hormone tests, standard diagnostics for diabetes (fasting glucose and insulin, oral glucose tolerance test, HbA1c), and transvaginal pelvic ultrasound may provide differential diagnosis.

Dietary management of PCOS should emphasize low saturated fat and high fiber, and low glycemic-index carbohydrate sources spread throughout the day in 4–6 meals/snacks. In addition, *n*–3 fats, cinnamon, and chromium rich foods or supplements may improve metabolic parameters *(16)*. Orlistat or metformin may be helpful to assist with testosterone reduction, improved insulin sensitivity, and weight loss and maintenance *(17)*. Oral contraceptives and androgen-reducing medications, such as spironolactone, may also be helpful to stabilize sex hormone levels and improve menses. Regular exercise, including both strength-building (resistance) and endurance components, can be helpful for weight loss, improvement of insulin sensitivity, and self-esteem. Counseling may also be indicated for mood disorder, help with body image and acceptance, and disordered eating if present *(16)*. Early detection of PCOS, or the proposed male equivalent (androgenic alopecia), can improve physical and mental health outcomes and reduce the risks of chronic diseases and infertility later in life.

6. MENOPAUSE AND NUTRITIONAL SUPPLEMENTS

The peri- and postmenopausal periods may pose challenging issues for women's nutrition. This can spark an interest in the use of complementary and alternative medicine (CAM). The use of hormone replacement therapy (HRT) to alleviate symptoms associated with menopause declined sharply after the Women's Health Initiative (WHI) showed that HRT poses an increased risk-to-benefit ratio *(1)*. Many women have turned to nutritional supplements and CAM for relief of symptoms.

Research completed in several countries has found phytoestrogens, particularly soy isoflavone extracts, may relieve menopausal symptoms such as hot flashes *(1)*. However, a recent review of studies found that hot flashes are only slightly influenced by isoflavones, and many times not at all *(18)*. Several studies have also suggested soy isoflavones have cancer-preventing properties in multiple organs including the mammary gland. However, recent studies have shown that the cancer-preventing properties may be related to soy consumption earlier in life *(18)*. In general, isoflavone administration is not recommended in women without childhood exposure to isoflavones due to isoflavones' inconsistent effects on the mammary gland and uterus, which may increase the risk of developing malignancies *(18)*. Caution should be taken in application of these findings due to limitations in dietary recall in these studies. Women who have had or are at increased risk of breast, uterine, or ovarian cancer; endometriosis; or uterine fibroids should be aware of the potential risks of using phytoestrogens to reduce unpleasant peri- and postmenopausal symptoms *(19)*.

Black cohosh is another nutritional supplement that has been reported to reduce menopausal-related hot flashes and improve mood *(20)*. However, a 12-mo study published in 2006 showed benefit for reducing hot flashes with estrogen therapy, but no benefit of black cohosh, a multibotanical, or multibotanical with dietary soy counseling above placebo *(21)*. Other supplements women commonly use to reduce menopausal symptoms include flaxseed, *Ginkgo biloba*, and red clover. Moreover, St. Johns Wort may be taken and is mildly effective for mood improvement *(20)*. However, few high-quality studies have been completed on the safety and efficacy of these treatment options *(1, 19–22)*. Of importance, up to 70% of women taking supplements may not inform their health-care provides and may thus risk drug interactions or unrecognized adverse reactions *(20)*.

Eighty percent of those affected by osteoporosis are women. During menopause, bone losses of 3–5% occur per year. Adequate calcium and vitamin D intake during childhood and the early reproductive years promotes bone build up that will extend the time until postmenopausal signs of osteoporosis appear *(1)*. Little evidence supports the claim that isoflavones have an anti-osteoporotic effect *(18)*. A European study found that postmenopausal women consuming fortified dairy products with 1,200 mg per day for 12 months had more positive changes in biochemical indexes of bone metabolism and BMD than those women taking the same amount of calcium in supplement form. Reasons for greater bioavailability of calcium from dairy products may be due to the role of magnesium and milk protein in bone metabolism *(22)*. A healthy diet, weight-bearing exercise, avoiding smoking, and limiting alcohol intake can further prevent bone loss *(1)*.

7. SUMMARY

The unique physiology of females and significant changes in anatomy directed by sex hormones across the lifespan pose nutritional challenges that may require assessment and intervention. Anthropometrics, diet and eating pattern analyses, and questions about body image and satisfaction should be routine aspects of annual physical examinations, especially coincident with puberty, pregnancy, and postpartum and peri-menopausal periods. These may help detect and monitor conditions that warrant nutritional, medical, and/or exercise interventions that will improve girls' and women's health and well-being.

SUGGESTED FURTHER READING

Position of the American Dietetic Association and Dietitians of Canada: Nutrition and women's health. J Am Diet Assoc 2004; 104:984–1001. Available at:http://www.eatright.org/cps/rde/xchg/ada/hs.xsl/advocacy_3780_ENU_HTML.htm – Last accessed: December 20, 2008.

Nattiv A, Loucks AB, Manore MM, Sanborn CF, Sungodt-Borgen J, Warren MP. American College of Sports Medicine Position Stand: The female athlete triad. Med Sci Sports Exerc 2007; 39:1867–1881. May be ordered at:http://www.acsm.org/Content/NavigationMenu/News/Pronouncements Statements/PositionStands/Position_Stands1.htm – Last accessed: December 20, 2008.

Menopausal Symptoms and CAM. National Institutes of Health: National Center for Complimentary and Alternative Medicine. Available at:http://nccam.nih.gov/health/menopauseandcam/. – Last accessed: December 20, 2008.

Mayo Clinic: Tools for Healthier Lives: Women's Health: Polycystic Ovary Syndrome. Available at:http://www.mayoclinic.com/health/polycystic-ovary-syndrome/DS00423. – Last accessed: December 20, 2008.

National Eating Disorders Association. Available athttp://www.NationalEatingDisorders.org. – Last accessed: December 20, 2008.

REFERENCES

1. Position of the American Dietetic Association and Dietitians of Canada: Nutrition and women's health. J Am Diet Assoc 2004; 104:984–1001.

2. Mumford SL, Siega-Riz AM, Herring A, Evenson KR. Dietary restraint and gestational weight gain. J Am Diet Assoc 2008; 108:1646–1653.

3. Teegarden D, Legowski P, Gunther C, McCabe G, Peacock M, Lyle R. Dietary calcium intake protects women consuming oral contraceptives from spine and hip bone loss. J Clin Endocrinol Metab 2005; 90:5127–5133.

4. Pitts SA, Emans SJ. Controversies in contraception. Curr Opin Pediatr 2008; 20: 383–389.

5. Peeling P, Dawson B, Goodman C, Landers G, Trinder D. Athletic induced iron deficiency: new insights into the role of inflammation, cytokines and hormones. Eur J Appl Physiol 2008; 103:381–391.

6. Tamura T, Pacciano MF. Folate and human reproduction. Am J Clin Nutr 2006; 83: 993–1014.

7. Yang TL, Hung J, Caudill MA, et al. A long-term controlled folate feeding study in young women supports that validity of the 1.7 multiplier in the dietary folate equivalency equation. J Nutr 2005; 135:1139–1145.

8. Tiggemann M. Body image across the adult life span: stability and change. Body Image 2004; 1(1):29–41.

9. Neumark-Sztainer D, Croll J, Story M, Hannan PJ, French SA, Perry C. Ethnic/racial differences in weight-related concerns and behaviors among adolescent girls and boys: findings from Project EAT. J Psychosom Res 2002; 53:963–974.

10. Lovejoy JC, Sainsbury A; the Stock Conference 2008 Working Group. Sex differences in obesity and the regulation of energy homeostasis. Obes Rev 2008 (Epub abstract only).

11. Sayegh R, Schiff I, Wurtman J, Spiers P, McDermott J, Wurtman R. The effect of a carbohydrate-rich beverage on mood, appetite, and cognitive function in women with premenstrual syndrome. Obstet Gynecol 1995; 86:520–528.

12. Bacon, L, Stern, JS, Van Loan MD, Keim NL. Size acceptance and intuitive eating improve health for obese, female chronic dieters. J Am Diet Assoc 2005; 105: 929–936.

13. Nattiv A, Loucks AB, Manore MM, Sanborn CF, Sungodt-Borgen J, Warren MP. American College of Sports Medicine Position Stand: The female athlete triad. Med Sci Sports Exerc 2007; 39:1867–1881.

14. Torstveist MK, Sundgot-Borgen J. The female athlete triad exists in elite athlete and controls. Med Sci Sports Exerc 2005; 37:1449–1459.

15. Berland NW, Thompson J, Linton PH. Correlation between the EAT-26 and the EAT-40, the Eating Disorders Inventory, and the Restrained Eating Inventory. Int J Eating Disorders 2006; 5:569–574.

16. Grassi A. Dietitian's Guide to PCOS. Luca Publishing, Haverfield, PA, 2007.

17. Jayagopal V, Kilpatrick ES, Holding S, Jennings PE, Atkin SL. Orlistat is as beneficial as metformin in the treatment of polycystic ovarian syndrome. J Clin Endocrinol Metab 2005; 90:729–733.

18. Wuttke W, Jarry H, Seidlova-Wuttke D. Isoflavones- safe food additives or dangerous drugs? Ageing Res Rev 2007; 6:150–188.

19. Menopausal Symptoms and CAM. National Institutes of Health: National Center for Complimentary and Alternative Medicine. Available at:http://nccam.nih.gov/health/menopauseandcam/. Last accessed: November 13, 2008.

20. Geller SE, Studee L. Botanical and dietary supplements for menopausal symptoms: what works, what doesn't. J Womens Health 2005; 14:634–649.

21. Newton KM, Reed SD, LaCroix AZ, Grothaus LC, Ehrlich K, Guiltinan J. Treatment of vasomotor symptoms of menopause with black cohosh, multibotanicals, soy, hormone therapy, or placebo. A randomized trial. Ann Int. Med 2006;145:869–879.

22. Manios Y, Moschonis G, Trovas G, Lyritis G. Changes in biochemical indexes of bone metabolism and bone mineral density after a 12-mo dietary intervention program: Post-menopausal Health Study. Am J Clin Nutr 2007; 86:781–789.

33 Diet, Physical Activity, and Cancer Prevention

Cindy D. Davis and John A. Milner

Key Points

- Maintain a healthy weight throughout life; this is one of the most important ways to reduce cancer risk. A healthy weight can be promoted by limiting consumption of high-calorie foods and sugary drinks and by being physically active throughout life.
- Eat mostly foods of plant origin. This includes at least five portions/servings (at least 400 g or 14 oz) of a variety of vegetables and fruits everyday; eating whole grains and/or pulses (legumes) with every meal; and limiting refined starchy foods.
- Limit red meat intake to 60 g per week and limit processed meat consumption.
- Limit daily alcoholic drink consumption. Although there is no consumption that is not associated with an increased cancer risk, modest amounts of alcohol (two drinks a day for men or one drink a day for women) can protect against coronary heart disease.
- Limit consumption of salt-preserved or salty foods.
- Cancer survivors should follow the recommendations for cancer prevention regarding diet, healthy weight, and physical activity.

Key Words: Cancer; diet and prevention; body mass index; phytochemicals; meat; alcohol

1. INTRODUCTION

Cancer is a leading cause of death in the United States. "Cancer" is a general term that represents more than 100 diseases, each with their own etiology. Cancer risk is influenced by both genetic and environmental factors including dietary habits. While each type of cancer has unique characteristics, they share one common feature, namely unregulated cell division. All cancers begin when a single cell acquires multiple genetic changes and loses

From: *Nutrition and Health: Nutrition Guide for Physicians*
Edited by: T. Wilson et al. (eds.), DOI 10.1007/978-1-60327-431-9_33,
© Humana Press, a part of Springer Science+Business Media, LLC 2010

control of its normal growth and replication processes *(1)*. The cancer process, which can occur over decades, includes fundamental, yet diverse, wide cellular processes that can be influenced by diet, such as carcinogen bioactivation, cellular differentiation, DNA repair, cellular proliferation/signaling, and apoptosis *(2)*.

Evidence continues to mount that altering dietary habits is an effective and cost-efficient approach for both reducing cancer risk and modifying the biological behavior of tumors *(3)*. The importance of diet was emphasized more than a quarter century ago when Doll and Peto *(4)* suggested that approximately 35% (10–70%) of all cancers in the United States might be attributable to dietary factors. In 2007, similar conclusions were reached by The World Cancer Research Fund/American Institute of Cancer Research (WCRF/AICR) after evaluating over 7,000 studies. Their report concluded that diet and physical activity were major determinants of cancer risk *(3)*. On a global scale, this could represent over 3–4 million cancer cases that can be prevented each year *(3)*.

The North American Association of Central Cancer Registries provides evidence that death rates from cancer have been dropping by about 2.1% a year in the United States since 2002 *(5)*. This trend is thought not to be a result of miraculous medical breakthroughs but a result of improvements in prevention, early detection, and treatment of some of the leading causes of cancer death. Greater attention to environmental factors, such as dietary habits and smoking, holds promise to make even greater reductions in cancer rates. Cancer is no longer being viewed as an inevitable consequence of aging. Only about 5–10% of cancers can be classified as familial. The capability of utilizing smoking cessation, food and nutrition strategies, and the promotion of physical activity points to cancer as a largely preventable disease.

While considerable evidence points to diet as a critical factor in determining cancer risk, there are numerous inconsistencies in the literature. Much of this variation in response may relate to the genetic background of the individual. Recent studies provide important proof that genetic polymorphisms can markedly influence the response to specific foods *(6, 7)*. By utilizing genetic information, we may be able to identify those individuals who must assure an adequate intake of a particular nutrient for cancer prevention. For example, dietary calcium can interact with a polymorphism in the vitamin D receptor (the *Fok 1* restriction site) to affect colon cancer risk. Whereas dietary calcium is not important in determining colon cancer risk in individuals who are homozygous for the capital F genotype for the vitamin D receptor, low dietary calcium increases colon cancer risk with increasing copies of the little f allele for the vitamin D receptor *(6)*. Selected polymorphisms may also be useful as surrogate markers for those who might be placed at risk from excessive exposures *(8)*. Colorectal adenoma risk is modified by the interplay between polymorphisms in PPAR delta and fish consumption. In individuals with the variant allele for PPAR delta (<10% of the population), increased fish consumption actually increases the risk of developing colorectal adenomas *(8)*. However, the existence of about 30,000 genes and many million single nucleotide polymorphisms indicate that understanding individual responses to foods or components will be extremely complicated.

2. BODY FATNESS

Today nearly two-thirds of the US population is considered overweight or obese. While these conditions have been linked to heart disease, only recently has evidence pointed to excess body weight as a risk factor for many cancers. Typically, obesity, defined as a body mass index (BMI) greater than 30, is associated with about a 20% increase in risk for most, but not all, cancers *(8)*. This lack of association across all cancers may simply reflect the imprecision in using BMI as a surrogate risk marker. The use of biomarkers of the metabolic syndrome holds promise for determining which shifts in body energetics are likely contributing to increased cancer risk or changes in the behavior of tumors *(9)*. Regardless, the WCRF/AICR panel judged the evidence as convincing that greater body fatness is a cause of cancers of the esophagus, pancreas, colorectum, breast (postmenopausal), endometrium, and kidney *(3)*. Greater body fatness is probably a cause of cancer of the gallbladder, both directly and indirectly, through the formation of gallstones *(3)*. In terms of weight-related factors, body weight alone does not completely determine an individual's ability to avoid or survive cancer. Location also appears important since abdominal fat accumulation may be more detrimental than visceral fat accumulations. For that reason a high waist circumference may be especially hazardous.

The term "energy balance" has often been used to describe the complex interaction between diet, physical activity, and genetics on growth and body weight over an individual's lifetime, and how these factors may influence cancer risk (Fig. 1). There are many potential interrelated mechanisms linking obesity to increased cancer risk, including insulin resistance, altered sex hormone metabolism, and increased inflammation (Fig. 1).

Early in the 20th century, research began to emerge that caloric restriction was an effective strategy for increasing longevity and decreasing cancer risk. Caloric restriction has several favorable effects on cancer processes including decreased mitogenic response, increased rates of apoptosis, reduced inflammatory response, induction of DNA repair enzymes, altered drug-metabolizing enzyme expression, and modified cell-mediated immune function *(9)*. At least parts of these anticancer properties associated with

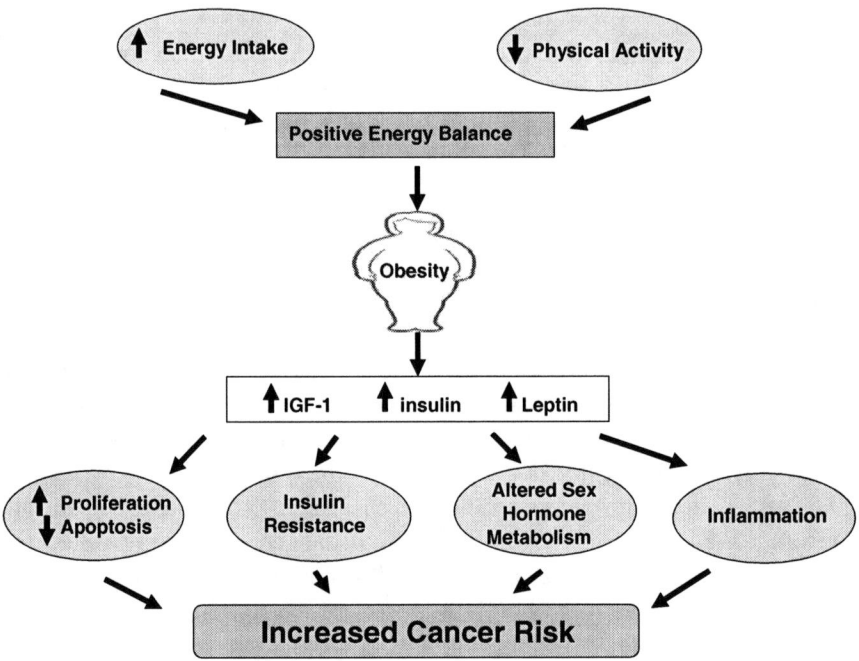

Fig. 1. Long-term positive energy balance due to excessive energy intake and/or low levels of energy expenditure can lead to obesity. The metabolic consequences of long-term positive energy balance and the accumulation of excessive body fat include increased IGF-1, insulin, and leptin concentrations which can stimulate cellular proliferation, inhibit apoptosis, increase insulin resistance, alter steroid hormone metabolism, and stimulate inflammatory/oxidative stress processes, all of which can contribute to increased cancer risk.

caloric restriction likely involve changes in the IGF-1 pathway (Fig. 1) *(9)*. Maintenance of a healthy weight throughout life may be one important way to protect against cancer, as well as a number of other common chronic diseases including hypertension and stroke, type 2 diabetes, and coronary heart disease.

3. PHYSICAL ACTIVITY

A key variable in the energy balance equation is energy expended via physical activity. Despite the circulatory benefits associated with physical activity, Americans are not incorporating enough physical activity into their daily routines. The Centers for Disease Control and Prevention (CDC) estimates that more than 50% of American adults do not get enough physical activity to prove beneficial to their health, and more than 25% are not active even during leisure time *(10)*. Unfortunately, statistics with children and adolescents are no more encouraging. Overall, industrialization, urbanization, and mechanization have fostered a largely sedentary population in many parts of the world.

Regular, sustained physical activity protects against cancer of some sites independent of its effects on body fatness *(3)*. The WCRF/AICR panel judged that the evidence that physical activity protects against colon cancer is convincing *(3)*. Physical activity probably protects against endometrial and postmenopausal breast cancer; however, the evidence suggesting that it protects against premenopausal breast cancer is limited *(3)*. Because physical activity promotes a healthy weight, it would be anticipated that exercise also protect against those cancers whose risk is increased by obesity.

Physical activity most likely influences the development of cancer through multiple, perhaps overlapping, biological pathways, several of which are mentioned in Fig. 1. Many researchers believe physical activity aids in regular bowel movements, which may decrease the time the colon is exposed to potential carcinogens; causes changes in insulin resistance, metabolism, and hormone levels, which may help prevent tumor development; and alters a number of inflammatory and immune factors *(11)*.

The WCRF/AICR report recommended that individuals should be moderately physically active, equivalent to brisk walking for at least 30 min everyday. As fitness improves, individuals should aim for at least 60 min of moderate activity, or 30 min of more vigorous physical activity, everyday *(3)*.

4. PLANT FOODS

Evidence that plant foods protect against cancer comes principally from epidemiological investigations and from a host of animal and cell culture studies. Plant-based diets will typically be high in nutrients and dietary fiber, but low in energy density. Recommendations for consumption tend to exclude starchy vegetables such as potato, yam, sweet potato, and cassava. Non-starchy vegetables probably protect against cancers of the mouth, pharynx, and larynx, and those of the esophagus and stomach *(3)*. Limited evidence also suggests that they may protect against cancers of the nasopharynx, lung, colorectum, ovary, and endometrium *(3)*. Fruit probably protect against cancers of the mouth, pharynx, and larynx, and those of the esophagus, lung, and stomach *(3)*. The possibility has also surfaced that fruit may also protect against cancers of the nasopharynx, pancreas, liver, and colorectum *(3)*. While these relationships are based on the epidemiologic literature, it must be pointed out that there are a number of limitations/considerations that are specific to the analysis of dietary intake of fruit and vegetables. These include the following: most studies of consumption of dietary fruit and vegetables have been conducted in populations with relatively homogeneous diets; smokers consume less fruit and vegetables than non-smokers; fat intake inversely correlates with fruit and vegetable intake in the United States; and studies using self-reporting tend to over-report vegetable and fruit consumption. Thus, it is not surprising that many uncertainties exist about the relationship between plant-based diets and cancer prevention.

Plants contain a wide range of bioactive food components including both essential micronutrients (e.g., vitamins C, E, and folic acid and the minerals selenium, zinc, iodine, and calcium) and non-essential substances (Table 1). The term phytochemicals is used as a collective term for a variety of plant components that often perform important functions in the plant, such as providing color, flavor, or protection. The phytochemical composition of fruits and vegetables depends on both the species and the subtype, as well as the environmental, cultivation, growing, harvesting, and storage conditions. It is widely believed that many of the health benefits, including cancer prevention, of diets enriched in fruits and vegetables are due, in part, to the presence of multiple phytochemicals. For example, allium vegetables, which include onions and garlic, are a rich source of organosulfur compounds; they appear to have protective effects against stomach and colorectal cancer *(3)*. Folate-rich foods may protect against pancreatic cancer, and at least

Table 1

Examples of Dietary Phytochemicals That May Be Protective Against Cancer

Phytochemical	Dietary Sources
Allyl sulfur compounds	Onions, garlic, leeks
Anthocyanidins	Berries, grapes
β-Carotene [a]	Citrus fruit, carrots, squash, pumpkin
Catechins	Tea, berries
Ellagic acid	Grapes, strawberries, raspberries, walnuts
Indoles	Cruciferous vegetables
Isoflavones	Soybeans and other legumes
Isothiocyanates	Cruciferous vegetables
Lycopene	Tomatoes and tomato products, guava, watermelon
Quercetin	Onion, red grapes, citrus fruit, broccoli
Resveratrol	Grapes (skin), red wine
Terpenes	Citrus fruits
Thioethers	Garlic, onions

[a] In some cases supplemental β-carotene may increase risk in humans *(19–21)*.

some evidence suggests that these foods also protect against esophageal and colorectal cancers *(3)*. Foods with higher amounts of carotenoids may reduce the risk of mouth, pharynx, and larynx and lung cancer *(3)*. Food containing β-carotene or vitamin C seems to protect against esophageal cancer; and foods containing lycopene possibly protect against prostate cancer *(3)*. There is limited evidence to suggest that foods containing quercetin protect against lung cancer *(3)*. Similarly, foods containing selenium are linked to reduced prostate cancer and there is some evidence suggesting that they also protect against stomach and colorectal cancers *(3)*. Food sources of pyridoxine and/or vitamin E may also protect against esophageal and prostate cancers *(3)*.

The magnitude of the response to fruit and vegetables is probably influenced by many factors, including the consumer's genetic background and a host of environmental factors, as well as the type, quantity, and duration of consumption of these foods, and interactions among food components. In data from 17 cohort studies that reported comparisons of the highest and lowest intake groups of fruit and vegetables and colorectal cancer, 11 out of 20 estimates were in the direction of reduced risk from higher intake, three of which were statistically significant *(3)*. Since a comprehensive review of the interactions between bioactive food components and cancer is beyond the scope of this chapter and has been published elsewhere *(12)*, only a couple of examples are provided to illustrate the principle that these food components are capable of modifying a variety of cancer processes. These examples have been chosen to demonstrate the magnitude and complexity of the potential interactions.

Food is generally complex as illustrated by the allium family; it contains about 500 species including garlic, onion, leeks, chives, and scallions. Allyl sulfur compounds arising from these foods are thought to be a primary factor in their anticancer properties. However, it is also clear that they contain many other constituents which may provide protection, including amino acids, carbohydrates, and flavonoids. Similarly, the health benefits of other foods cannot typically be related to a single component.

Epidemiologic findings and preclinical studies provide evidence that garlic and related sulfur constituents can suppress cancer risk and alter the biological behavior of tumors *(13, 14)*. One randomized controlled trial reported a statistically significant 29% reduction in both size and number of colon adenomas in colorectal patients taking aged garlic extract, while five of eight case–control/cohort studies suggested a protective effect of high intake of raw/cooked garlic *(14)*. Preclinical studies have shown that garlic and/or its related organosulfur compounds suppress mammary, colon, skin, uterine, esophagus, lung, renal, forestomach, and liver cancer incidence in animal models *(12)*.

Similar to other foods, the anticancer protection provided by garlic may involve changes in several biological targets. Garlic and its sulfur constituents have been reported to suppress formation and bioactivation of carcinogens, enhance DNA repair, reduce cell proliferation, enhance apoptosis, decrease inflammation, and block angiogenesis (14). It is likely that many of these processes are modified simultaneously. There is evidence that some garlic constituents can influence histone homeostasis and thus shifts in cancer-related processes may relate to shifts in epigenetic homeostasis. Druesne et al. (15) reported that diallyl disulfide increased histone H3 acetylation in cultured Caco-2 and HT-29 cells and normal rat colonocytes by reducing histone deacetylase activity. This hyperacetylation was accompanied by an increase in tumor promoter p21 (waf1/cip1) expression demonstrating that epigenomic events can influence subsequent gene expression patterns which culminates in cells being blocked in the G2 phase of the cell cycle. A variety of constituents in foods have also been reported to influence epigenetics and vice versa.

It is not currently known whether additive or antagonistic responses occur among dietary components that have the same molecular target. For example, both garlic organosulfur compounds and sulforaphane, which is present in broccoli, induce expression of detoxifying enzymes via the binding of the transcription factor Nrf2 to the antioxidant response element (ARE), which is located in the promoter region of related genes. Can these findings be interpreted to mean that if an individual consumes sufficient organosulfur compounds then sulforaphane will no longer have any anticancer effects? Or, might other molecular targets be important?

Folate nutriture serves as another example for the importance of diet–gene interactions. The mechanisms by which dietary folate can modulate carcinogenesis are related to the sole biochemical function of folate – mediating the transfer of one-carbon moieties. In this role, folate is an important factor in DNA synthesis, stability, integrity, and repair. A growing body of evidence from cell culture, animal, and human studies indicates that folate deficiency is associated with DNA strand breaks, impaired DNA repair, and increased mutations and that folate supplementation can correct some of these defects induced by folate deficiency. A large number of epidemiologic and intervention studies support the role of folate in reducing the risk of colorectal cancer (3). However, a common polymorphism in methylenetetrahydrofolate reductase (MTHFR) can potentially modify this relationship. Since there is no clear relationship between plasma folate and colorectal adenomas among those with the CC or CT genotype for MTHFR, only a subset of the population (i.e., those with the TT genotype) may benefit from an increased folate intake (16). These results demonstrate that not all individuals should be expected to respond identically to bioactive food components. Furthermore, mutations in another folate-metabolizing enzyme, thymidylate synthase, appear to modulate folate intake and colon cancer risk *(17)*. Possibly 50–100 genes, either directly or indirectly, are involved with folate metabolism; these include receptors, binding proteins, enzymes, tissue-specific gene products, and downstream factors that rely on folate-derived metabolites. These various factors may determine if folate is an important dietary variable. When one takes into account the variability that is known to occur within the human genome, literally thousands of polymorphisms may be determinants of the biological response to folate.

Folate also serves as an excellent example that dietary components may have different biological effects in normal compared to transformed cells. Animal studies and clinical observations suggest that folate possesses dual modulatory effects on carcinogenesis depending on the timing and dose of folate intervention *(18)*. Folate deficiency has an inhibitory effect, whereas folate supplementation has a promoting effect, on progression of established neoplasms. Conversely, folate deficiency in normal epithelial tissues appears to predispose them to neoplastic transformation, while modest levels of folate supplementation suppress the development of tumors in normal tissues *(18)*. These types of observations suggest that the optimal timing and dose of nutrient intervention need to be established for safe and effective cancer prevention in humans.

Common green, yellow/red, and yellow/orange vegetables and fruits contain a host of carotenoids. These include lutein, zeaxanthin, cryptoxanthin, lycopene, β-carotene, α-carotene, and zeaxanthin. Many epidemiological studies have reported that high intakes of β-carotene-rich fruits and vegetables or high plasma concentrations of the nutrient have a significant inverse association with lung cancer risk *(3)*. The epidemiological data linking high intakes of β-carotene-rich fruits and vegetables to reduced lung cancer risk, along with animal data demonstrating that β-carotene inhibits cancer-related events, such as the induction of stimulation of intercellular communication via gap junctions, which can have a role in the regulation of cell growth, differentiation, and apoptosis, provide strong support for testing the effect of β-carotene supplements on lung cancer in randomized intervention trials, as was done in the α-Tocopherol β-Carotene Study (ATBC) *(19)*, the Physician's Health Study (PHS) *(20)*, and the β-Carotene and Retinol Efficacy Trial (CARET) *(21)*. Unexpectedly, results from the ATBC and CARET studies showed adverse treatment effects, namely increased lung cancer incidence in high-risk subjects. The different results obtained in supplementation trials compared to cohort studies may reflect that fruits and vegetables contain, in addition to β-carotene, many other compounds that may be protective against cancer. In fact, β-carotene may simply be a marker for the actual protective substances in fruit and vegetables. Alternately, β-carotene may have different effects when consumed as a supplement rather than in the food supply. It is possible that a protective association present at dietary intake amounts of carotenoids is lost or reversed by the pharmacological levels present in supplementation trials. The ATBC, CARET, and PHS studies illustrate that definitive evidence of both safety and efficacy is required for individual fruit and vegetable constituents before dietary guidelines beyond simply greater consumption can be proposed. Thus, consumption of supplements for cancer prevention might have unexpected adverse effects; consumption of the relevant nutrients through the diet is preferred.

Enhanced whole grain intake has also been linked to a reduction in cancer risk. Jacobs et al. (22) concluded, based on a meta-analysis of 40 case-control studies, that whole grain intake was associated with decreased risk for various cancers, particularly those of the colon/rectum (pooled OR [odds ratio] = 0.79) and stomach (pooled OR = 0.57). Benefits attributed to whole grain consumption are observed at relatively low intakes (between 2 and 3 servings per day). However, typical consumption of whole grain foods in some Western countries is less than one serving per day. The main sources of whole grains are wholemeal and rye breads and whole grain breakfast cereals. Unraveling the effects of grains is complicated by the fact that those consuming enhanced quantities in the United States tend to be older, from a high socioeconomic group, are less likely to smoke, and are more likely to exercise than those consuming low quantities (23). Several compounds, including phytate, phytoestrogens such as lignan, plant stanols, and sterols, and several vitamins and minerals, present in whole grains may contribute to the observed lower risk of cancer. Another feature of whole grains, and also of fruit and vegetables, which may explain their anticarcinogenic action is that the high-fiber content is satiating and therefore helps prevent over-consumption of energy. The importance of fiber is examined in Chapter 2.

5. MEAT INTAKE

Meat, including all animal flesh apart from fish and seafood, can be further classified as either red (beef, pork, lamb, and goat) or poultry, which usually has more white than red muscle fibers. The term processed meat refers to meats preserved by smoking, curing, or salting, or addition of chemical preservatives (3). The WCRF/AICR report suggests that there is convincing evidence that red meats and processed meats are causally related to about a 20% increase in colorectal cancer (3). Moreover, recent evidence suggests that a combination of multiple SNPs in four cytochrome P-450 enzymes, which is present in almost 5% of the population, is associated with over a 40-fold increased risk of colorectal cancer with high red meat consumption (>5 times/week) (24). A range of mechanisms may account for this observed relationship between meat consumption and colorectal cancer risk. Cooking methods may foster the formation of carcinogens including polycyclic aromatic hydrocarbons (PAH) and heterocyclic amines. Carcinogenic nitroso compounds may occur in some processed meats. Recent evidence suggests that heme iron in meat may foster the generation of free radicals *(25)*.

Over 100 distinct PAH are formed when organic substances like meat or tobacco burn incompletely. These compounds are formed from the pyrolysis of fats that occurs when fat drips from meat onto hot coal, forming smoke that is redeposited on the meat surface. Eleven PAH compounds have been classified as carcinogenic to laboratory animals and as suspect carcinogens in humans *(26)*. The second class of compounds found in cooked meats is the heterocyclic amines (HCA). These are formed during high-temperature cooking by pyrolysis of proteins, amino acids, or creatinine. The amount in the diet can be substantial and is influenced by cooking habits such that prolonged high-temperature cooking of meats results in the greatest content. Epidemiologic studies have linked HCA with cancers of the colorectum, breast, prostate, lung, and pancreas *(27)*. Polymorphisms in specific genes associated with metabolism or detoxification of HCA (e.g., *CYP1A1, CYP1A2, GSTM1,* and *NAT2*) may explain variations in genetic susceptibility among individuals *(28)*. In view of the possible role of HCA in human carcinogenesis, minimizing exposure seems prudent, i.e., avoiding overheating and overcooking.

Nitrites and nitrates are often used as preservatives in meats and other "cured" products. These additives are not carcinogenic in experimental animals. However, nitrate can interact with dietary substances such as amines or amides to produce N-nitroso compounds (nitrosamines and nitrosoamides) which are potent carcinogens in animals and probably humans *(29)*. Epidemiologic studies have demonstrated a direct relationship between nitrosamine exposure and cancer of the stomach, esophagus, nasopharynx, urinary bladder, liver, and brain *(29)*. Several naturally occurring foods and their constituents, including tea, garlic, and cruciferous vegetables, may inhibit the formation of endogenous nitrosamines. This reduction in carcinogen formation may contribute to the generally protective effect of fruit and vegetables on cancer risk since vitamin C may reduce the formation of nitrosamines while other compounds, such as allyl sulfur, may reduce their bioactivation to agents which bind to DNA and thereby lead to the initiation phase of cancer.

Iron deficiency is the most common and widespread nutritional deficiency in the world. Heme iron from animal sources is better absorbed than iron from plant sources, and thus animal food is important in minimizing this nutritional deficiency. However, excess heme iron in the colon may irritate the mucosa and alter the normal rates of proliferation/exfoliation, circumstances that increase the risk for the development of colon cancer *(30)*.

Furthermore, free iron can catalyze the generation of free radicals which may also contribute to the increased colon cancer risk with high meat consumption *(25)*.

We need to bear in mind that meat can be a valuable source of many nutrients, including protein, iron, zinc, selenium, and vitamins B_6 and B_{12}. Therefore, consumption of red meat should be limited rather than avoided. Also, it is important to look at the whole diet and look at interactions among different food groups; for example, fruit and vegetables decreasing the formation of nitrosamines.

6. ALCOHOL

Dietary alcohol (ethanol) has been classified by the International Agency for Cancer Research (IARC) as a human carcinogen. This topic is also examined in Chapter 11. Alcohol is both a source of dietary energy and a drug, and thus can influence both mental and physical performance. The WCRF/AICR panel judged that there is convincing evidence that alcoholic drinks increase cancer of the mouth, pharynx and larynx, esophagus, colorectum (men), and breast *(3)*. Alcoholic drinks are probably also a cause of liver and colorectal cancers in women *(3)*. The type of beverage consumed does not appear to influence risk and thus total alcohol appears to be the primary agent leading to the transformation of cells to neoplastic lesions.

Acetaldehyde, the first and most toxic metabolite of alcohol metabolism, is particularly damaging to cells. In experimental animals it reacts with DNA to form cancer-promoting compounds *(31)*. In addition, highly reactive, oxygen-containing molecules formed during alcohol metabolism can damage DNA, thus promoting tumor development *(31)*. Experimentally, chronic alcohol consumption has been reported to promote tumor proliferation via increased VEGF expression and tumor angiogenesis *(32)*. Considerable evidence also points to the ability of alcohol to alter retinoid metabolism and thus interfere with differentiation *(33)*. A change in DNA methylation may be an overarching factor accounting for changes in multiple cancer-related processes *(33)*. The response to alcohol may depend on multiple factors including smoking, adequacy of the diet, and genetic susceptibility *(33)*. A true understanding of the effect of dietary alcohol may be clouded because of the compounds found in alcohol, which can both promote and potentially suppress tumorigenesis.

7. CONCLUSIONS

Mounting evidence continues to demonstrate that the foods we eat can have a profound effect on cancer risk and tumor behavior. The overall response is likely dependent on literally thousands of bioactive components that occur in the foods consumed and their interactions with other environmental factors and the consumer's genetics. These effects, which may be inhibitory or stimulatory depending on the specific bioactive food component, are surely mediated through diverse biological mechanisms. The identification and elucidation of the specific molecular sites for food components is critical for identifying those who will benefit maximally or be placed at risk from excess exposures. Until this information is available it remains prudent to eat a variety of foods and to maintain a healthy weight through controlling caloric intake and exercise.

Expanding knowledge about the physiological consequences of nutrigenomics – which includes nutrigenetic (genetic profiles that modulate the response to food components), nutritional transcriptomics (influence of food components on gene expression profiles), and nutritional epigenomics (influence of food components on DNA methylation and other epigenetic events and vice versa) – should help identify those who will and will not respond to dietary interventions. New reports are constantly surfacing that population studies are under-estimating the significance of diet in overall cancer prevention and therapy and that subpopulations may be particularly sensitive to subtle changes in eating behaviors. To identify those who will benefit most from dietary change more attention needs to be given to the identification of three types of biomarkers: (1) those reflecting exposures needed to bring about a desired response, (2) those which indicate a change in a physiologically relevant biological process which is linked to cancer, and (3) those which can be used to predict a personalized susceptibility based on nutrient–nutrient interactions and gene–nutrient interactions. As the science of nutrition unfolds, a clearer understanding will surely emerge about how food components modulate cancer, and how the food supply might be modified through agronomic approaches and/or biotechnology. While the challenges to unraveling the relationships between diet and cancer prevention are enormous, so is the societal and health benefits that will occur because of these discoveries.

SUGGESTED FURTHER READING

World Cancer Research Fund/American Institute for Cancer Research. Food, Nutrition, Physical Activity, and the Prevention of Cancer: a Global Perspective. American Institute for Cancer Research, Washington, DC, 2007.

Davis CD. Mechanisms for cancer-protective effects of bioactive dietary components in fruits and vegetables. In: Berdanier CD, Dwyer J, Feldman EB, eds. Handbook of Nutrition and Food, second edition. CRC Press, Boca Raton, FL, 2007, pp. 1187–1210.

http://www.aicr.org/site/PageServer

http://www.cancer.gov/

Current Cancer Drug Targets, August 2007, special issue on Nutritional Preemption of Cancer.

REFERENCES

1. Heron M. Deaths: leading causes for 2004. Natl Vital Stat Rep 2007; 56:1–95.
2. Hanahan D, Weinberg RA. The hallmarks of cancer. Cell 2000; 100:57–70.
3. World Cancer Research Fund/American Institute for Cancer Research. Food, Nutrition, Physical Activity, and the Prevention of Cancer: A Global Perspective, Washington, DC, 2007.
4. Doll R, Peto R. The causes of cancer: quantitative estimates of avoidable risk of cancer in the United States today. J Natl Cancer Inst 1981; 66:1191–1308.
5. Espey DK, Wu XC, Swan J, et al. Annual report to the nation on the status of cancer, 1975–2004, featuring cancer in American Indians and Alaska Natives. Cancer 2007; 110:2119–2152.
6. Wong HL, Seow A, Arakawa K, Lee HP, Yu MC, Ingles SA. Vitamin D receptor start codon polymorphism and colorectal cancer risk: effect modification by dietary calcium and fat in Singapore Chinese. Carcinogenesis 2003; 24:1091–1095.
7. Siezen CL, van Leeuwen AI, Kram NR, Luken ME, van Kranen HJ, Kampman E. Colorectal adenoma risk is modified by the interplay between polymorphisms in arachidonic acid pathways genes and fish consumption. Carcinogenesis 2005; 26:449–457.
8. Calle EE, Rodriquez C, Walker-Thurmond K, Thun MJ. Overweight, obesity and mortality from cancer is a prospectively studied cohort of U.S. adults. N Engl J Med 2003; 348:1625–1638.
9. Powolny AA, Wang S, Carlton PS, Hoot DR, Clinton SK. Interrelationships between dietary restriction, the IGF-1 axis, and expression of vascular endothelial growth factor by prostate adenocarcinoma in rats. Mol Carcinog 2008; 47:458–465
10. Centers for Disease Control and Prevention (CDC). Prevalence of regular physical activity among adults- United States, 2001 and 2005. MMWR Morb Mortal Wkly Rep 2007; 56:1209–1212.
11. Rogers CJ, Berrigan D, Zaharoff DA, et al. Energy restriction and exercise differentially enhance components of systemic and mucosal immunity in mice. J Nutr 2008; 138: 115–122.
12. Davis CD. Mechanisms for cancer-protective effects of bioactive dietary components in fruits and vegetables. In: Berdanier CD, Dwyer J, Feldman EB, eds. Handbook of Nutrition and Food, 2nd ed. CRC Press, Boca Raton FL, 2007, pp. 1187–1210.
13. Ngo SN, Williams DB, Cobiac L, Head RJ. Does garlic reduce risk of colorectal cancer? A systematic review. J Nutr 2007; 137:2264–2269.
14. Shukla Y, Kaira N. Cancer chemoprevention with garlic and its constituents. Cancer Lett 2007; 247:167–181.
15. Druesne-Pecollo N, Chaumonetet C, Pagniez A, et al. In vivo treatment by diallyl disulfide increases histone acetylation in rat colonocytes. Biochem Biophys Res Commun 2007; 354:140–147.
16. Marugame T, Tsuji E, Kiyohara C, et al. Relation of plasma folate and methylenetetrahydrofolate reductase C677T polymorphism to colorectal adenomas. Int J Epidemiol 2003; 32:64–66.
17. Ulrich CM, Curtin K, Potter JD, Bigler J, Caan B, Slattery ML. Polymorphisms in the reduced folate carrier, thymidylate synthase, or methionine synthase and risk of colon cancer. Cancer Epidemiol Biomarkers Prev 2005; 14:2509–2516.
18. Kim YI. Role of folate in colon cancer development and progression. J Nutr 2003; 133:3731s–3739s.
19. Heinonen OP, Huttunen IK, Albanes D, et al. for the Alpha- Tocopherol Beta-Carotene Cancer Prevention Study Group. The effect of vitamin E and beta carotene on the

incidence of lung cancer and other cancers in male smokers. N Engl J Med 1994; 330: 1029–1035.

20. Hennekens CH, Buring IE, Manson IE, et al. Lack of effect of long-term supplementation with beta carotene on the incidence of malignant neoplasms and cardiovascular disease. N Engl J Med 1996; 334:1145–1149.

21. Omenn OS, Goodman GE, Thomquist MD, et al. Effects of a combination of beta carotene and vitamin A on lung cancer and cardiovascular disease. N Eng J Med 1996; 334:1150-1155.

22. Jacobs DR, Jr, Marquart L, Slavin J, Kushi LH. Whole-grain intake and cancer: an expanded review and meta-analysis. Nutr Cancer 1998; 30:85-96.

23. Lang R, Jebb SA. Who consumes whole grains, and how much? Proc Nutr Soc 2003; 62:123-127.

24. Kury S, Buecher B, Robiou-du-Pont S, et al. Combinations of cytochrome P450 gene polymorphisms enhancing the risk for sporadic colorectal cancer related to red meat consumption. Cancer Epidemiol biomarkers Prev 2007; 16:1460–1467.

25. Tappel A. Heme of consumed ret meat can act as a catalyst of oxidative damage and could initiate colon, breast and prostate cancers, heart disease and other diseases. Med Hypothesis 2007; 68:562–564.

26. Goldamn R, Shields PG. Food mutagens. J Nutr 2003; 133:965S-973S.

27. Snyderwine EG, Sinha R, Felton JS, Ferguson LR. Highlights of the eighth international conference on carcinogenic/mutagenic N-substituted aryl compounds. Mutation Res 2002; 506–507:1–8.

28. Murtaugh MA, Ma K, Sweeney C, Caan BJ, Slattery ML. Meat consumption patterns and preparation, genetic variants of metabolic enzymes, and their association with rectal cancer in men and women. J Nutr 2004; 134:776–784.

29. Ferguson LR. Natural and human-made mutagens and carcinogens in the human diet. Toxicology 2002; 181–182:79–82.

30. Sesnick AL, Termont DS, Kleibeuker JH, Van der Meer R. Red meat and colon cancer: the cytotoxic and hyperproliferative effects of dietary heme. Cancer Res 1999; 59: 5704–5709.

31. Seitz HK, Becker P. alcohol metabolism and cancer risk. Alcohol Res Health 2007; 30:44–47.

32. Tan W, Bailey AP, Shparago M, et al. Chronic alcohol consumption stimulates VEGF expression, tumor angiogenesis and progression of melanoma in mice. Cancer Biol Ther 2007; 6:1211–1217.

33. Seitz HK, Stickel F. Molecular mechanisms of alcohol-mediated carcinogenesis. Nat Rev Cancer 2007; 7:599–612.

34 Food Allergy and Intolerance: Diagnoses and Nutritional Management

Kathy Roberts

Key Points

- Adverse food reactions (hypersensitivity) can be either immune mediated (food allergy) or nonimmune mediated (intolerance).
- Nonimmune mediated reactions (intolerance) are classified as enzymatic, pharmacologic, or undefined food intolerance; together they account for the majority of food hypersensitivity reactions.
- Diagnosis of food allergy is based on medical history, physical examination, and diagnostic tests; the oral food challenge is considered the "gold standard" for diagnosis.
- Therapy for food allergy is complete exclusion of the allergen-containing food(s).
- It is recommended that practitioners consider patient referral to a registered dietitian for education on elimination diets and monitoring for nutritional adequacy.
- Initiating early intervention in high-risk infants may decrease prevalence.

   Key Words: Food allergy; food intolerance; lactose intolerance; diagnostic tests; oral food challenge; elimination diets; pharmacologic food intolerance; dietary management

1. INTRODUCTION

Food hypersensitivity (FHS) is an adverse food reaction caused by a mechanism that is either immune mediated (*food allergy*) or nonimmune mediated (*nonallergic food hypersensitivity*). The prevalence of food-induced allergy responses has been increasing in the United States over the past few decades, particularly in the pediatric population. It is estimated that 6–8% of children less than 4 years of age and 3.7% of adults have food

From: *Nutrition and Health: Nutrition Guide for Physicians*
Edited by: T. Wilson et al. (eds.), DOI 10.1007/978-1-60327-431-9_34,
© Humana Press, a part of Springer Science+Business Media, LLC 2010

allergy *(1)*. A few foods cause approximately 90% of food allergies: milk, eggs, soy, wheat, peanuts, fish, shellfish, and tree nuts.

Nonallergic food hypersensitivity, also known as food intolerance, accounts for the majority of adverse reactions. The most common food intolerance, lactose intolerance, affects from 30 to 50 million adults in the United States, yet is often misdiagnosed as an allergy *(2, 3)*. When assessing patients with food hypersensitivity, it is important for clinicians to determine whether the reaction is food allergy or nonallergic food hypersensitivity, as subsequent evaluation will differ between the two.

2. FOOD ALLERGY

2.1. Pathophysiology

Food allergy is caused by a malfunction of the gastrointestinal (GI) mucosal immune response to dietary proteins. The mucosal immune system is continually exposed to an antigen load consisting of dietary antigens and commensal bacteria, as well as harmful pathogens. Unlike the systemic immune system that functions by activating an immediate response in the presence of antigens, the GI immune system requires a mechanism that will suppress the response to harmless antigens while also protecting against harmful pathogens *(oral tolerance)* *(4)*. Food allergy develops in individuals with a genetic predisposition when oral tolerance breaks down allowing an immune response to occur. An acute response is generally immunoglobulin E (IgE) mediated; responses that are subacute or chronic are more likely cell (mainly T-cell) mediated. Clinical manifestations of the allergic reaction typically involve the skin (urticaria, angioedema), respiratory system (asthma, runny nose, tightening of the throat), GI tract (nausea, vomiting, diarrhea, abdominal pain), or systemic (cardiac arrhythmia, anaphylactic shock) *(5–7)* (Table 1).

2.2. Diagnosing Food Allergy

2.2.1. MEDICAL HISTORY

Diagnosis of a food allergy starts with a thorough history. Questions should include (1) what is the clinical reaction, (2) suspected food(s), (3) the amount of food that provokes the reaction, (4) timing between ingestion and occurrence of symptoms, (5) how often has the response occurred, and (6) were other factors (exercise, illness) involved in triggering the response *(8, 9)*. Diet diaries recording all foods ingested over a specific time period and documenting type and timing of adverse response can be an effective complement to the diet history.

Table 1
Food Hypersensitivity Disorders

IgE Mediated	
Gastrointestinal	Oral allergy syndrome, gastrointestinal anaphylaxis
Cutaneous	Urticaria, angioedema, morbilliform rashes and flushing
Respiratory	Acute rhinoconjunctivitis, bronchospasm
Generalized	Anaphylactic shock
Mixed IgE and cell mediated	
Gastrointestinal	Allergic eosinophilic esophagitis, allergic eosinophilic gastroenteritis
Cutaneous	Atopic dermatitis
Respiratory	Asthma
Cell mediated	
Gastrointestinal	Food protein-induced enterocolitis, food protein-induced proctocolitis, food protein-induced enteropathy syndromes, celiac disease
Cutaneous	Contact dermatitis, dermatitis herpetiformis
Respiratory	Food-induced pulmonary hemosiderosis (Heiner syndrome)

Reprinted from Ref. *(14)* with permission from Elsevier.

2.2.2. PHYSICAL EXAMINATION

There are no physical or clinical symptoms that are distinctly characteristic of food allergy. The presence of symptoms at the time of the exam may or may not be related to allergy *(9, 10)*. Height and weight should be evaluated, especially in the pediatric population, as factors such as food avoidance or GI symptoms may result in growth restriction or weight loss.

2.2.3. DIAGNOSTIC TESTS

Diagnostic tests to detect food-induced allergy response are often necessary to rule out differential diagnoses. Skin-prick testing (SPT) is a rapid means to detect the presence of specific IgE antibodies. A negative SPT is highly predictive (>95%) in confirming the absence of IgE-mediated food allergies, while a positive response is much less definitive (<50%)

in confirming this diagnosis *(8, 11)*. Serum IgE antibody testing (radioal-lergosorbent tests [RAST]) is an alternate means to detect the presence of food-specific IgE antibodies. Similar to the SPT, a negative result on RAST testing is more predictive in ruling out an IgE response then a positive result is to diagnoses of food allergy *(11)*. No laboratory tests are conclusive for identifying foods responsible for non-IgE-mediated disorders (food hyper-sensitivity reactions) such as eosinophilic gastroenteritis or protein-losing enteropathy *(10)*. Food-specific IgG antibodies are typically elevated in patients presenting with food allergies, affecting the GI tract; however, this only reflects exposure. Diagnosis is typically substantiated with endoscopy and biopsy findings.

2.2.4. ELIMINATION DIET AND ORAL FOOD CHALLENGE

In the first stage of the elimination diet, food(s) that have been identified by diet history and/or positive SPT/RAST testing are eliminated simulta-neously. In formula-fed infants this involves switching to a hypoallergenic formula. For breastfed infants either the maternal diet is restricted or the infant is fed a hypoallergenic formula. In both children and adults, all forms of the suspected allergen(s) must be completely eliminated. The length of the trial is typically 7–14 days for IgE-mediated responses and for up to 12 weeks in some food hypersensitivity reactions. Patients presenting with sig-nificant improvement in symptoms on the elimination diet typically undergo a subsequent food challenge to confirm the diagnosis of food allergy. The double-blind, placebo-controlled food challenge (DBPCFC) is considered the "gold standard" for diagnosing food allergy *(12)*. This should be admin-istered in a facility with trained staff, and with medical equipment available to manage an anaphylactic response, and should be avoided in patients where confirmed severe anaphylaxis has occurred. The food to be tested is given at an initial dose that is below the patient's threshold dose, determined by patient's history and established data. Dosing is increased over a time inter-val sufficient to monitor for reactions until the amount of a typical serving for that food is reached.

2.3. Nutritional Management

The only completely effective therapy for food allergy is elimination of the proven allergen. If not properly monitored for adequacy, elimination diets can lead to nutritional deficiency, especially if the diet excludes a large number of foods and is prescribed for a long period. Practitioners should consider a patient referral to a registered dietitian for extensive education on the multiple issues impacting adherence to the diet *(11, 13)*.

Infants and children with food allergy have the same nutrient requirements as healthy children, with emphasis on adequate energy, protein, fat, and micronutrients to support growth and development. When a food or food group is eliminated, it is important to consider the nutritional impact, especially if the avoidance of a single allergen requires the removal of a large number and variety of foods. The individual's diet will require modification to include alternate dietary sources of the nutrients or supplementation if indicated. Monitoring growth velocity and weight-to-length ratio on a pediatric growth charts is effectual in identifying infants and children presenting with possible nutritional deficiency.

Patients should be taught label reading to identify allergens found in the food ingredients. Effective 2006, the Food and Drug Administration requires food labels to clearly state if food products contain any ingredients containing protein derived from the eight major allergenic foods: milk, eggs, fish, shellfish, tree nuts, peanuts, wheat, or soybeans. This should reduce the occurrence of exposure to these foods through previously unidentified ingredients in fillers or certain additives, such as flavors.

A further consideration is the management of "high-risk" situations. Dining out, especially at restaurants, buffets, and school cafeterias, can increase the possibility of exposure to allergens from either unknown ingredients or through cross-contamination. In addition to ingestion, skin contact or inhalation of airborne food particles can induce an allergic response in individuals who are extremely sensitive.

Individuals at risk of anaphylaxis require education on the management of this life-threatening reaction. Recommendations include

- Prescription for self-injectable epinephrine with instructions for patient and/or caregivers on its use.
- Provide the patient and/or caregivers, teachers, coaches, etc. with a written emergency plan describing the allergy, appropriate avoidance measures, symptoms, and medications to be given in case of accidental exposure.
- Stress importance of immediate response to accidental exposure in high-risk patients.

Children with food allergies should be continually reevaluated over time to determine if they have developed a tolerance to the allergen (8, 14). The process of outgrowing a food allergy varies depending on the food itself, age, and the severity of the individual's response. Up to 90% of infants with cow's milk allergy may tolerate milk after 3 years of age, while, conversely, up to 80% of children allergic to peanuts, tree nuts, and seafood never develop tolerance (15). Although younger children are more likely to develop tolerance over time, older children and adults may also lose their reactivity. Periodic food challenges in the controlled environment of a physician or allergist is warranted to determine whether an individual has acquired tolerance.

2.4. Prevention

The American Academy of Pediatrics identifies a family history of atopy as a significant risk factor for developing food allergy in newborns and infants. It is recommended that intervention should be started early in the perinatal period for optimal outcome and includes the following:

- Exclusive breastfeeding for the first 4–6 mo
- No allergen avoidance diet during pregnancy with the exception of peanuts
- Avoidance diets during lactation to be determined on an individual basis, with the exception of avoidance of peanuts
- Avoid introduction of solid foods until 6 mo of age, adding the least allergenic first
- Major allergens such as peanuts, nuts, and seafood introduced only after 3 years of age *(16)*.

3. FOOD INTOLERANCE

3.1. Pathology

Nonallergic food hypersensitivity (food intolerance) is an adverse food-induced reaction that does not involve the immune system (Table 2). Causes of food intolerance include an anatomical problem, enzymatic deficiency, metabolic disorder, toxins, or the effect of pharmacological substances found in the food *(8, 17)*. Adverse reactions for which the mechanism is unknown, such as food additive reactions, are considered an undefined

Table 2
Nonallergic Food Hypersensitivity

Anatomical	Hiatal hernia; pyloric stenosis; tracheoesophageal fistula
Metabolic	Enzyme deficiencies (lactase, sucrose–isomaltase, glucose–galactose); galactosemia; PKU
Digestive	Gallbladder disease; peptic ulcer disease
Infection	Bacteria; virus; parasitic
Toxins	Bacterial; fungal; scombroid fish poisoning; saxitoxin
Pharmacologic agents	Caffeine (coffee, soft drinks); histamine (fish, sauerkraut); serotonin (banana, tomato); tyramine (cheese, yeast extract, wine, pickled herring, soy sauce)
Undefined intolerance	Food additives: sulfites; nitrites; nitrates; monosodium glutamate; dyes

Adapted from Ref. *(8)*.

food intolerance. Susceptible individuals may show intolerance to agents such as sulfites, nitrates, monosodium glutamate (MSG), and some food colorings *(17)*.

3.2. Enzymatic Food Intolerance

Enzymatic food intolerance is a food hypersensitivity that is caused by enzyme deficiency. The most common is lactose intolerance, which results from a deficiency of lactase, the enzyme responsible for the digestion of lactose in milk. The nonhydrolyzed lactose is fermented by bacteria in the gut producing lactic acid, carbon dioxide, and hydrogen gas that trigger symptoms of nausea, cramps, bloating, flatulence, and diarrhea. These symptoms range in severity and typically appear from 30 min to 2 h after ingesting lactose. The condition is associated with the natural decline in lactase production with age. It is more prevalent in certain ethnic groups: 50–80% of Latinos, 60–80% of Africans and African-Americans, 80–100% of American Indians, 85–100% of Asians, 60–80% Ashkenazi Jews, and 2–15% of Northern Europeans *(18)*.

Lactase deficiency is diagnosed based on presentation of symptoms that occur following milk digestion and with positive results in lactose breath hydrogen test or lactose tolerance test. The stool acidity test is used as a diagnostic tool in infants younger than 6 mo for whom a large lactose load can lead to complications of dehydration.

Nutrition intervention for lactose intolerance includes restricting lactose intake to <12 g/day, instruction on use of lactase enzyme supplements, and nutrition education to promote adequate consumption of all nutrients, especially nondairy sources of calcium and vitamin D *(18)*. Some individuals may tolerate ingestion of low-lactose dairy foods (e.g., aged cheeses) or cultured milk products (e.g., yogurt, buttermilk). Others can improve tolerance by introducing small amounts of lactose-containing foods with a meal or snack and gradually increasing the amount over time.

3.3. Pharmacologic Food Intolerance

Pharmacologic food intolerance is an adverse response to naturally occurring substances, such as vasoactive amines commonly found in foods. Tyramine and phenylethylamine may trigger migraines in susceptible individuals by initiating a series of reactions that causes vasoconstriction followed by rebound dilation of the cranial blood vessels *(19)*. Consumption of foods with a high tyramine and phenylethylamine content has also been associated with adverse reactions in persons taking monoamine oxidase (MAO) inhibitors. Tyramine and phenylethylamine are normally metabolized by MAO in the gut; reduced levels of this enzyme can lead to abnormal concentration of the amines in the blood resulting in symptoms such as tachycardia, hypertension crisis, and migraine *(17, 19)*.

Potential dietary triggers for pharmacologic food intolerance include *(19)*

- tyramine: aged cheeses; aged/fermented/pickled meats, fish, or poultry; fermented alcoholic beverage such as wine, sherry, ale, and beer; and fermented soy products like miso and soy sauce; snow peas, lima, and fava beans; all tree nuts and peanuts
- phenylethylamine: chocolate, champagne, red wine, yellow cheeses, and citrus fruits
- histamine: fish (tuna, mackerel, herring, sardine), wine, spinach, and eggplant
- caffeine: coffee, some soft drinks, and some energy drinks
- phenolic amines: citrus fruit.

3.4. Undefined Intolerance

Food additives such as sulfites, salicylates, benzoates and parabens, tartrazine, butylated hydroxyanisole (BHA), butylated hydroxytoluene (BHT), nitrates, nitrites, aspartame, and monosodium glutamate (MSG) have been identified as contributing agents to adverse responses to foods *(20)*. Several possible causal mechanisms have been examined; however, further studies are needed to identify the exact etiology of these reactions *(21)*.

3.5. Diagnosing Food Intolerance

With the exception of some enzymatic nonallergic food intolerances (see lactose intolerance above), no specific laboratory tests are available to identify foods responsible for non-IgE-mediated reactions *(8, 11, 22)*. Initial evaluation of patients with suspected food intolerance should include a detailed history of reported symptoms, frequency of occurrence, suspected food and quantity ingested, and time between ingestion and development of symptoms. When specific food(s) are suggested by diet history, they are eliminated from the diet for a period of 1–2 weeks, or more, depending on the chronicity of the condition. If symptoms resolve during this period, the food is reintroduced in either an open challenge using the unmasked food or with double-blind placebo-controlled food challenge (DBPC).

When diet history does not identify a specific trigger food, an oligoantigenic diet (OAD) may be used. This is a highly restrictive diet in which the majority of known food allergens are eliminated, including milk, wheat, eggs, soy, nuts, corn, citrus, chocolate, and processed foods with additives and preservatives.

The diet is typically followed for a period of 4 weeks, after which individual foods are reintroduced one at a time over a specified period. Food intolerance is suspected if a person is symptom free on the OAD and relapses with the addition of specific foods. The diagnosis can be confirmed with a DBPC *(23)*.

3.6. Nutritional Management

Dietary management of food intolerance should be individualized based on the type of intolerance and the severity of the reaction. In some instances occasional consumption of small servings of the trigger food may be tolerated *(24)*. For others, complete elimination of the food or substance is required. In cases where multiple substances need to be avoided (e.g., food additives and preservatives) the diet can be quite restrictive and may pose a challenge for long-term adherence *(25)*.

4. SUMMARY

The prevalence of food hypersensitivity, both immune and nonimmune mediated, has been increasing in the United States. Examining reactions of the immune system to specific components of the allergens has increased understanding of the pathophysiology of food hypersensitivities. Diagnosis includes screening techniques to differentiate between IgE-mediated and non-IgE-mediated responses. Treatment for food allergy is complete exclusion of the allergen-containing food(s). Practitioners should consider a patient referral to a registered dietitian for education on issues impacting adherence to the diet and to monitor diet for nutritional adequacy. In some cases, tolerance to food allergens may develop in some individuals over time; therefore periodic oral food challenges in the controlled environment of a physician or allergist are warranted. Finally, initiating early intervention in high-risk infants may decrease prevalence of food hypersensitivities.

SUGGESTED FURTHER READING

American Academy of Allergy, Asthma, and Immunology. Available at: http://www.aaaai.org. Last accessed March 27, 2008.

Food Allergy and Anaphylaxis Network. Available at: http://www.foodallergy.org. Last accessed March 27, 2008.

Metcalfe DD, Sampson HA, Simon RA. Food Allergy: Adverse Reactions to Foods and Food Additives, 4th ed. Blackwell Publishing, Malden, MA, 2008.

Sampson HA. Update on food allergy. J Allergy Clin Immunol 2004; 113:805–819.

U.S. Department of Health and Human Services, National Institutes of Health, National Institute of Allergy and Infectious Diseases. Food Allergy an Overview. NIH Publication No. 07-5518. July 2007. Available at: www.niaid.nih.gov. Last accessed March 27, 2008.

REFERENCES

1. U.S. Department of Health and Human Services. National Institutes of Health. Food Allergy. Publication No. 07-5518, July 2007.
2. National Institute of Diabetes and Digestive and Kidney Diseases, NIH, DHHS. Digestive Disease Statistics. Available at: http://digestive.niddk.nih.gov/statistics/statistics.htm. Last accessed March 27, 2008.
3. Bahna SL. Cow's milk allergy versus cow milk intolerance. Ann Allergy Asthma Immunol 2002; 89(6 Suppl 1):56–60.
4. Strobel S, Mowat AM. Immune responses to dietary antigens: oral tolerance. Immunol Today 1998; 19:173–181.
5. Fasano MB. Dermatologic food allergy. Ped Annals 2006; 35:727–731.
6. Assa'ad AH. Gastrointestinal food allergy. Pediatr Ann 2006; 35:718–726.
7. El-Gamal YM, Hossny EM. Respiratory food allergy. Ped Annals 2006; 35:733–740.
8. Sampson HA. Food allergy. Part 2: Diagnosis and management. J Allergy Clin Immunol 1999; 103:981–989.
9. Knight AK, Bahna SL. Diagnosis of food allergy. Pediatr Ann 2006; 35:709–714.
10. Bahna SL. Diagnosis of food allergy. Ann Allergy Asthma Immunol 2003; 90(Suppl 3):77–80.
11. Sicherer SH. Manifestations of food allergy: Evaluation and management. Am Fam Physician 1999; 59:415–424.
12. Sampson HA. Food allergy. J Allergy Clin Immunol 2003; 111:540–547.
13. Mofidi S. Nutritional management of pediatric food hypersensitivity. Pediatrics 2003; 111:1645–1653.
14. Sampson HA. Update on food allergy. J Allergy Clin Immunol 2004; 113:805–819.
15. Fiocchi A, Martelli A. Dietary management of food allergy. Pediatr Ann 2006; 35:10:755–763.
16. Zeiger RS. Food allergen avoidance in the prevention of food allergy in infants and children. Pediatrics 2003; 111:1662–1671.
17. Ortolani C, Pastorello EA. Food allergies and food intolerances. Best Pract Res Clin Gastroenterol 2005; 20:467–483.
18. American Dietetic Association Nutrition. Care Manual. Available from: www.nutritioncaremanual.org . Last accessed August 5, 2008.
19. Millichap JG. The diet factor in pediatric and adolescent migraine. Pediatr Neurol 2003; 28:9–15.
20. Fraser O, Sumar S, Sumar N. Adverse reaction to foods. Nutr Food Sci 2000; 30:236–243.
21. Bruijnzeel-Koomen C, Ortolani C, Aas K, et al. Adverse reactions to food. Allergy 1995; 50:623–635.
22. Muraro MA. Diagnosis of food allergy: the oral provocation test. Pediatr Allergy Immunol 2001; 12(Suppl 14):31–36.
23. Cruz NV, Bahna S. Do foods or additives cause behavior disorders? Pediatr Ann 2006; 35:744–754.

24. U.S. Department of Health and Human Services, National Institutes of Health. Lactose Intolerance: Information for Health Care Providers. NIH Publication No 05-5305B, January 2006.
25. Cormier E, Elder JH. Diet and child behavior problems: Fact or Fiction? J Pediatr Nurs 2007; 33:138–143.

35 Drug Interactions with Food and Beverages

Garvan C. Kane

Key Points

- Vitamin K-rich foods impair anticoagulant effects of warfarin
- Acidic beverages aid absorption of antifungal drugs
- Grapefruit juice, alcohol, and caffeine may interfere with drug metabolism

Key Words: Drug metabolism; tyramine; CYP3A4; grapefruit; HMG-CoA reductase inhibitor; alcohol; caffeine

1. INTRODUCTION

"Take your medication on an empty stomach with a glass of water" – the ideal advice for most patients. Yet for many reasons, this is rarely done, because of patient preference or convenience. In some instances, patients will be instructed to take their medication with a particular food or beverage to aid palatability (and hence compliance), minimize local irritation to the gastrointestinal tract, or aid in drug absorption. Importantly, there are incidences when the consumption of certain foods in combination with certain medications presents a problem by interfering with the absorption, metabolism, or excretion of a drug. If these instances go unrecognized, there may be significant divergence of expected drug levels and hence expected clinical drug effects. This chapter highlights some of the main instances where concomitant ingestion of particular foods or beverages can interfere with medication action and review how these interactions can sometimes be used to aid in patient management.

From: *Nutrition and Health: Nutrition Guide for Physicians*
Edited by: T. Wilson et al. (eds.), DOI 10.1007/978-1-60327-431-9_35,
© Humana Press, a part of Springer Science+Business Media, LLC 2010

2. MEDICATIONS TO BE TAKEN ON AN EMPTY STOMACH

In general, food will slow absorption by reducing the drug's concentration; however, in the majority of cases the overall degree of final absorption is largely unaffected, with modest if any clinical effects. Food intake may have other effects on drug absorption: stimulation of gastric and intestinal secretions may aid drug dissolution, and fat-stimulated release of bile salts promotes the uptake of lipophilic compounds. However, in certain cases, for example with levothyroxine, bisphosphonates, alendronate, and risedronate, the drugs should be taken first thing in the morning on an empty stomach with plain water.

While not technically a drug, iron supplements will also have much better absorption if taken on an empty stomach. However, while food will typically cut in half the amount of iron absorbed, it may be needed to minimize gastric irritation. Readers may wish to consult Chapter 7 for a more in-depth discussion of this topic.

3. SPECIFIC EXAMPLES OF FOOD-DRUG INTERACTIONS

3.1. Effects of Vitamin K on Warfarin Anticoagulation

The anticoagulant effect of warfarin is mediated through inhibition of the vitamin K-dependent coagulation factors II, VII, IX, and X. A key feature in the stability of the warfarin anticoagulant effect is week-to-week differences in the content of vitamin K in the diet. Foods particularly high in vitamin K include vegetable oils, asparagus, broccoli, brussel sprouts, cabbage, lettuce, parsley, peas, pickles, and spinach. Many multivitamin preparations, dietary supplements, and herbal products are also high in vitamin K. While the clinical effect of increased dietary vitamin K can be overcome with increased warfarin, it is the variability of the clinical anticoagulant effect that is of greatest importance. Indeed, in cases where a patient's warfarin control is quite unstable, a supplement of modest dietary daily vitamin K (e.g., 60–80 μg/day) may help in achieving a more stable warfarin effect.

3.2. Monoamine Oxidase Inhibitors and Tyramine

Monoamine oxidase (MAO) inhibitors used in the treatment of depression and phobic anxiety disorders are being increasingly replaced by safer alternatives due a number of potentially dangerous interactions with foods containing high levels of tyramine (e.g., beer, ale, red wine, soy, aged cheeses, smoked or pickled fish or meat, anchovies, yeast, and vitamin supplements). Ingested tyramine is normally metabolized by MAO in the bowel wall and liver. However, when MAO is inhibited, tyramine reaches the circulation where it leads to a sudden and significant release of norepinephrine, leading to severe systemic hypertension.

3.3. Calcium Impairs Certain Antibiotic Absorption

Calcium-rich foods, such as dairy products and tofu, even milk added to tea or coffee, are sufficient to significantly impede the absorption of several antibiotics, including tetracycline, minocycline, doxycycline, levofloxacin, and ciprofloxacin (1). To improve their absorption these medications should be taken 1 h before or 2 h after calcium, magnesium, and iron supplements or dairy products.

4. SPECIFIC EXAMPLES OF FOOD–BEVERAGE INTERACTIONS

4.1. Use of Acidic Beverages to Aid Drug Absorption

The oral broad-spectrum antifungal drugs, ketoconazole and itraconazole, are dependent on an acidic environment for absorption. This is because an acidic pH induces a more fat-soluble charge on the carboxyl groups. If gastric acid production is low (achlorhydria), either due to a manifestation of the patient's medical condition (e.g., AIDS gastropathy) or their use of acid-suppression therapy, then the absorption of these drugs is compromised (2). These weakly alkaline drugs dissolve poorly in the relatively higher pH in the proximal small intestine and absorption is low. In such instances patients should be advised to take their ketoconazole or itraconazole with an acidic beverage to boost drug availability by as much as 50% (Table 1) (3).

Table 1
pH of Selected Commercially Available Beverage

Beverage[a]	pH	Beverage	pH
Coca-Cola Classic	2.5	Diet Coca-Cola	3.2
Pepsi	2.5	Diet Pepsi	3.2
Cranberry juice	2.8	Mountain Dew	3.3
Canada Dry ginger ale	2.7	Tropicana grapefruit juice	3.4
Dr. Pepper	2.9	7-Up	3.4
Sprite	2.9	Tropicana orange juice	3.8

[a]Those medications in the left column tend to aid in ketoconazole absorption.

4.2. Grapefruit Juice Inhibits Drug Metabolism

Grapefruit and grapefruit juice, unlike other citrus fruits, interact with a number of prescription drugs, interfering with their metabolism and

Table 2
Drug–Food Interactions[a]

Drug	Interaction	Drug	Interaction	Drug	Interaction
Artemether	Grapefruit ↑ DE	**Isoniazid**	Alcohol ↑ AE Dairy, Ca, Mg, Fe ↓ DE	**Simvastatin**	Grapefruit ↑ DE
Atorvastatin	Grapefruit ↑ DE	**Levofloxacin**	Dairy, Ca, Mg, Fe ↓ DE	**Sulfa drugs**	Alcohol ↑ AE
Buspirone	Grapefruit ↑ DE	**Lithium**	Caffeine ↓ DE	**Tacrolimus**	Grapefruit ↑ DE
Carbamazepine	Grapefruit ↑ DE	**Loratadine**	Grapefruit ↑ DE	**Terfenadine**	Grapefruit ↑ DE
Cefotetan	Alcohol ↑ AE	**Lovastatin**	Grapefruit ↑ DE	**Tetracycline**	Dairy, Ca, Mg, Fe ↓ effect
Cilostazol	Grapefruit ↑ DE	**Methadone**	Grapefruit ↑ DE	**Theophylline**	Caffeine ↑ DE
Ciprofloxacin	Dairy, Ca, Mg, Fe ↓ DE	**Metronidazole**	Alcohol, ↑ AE	**Thyroid hormone**	Food ↓ effect
Clomipramine	Grapefruit ↑ DE	**Midazolam**	Grapefruit ↑ DE	**Tranylcypromine**	Tyramine, ↑ AE
Clozapine	Caffeine ↑ DE	**Minocycline**	Dairy, Ca, Mg, Fe ↓ DE	**Triazolam**	Grapefruit ↑ DE
Cyclosporine	Grapefruit ↑ DE	**Nimodipine**	Grapefruit ↑ DE	**Warfarin**	Vitamin K-rich foods ↓ DE
Diazepam	Grapefruit ↑ DE	**Nisoldipine**	Grapefruit ↑ DE	**Zaleplon**	Grapefruit ↑ DE
Doxycycline	Dairy, Ca, Mg, Fe ↓ DE	**Nitrofurantoin**	Alcohol ↑ AE		
Ebastine	Grapefruit ↑ DE	**Phenelzine**	Tyramine ↑ AE		
Felodipine	Grapefruit ↑ DE	**Pranidipine**	Grapefruit ↑ DE		
Griseofulvin	Alcohol ↑ AE	**Saquinavir**	Grapefruit ↑ DE		
Fe supplements	Food ↓ effect	**Sertraline**	Grapefruit ↑ DE		
Isocarboxazid	Tyramine ↑ AE	**Sildenafil**	Grapefruit ↑ DE		

[a]This list is not meant to be exhaustive, but merely highlighting some of the main food and beverages that give may rise to a clinically significant interaction with particular drugs.

Ca, calcium; Mg, magnesium; Fe, Iron; AE, adverse effects; DE, drug effects increasing the risk of dose-dependent side effects *(4,5)*. The flavonoid compounds present in a typical glass of grapefruit juice (and which are also present in the whole fruit, the pulp, and the peel), act to irreversibly inhibit a key metabolizing enzyme (CYP3A4) in the intestinal wall, although no adverse effects are seen on the similar enzyme in the liver *(6)*. The extent to which an individual is affected by grapefruit juice is largely genetically predetermined, related to the extent and relative distribution of isoforms of this enzyme in the intestines of individuals. While there are broad ethnic differences (African Americans affected more than Caucasians), prediction of the scope of the effect in a particular individual is impossible in the clinic.

Only specific drugs - those that are significantly metabolized by CYP3A4 in the intestine - are affected by this food/beverage interaction. Responses are typically quite variable between individuals with patients with the highest intestinal expression of CYP3A4 experiencing the greatest grapefruit juice interaction. With this comes a range of dose-dependent effects, and both desirable and undesirable clinical effects can be observed.

The drugs most affected by grapefruit juice include the dihydropyridine calcium antagonists: felodipine, pranidipine, nisoldipine, and nimodipine. Any possible interactions with other agents, such as amlodipine, cardizem, and verapamil, are not likely to be of clinical significance. The HMG-CoA reductase inhibitors (statins, such as lovastatin and simvastatin, and to a lesser extent atorvastatin) can all undergo significant interaction with grapefruit juice. Fluvastatin and pravastatin are unaffected. Other medications undergoing a significant interaction with grapefruit juice include the immunosuppressants (cyclosporine and tacrolimus); the antihistamines (terfenadine, ebastine, and loratadine); the antimicrobials (artemether and saquinavir); the neuropsychiatric drugs (diazepam, midazolam, triazolam, buspirone, sertraline, carbamazepine, clomipramine, zaleplon, and methadone), cilostazol, and sildenafil.

To summarize, grapefruit juice inhibits the metabolism of many medications spanning a variety of clinical fields. In general, the subset of patients in whom grapefruit juice gives the greatest effect are those who at baseline display the greatest amounts of intestinal metabolism and hence the lowest rates of drug bioavailability. In day-to-day practice this group remains hard to identify and this inhibition of metabolism can lead to many-fold increases in circulating drug levels and place these patients at risk for dose-dependent side effects. Unfortunately, due to a variety of both patient and grapefruit factors (perhaps explained by changes in the constituents of grapefruit with different crops and preparations) this effect is unpredictable and cannot be used clinically. Until these issues are defined it seems prudent to dissuade patients from combining grapefruit juice with any of the above-mentioned medications, particularly when they are taking them for the first time or in high doses.

4.3. Effect of Alcohol on Drug Action

The effects of alcohol consumption on health are described elsewhere in the chapter by Wilson (Chapter 9). Alcohol imparts many effects on drug therapy, both acutely and with chronic excessive consumption *(7)*. Alcohol may delay gastric emptying and thus slow the onset of absorption of many medications. Over time, heavy alcohol consumption may also lead to chronic altered bowel motility. Chronic consumption of excessive quantities of alcohol may result in cirrhosis and an associated impairment of hepatic drug metabolism. Like caffeine and grapefruit juice, concomitant alcohol can also acutely and directly affect drug metabolism. CYP2E1 is one of the enzymes that is responsible for alcohol metabolism. In the acute setting, alcohol competes for this enzyme and may reduce the metabolism of medications normally metabolized by CYP2E1 (e.g., warfarin, phenytoin, and rifampicin). Chronic alcohol consumption, by inducing a 5- to 10-fold increase in CYP2E1 levels, may alternatively increase metabolism of these drugs over time.

CYP2E1 is one of the minor pathways of acetaminophen metabolism with the end-product being a toxic metabolite. Therefore, chronic alcohol use greatly predisposes to acetaminophen toxicity. Cefotetan, griseofulvin, isoniazid, metronidazole, nitrofurantoin, and sulfa drugs mimic disulfiram by also inhibiting acetaldehyde dehydrogenase, a key enzyme in the metabolism of alcohol. Hence, consumption of alcohol by many patients taking these antimicrobials is associated with greatly increased concentrations of acetaldehyde and symptoms of tachycardia, flushing, vomiting, confusion, and hypotension. Red wine has also been shown to cause inhibition of intestinal CYP3A4, albeit to a lesser extent than grapefruit juice. Hence, a clinically significant effect of red wine on medications normally metabolized in the intestine by CYP3A4 would likely be uncommon. However, in rare patients (those with the highest intestinal CYP3A4 concentrations) red wine may carry the same risks as grapefruit juice for dose-dependent side effects.

4.4. Effect of Caffeine on Drug Action

Caffeine is widely consumed through coffee, tea, and many carbonated beverages. Acting as a central nervous system stimulant, caffeine leads to elevation in mood, a reduction in fatigue, and an increased facility for work. In addition to these stimulant effects and its effects on the cardiovascular system, caffeine has specific actions on drug metabolism, interacting with the CYP1A2 enzyme system responsible for the metabolism of certain drugs *(8)*. However, it is likely that there are only a few medications which undergo a clinically significant interaction with usual doses of dietary caffeine; these are particularly medications with a narrow margin between when they are therapeutic and toxic (e.g., clozapine, lithium, and theophylline). The consumption of dietary caffeine should be minimized in patients taking these medications. Clozapine, an atypical antipsychotic used in the treatment of schizophrenia, is one such medication. There are a number of reported cases of the presence of dose-dependent clozapine side effects in patients consuming large quantities of caffeine (5–10 cups of coffee/d). It should be noted that this psychiatric population is one in which caffeine consumption is frequently high. Also noted is that ingestion of large quantities of caffeine may lead to a reduction in lithium levels and a decrease in its therapeutic effect.

5. CONCLUSION

This chapter has reviewed the common drug interactions with food and beverages. By acting on gastric motility, pH, and drug metabolism, food and beverages can have a variety of effects on the absorption and metabolism of medications, as well as many vitamins and minerals, with the clinical significance ranging from passing interest to concern for significant toxicity. Particularly for those medications such as grapefruit juice that affect drug metabolism, there is huge variability from one person to the next and the risks of dangerous interactions are only present in a few. With further understanding and perhaps profiling of patients for their gene expression of metabolic enzymes, it may be possible to identify those most at risk for both beverage-drug and drug-drug interactions. In the meantime it is best for patients to take their medications with a glass of water unless otherwise advised.

SUGGESTED FURTHER READING

Drug: Facts and Comparisons; Micromedex Drugdex System. http://www.thomsonhc.com

Brunton L, Lazo J, Parker K. Goodman & Gilman's The Pharmacological Basis of Therapeutics, 11th Ed. McGraw-Hill, New York, 2005.

Genser D. Food and drug interaction: consequences for the nutrition/health status. Ann Nutr Metab 2008; 52 S1:29–32.

Center for Food-Drug Interaction Research and Education. University of Florida. http://www.grove.ufl.edu/~ned/fdic

REFERENCES

1. Jung H, Peregrina AA, Rodriguez JM, Moreno-Esparza R. The influence of coffee with milk and tea with milk on the bioavailability of tetracycline. Biopharm Drug Dispos 1997; 18:459–463.

2. Lake-Bakaar G, Tom W, Lake-Bakaar D, et al. Gastropathy and ketoconazole malabsorption in the acquired immunodeficiency syndrome (AIDS). Ann Intern Med 1988; 109: 471–473.

3. Chin TW, Loeb M, Fong IW. Effects of an acidic beverage (Coca-Cola) on absorption of ketoconazole. Antimicrob Agents Chemother 1995; 39:1671–1675.

4. Bailey DG, Malcolm J, Arnold O, Spence JD. Grapefruit juice-drug interactions. Br J Clin Pharmacol 1998; 46:101–110.

5. Kane GC, Lipsky JJ. Drug-grapefruit juice interactions. Mayo Clin Proc 2000; 75: 933–942.

6. Lundahl JU, Regardh CG, Edgar B, Johnsson G. The interaction effect of grapefruit juice is maximal after the first glass. Eur J Clin Pharmacol 1998; 54:75–81.

7. Fraser AG. Pharmacokinetic interactions between alcohol and other drugs. Clin Pharmacokinet 1997; 33:79–90.

8. Carrillo JA, Benitez J. Clinically significant pharmacokinetic interactions between dietary caffeine and medications. Clin Pharmacokinet 2000; 39:127–153.

Appendix A: Aids to Calculations

WEIGHT

1 gram = 0.035 oz
1 kg = 2.20 lb
1 oz = 28.35 grams
1 lb = 454 grams

LENGTH

1 cm = 0.393 in
1 meter = 39.37 in
1 in = 2.54 cm
1 ft = 30.4 cm

VOLUME

1 pint (US) = 0.473 L = 16 oz
1 quart (US) = 0.946 L = 32 oz
1 fluid oz = 29.57 mL
1 L = 2.11 pints (US)
1 cup = 8 oz = 236 mL (commonly rounded to 250 mL)
1 teaspoon (tsp) = 5 mL
1 tablespoon (tbs or T) = 3 teaspoons = 15 mL

TEMPERATURE

To change Fahrenheit (°F) to Celsius (°C), subtract 32, then divide by 1.8
To change °C to °F, multiply by 1.8, then add 32
Boiling point 100°C = 212°F
Body temperature 37°C = 98.6°F
Freezing point 0°C = 32°F

From: *Nutrition and Health: Nutrition Guide for Physicians*
Edited by: T. Wilson et al. (eds.), DOI 10.1007/978-1-60327-431-9,
© Humana Press, a part of Springer Science+Business Media, LLC 2010

ENERGY

1 kcal = 4.2 kJ (kilojoules)
Energy in food components (kcal per gram)
Fat: 9
Carbohydrate: 4
Protein: 4
Alcohol: 7

BODY MASS INDEX (BMI)

BMI = weight (kg) divided by height $(m)^2$ *or* [weight (lb) x 703] divided by
   height $(in)^2$

Appendix B: Sources of Reliable Information on Nutrition

BOOKS

Willett W, Skerrett PJ. Eat, Drink, and Be Healthy: The Harvard Medical School Guide to Healthy Eating. Free Press, New York, 2005.

Duyff R, American Dietetic Association. American Dietetic Association Complete Food and Nutrition Guide. Wiley, Hoboken, NJ, 2006.

Nestle M. What to Eat. North Point Press, New York, 2007.

Temple NJ, Wilson T, Jacobs DR, Jr (eds). Nutritional Health: Strategies for Disease Prevention, 2nd ed. Humana Press, New Jersey, 2006.

JOURNALS AND MAGAZINES

Nutrition Action. A monthly magazine that provides up-to-date and reliable information on nutrition and health. The main target audience is the general public. It is published by the Center for Science in the Public Interest. A subscription may be purchased by sending an e-mail to: circ@spinet.org. Or visit their website at www.cspinet.org.

The Arbor Clinical Nutrition Updates. This e-journal provides regular detailed summaries on diverse topics in the area of nutrition and health. The main target audience are health professionals. A subscription may be purchased at their website: http://www.nutritionupdates.org.

INTERNET WEBSITES

http://www.mayoclinic.com
This is operated by the Mayo Clinic and provides much information on health and disease, including diet and supplements. It also sells books written by Mayo Clinic experts.

http://www.healthfinder.gov
A source of health information on many topics. The website is run by the U.S. Department of Health and Human Services.

http://medlineplus.gov
This website is operated by agencies of the U.S. government and provides extensive information on many aspects of health and medicine. (Also in Spanish)

http://www.ncbi.nlm.nih.gov/PubMed.
MEDLINE. This is the "big brother" of MedlinePlus. It provides direct access to a database of more than ten million articles published in thousands of scholarly journals in all areas of the biomedical sciences.

http://www.eatright.org
American Dietetic Association. Resource for nutrition information. (Also in Spanish)

http://www.nhlbi.nih.gov

National Heart, Lung, and Blood Institute. Provides much valuable information on heart disease and related subjects. (Also in Spanish)

http://www.amhrt.org

American Heart Association. Another resource on heart disease. (Also in Spanish)

http://www.cancer.gov

National Cancer Institute. This provides extensive information on all aspects of cancer. (Also in Spanish)

http://www.diabetes.org

American Diabetes Association. Extensive information on all aspects of diabetes. (Also in Spanish)

http://www.aap.org

American Academy of Pediatrics. Information on all aspects of pediatrics, including nutrition.

http://win.niddk.nih.gov

The Weight-control Information Network (WIN). Information on all aspects of weight control. (Also in Spanish)

The following two organizations run websites that give reliable information on various health frauds: National Council Against Health Fraud (NCAHF)

http://www.ncahf.org

Quackwatch http://www.quackwatch.org

People can obtain an analysis of their diet, at no cost, at the following websites. In each case a diet record is entered and the website provides extensive information on nutrient content.

http://www.mypyramidtracker.gov.

This is provided by MyPyramid (the American food guide).

http://www.nutritiondata.com. Operated by NutritionData

A Canadian website can be found by doing a Google search for "nutrient value of some common foods". This provides detailed information on the nutrition content of large numbers of foods.

Appendix C: Dietary Reference Intakes (DRI)

Dietary Reference Intakes (DRI) are composed of four tables. These include Recommended Dietary Allowances (RDA) and Adequate Intakes (AI), as explained in Chapter 5. A simplified version of these tables indicating appropriate target RDA or AI values is included below. The values indicate a target amount (quantity per day) for each nutrient, depending on age and sex. The full tables include: values for people aged from birth to 18 yr; values for energy, fat, carbohydrate, water, and 11 other nutrients; and values for Tolerable Upper Intake Levels. For the full tables go to the following website: http://fnic.nal.usda.gov, then click on "Dietary Guidance".

RDA or AI Values for the Major Vitamins and Minerals

| | | Male | Female | | | | |
		>18 yr	19–50 yr	51–70 yr	>70 yr	Pregnancy	Lactation
Dietary fiber	g	38	25	21	21	28	29
Protein	g	56	46	46	46	71	71
Thiamin	mg	1.2	1.1	1.1	1.1	1.4	1.4
Riboflavin	mg	1.3	1.1	1.1	1.1	1.4	1.6
Niacin	mg	16	14	14	14	18	17
Vitamin B_6	mg	1.3*	1.3	1.5	1.5	1.9	2.0
Folate	μg	400	400	400	400	600	500
Vitamin B_{12}	μg	2.4	2.4	2.4	2.4	2.6	2.8
Vitamin C	mg	90	75	75	75	85	120
Vitamin A	μg ‡	900	700	700	700	770	1300
Vitamin D	μg ¶	5#	5	10	15	5	5
Vitamin E	mg	15	15	15	15	15	19
Potassium	mg	4700	4700	4700	4700	4700	5100
Calcium	mg	1000§	1000	1200	1200	1000	1000
Magnesium	mg	420	315	320	320	355	315
Iron	mg	8	18	8	8	27	9
Zinc	mg	11	8	8	8	11	12
Iodine	μg	150	150	150	150	220	290
Selenium	μg	55	55	55	55	60	70
Copper	μg	900	900	900	900	1000	1300

* 1.7 mg at age >50
\# 10 μg at age 51–70; 15 μg at age >70
§ 1200 mg at age >50
‡ 1000 μg of vitamin A = 3300 IU 5 μg of vitamin D = 200 IU

Subject Index

Editor Biographies

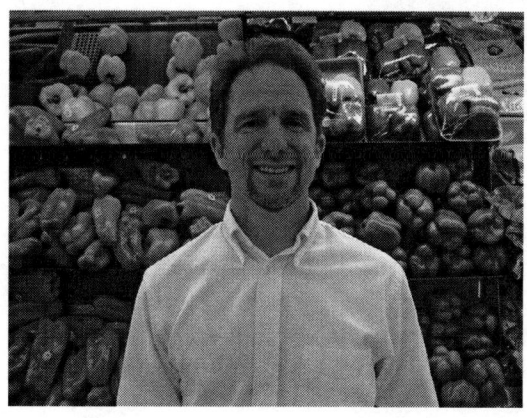

Dr. Ted Wilson, Ph.D. is an associate professor of biology at Winona State University in Winona, Minnesota. He teaches courses in nutrition, physiology, cardiovascular physiology, cell signal transduction, and cell biology. His research examines how diet affects human nutritional physiology and whether food/dietary supplement health claims can be supported by measurable physiological changes. He has studied many foods, dietary supplements. and disease conditions including low-carbohydrate diets, cranberries and cranberry juice, pomegranate juice, apple juice, grape juice, wine, resveratrol, creatine phosphate, soy phytoestrogens, tomatoes, eggplants, coffee, tea, energy drinks, heart failure prognosis, diabetes, and obesity. Diet-induced changes have included physiological evaluations of plasma lipid profile, antioxidants, vasodilation, nitric oxide, platelet aggregation, glycemic and insulinemic responses using in vivo and in vitro models. With Dr. N. Temple he has edited *Beverages in Nutrition and Health* (Humana Press, 2004) and *Nutritional Health: Strategies for Disease Prevention* (Humana Press, 2001 first and 2006 second edition).

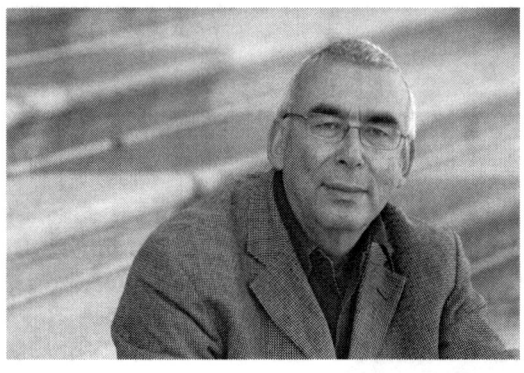

Norman J. Temple, Ph.D. is the professor of nutrition at Athabasca University in Alberta, Canada. Dr. Temple's specialty is nutrition in relation to health. He has published 10 previous books. Together with Denis Burkitt he coedited *Western Diseases: Their Dietary Prevention and Reversibility* (Humana Press, 1994). This continued and extended Burkitt's pioneering work on the role of dietary fiber in chronic diseases of lifestyle. With Dr. Ted Wilson he coedited the books mentioned above. He also coedited *Excessive Medical Spending: Facing the Challenge* (Radcliffe Publishing, 2007). He conducts collaborative research in Cape Town on the role of the changing diet in South Africa on the pattern of diseases in that country, such as obesity, diabetes, and heart disease.

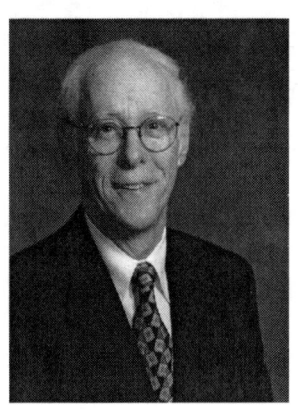

George A. Bray, M.D., MACP, MACE is a Boyd professor at the Pennington Biomedical Research Center of Louisiana State University in Baton Rouge, Louisiana, and professor of medicine at the Louisiana State University Medical Center in New Orleans. He was the first executive director of the Pennington Biomedical Research Center in Baton Rouge, a post he held from 1989 to 1999. He is a master in both the American College of Physicians and the American College of Endocrinology. Dr. Bray founded the North American Association for the Study of Obesity (NAASO now The Obesity Society), and he was the founding editor of its journal, *Obesity Research*, as well as co-founder of the *International Journal of Obesity* and the first editor of *Endocrine Practice,* the official journal of the American College of Endocrinologists. Dr. Bray has received many awards during his medical career. It include the Johns Hopkins Society of Scholars, honorary fellow, American Dietetic Association, Joseph Goldberger Award from the American Medical Association, the McCollum Award from the American Society of Clinical Nutrition, and the Osborne–Mendel Award from the American Society of Nutritional. Dr. Bray has also received the TOPS Award from NAASO, the Weight Watchers Award, the Bristol-Myers Squibb Mead Johnson Award in Nutrition, and the Stunkard Lifetime Achievement Award. During the past 40 years, Dr. Bray has authored or co-authored more than 1,700 publications, ranging from peer-reviewed articles to reviews, books, book chapters, and abstracts.

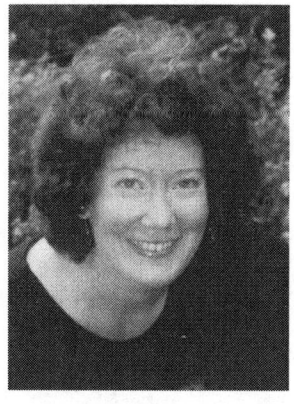

Marie Boyle Struble, Ph.D., R.D., is adjunct professor of nutrition for the Graduate Program in Nutrition at the College of Saint Elizabeth in Morristown, New Jersey, and is former professor and director of the Graduate Program in Nutrition at the college. She also teaches online distance courses for the master's in Public Health Nutrition Program at the University of Massachusetts in Amherst. She is co-author of the basic nutrition textbook *Personal Nutrition* and the senior level textbook *Community Nutrition in Action: An Entrepreneurial Approach* (both published by Wadsworth/Cengage Publishing, Belmont, CA). She is editor of the *Journal of Hunger and Environmental Nutrition*, published by Taylor & Francis Publishers, and co-authored the current position paper of the American Dietetic Association on World Hunger, Malnutrition, and Food Insecurity. Her research interests include global nutrition issues, nutrition and aging, and generational diversity and consumer food trends.

About the Series Editor

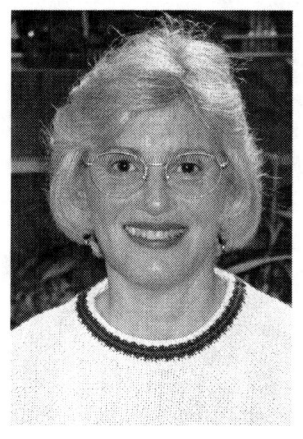

Dr. Adrianne Bendich is Clinical Director, Medical Affairs at GlaxoSmithKline (GSK) Consumer Healthcare, where she is responsible for leading the innovation and medical programs in support of many well-known brands, including TUMS and Os-Cal. Dr. Bendich had primary responsibility for GSK's support for the Women's Health Initiative (WHI) intervention study. Prior to joining GSK, Dr. Bendich was at Roche Vitamins, Inc. and was involved with the groundbreaking clinical studies showing that folic acid-containing multivitamins significantly reduced major classes of birth defects. Dr. Bendich has co-authored over 100 major clinical research studies in the area of preventive nutrition. Dr. Bendich is recognized as a leading authority on antioxidants, nutrition and immunity and pregnancy outcomes, vitamin safety and the cost-effectiveness of vitamin/mineral supplementation.

Dr. Bendich is the editor of nine books, including "Preventive Nutrition: The Comprehensive Guide For Health Professionals" coedited with Dr. Richard Deckelbaum, and is Series Editor of "Nutrition and Health" for Humana Press with 32 published volumes, including "Probiotics in Pediatric Medicine" edited by Dr. Sonia Michail and Dr. Philip Sherman; "Handbook of Nutrition and Pregnancy" edited by Dr. Carol Lammi-Keefe, Dr. Sarah Couch, and Dr. Elliot Philipson; "Nutrition and Rheumatic Disease" edited by Dr. Laura Coleman; "Nutrition and Kidney Disease" edited by Dr. Laura Byham-Grey, Dr. Jerrilynn Burrowes, and Dr. Glenn Chertow; "Nutrition and Health in Developing Countries" edited by Dr. Richard Semba and Dr. Martin Bloem; "Calcium in Human Health" edited by Dr. Robert Heaney and Dr. Connie Weaver, and "Nutrition and Bone Health" edited by Dr. Michael Holick and Dr. Bess Dawson-Hughes.

Dr. Bendich served as associate editor for "Nutrition," the International Journal, served on the editorial board of the Journal of Women's Health and Gender-Based Medicine, and was a member of the Board of Directors of the American College of Nutrition.

Dr. Bendich was the recipient of the Roche Research Award, is a *Tribute to Women and Industry* Awardee, and was a recipient of the Burroughs Wellcome Visiting Professorship in Basic Medical Sciences, 2000–2001. In 2008, Dr. Bendich was given the Council for Responsible Nutrition (CRN) Apple Award in recognition of her many contributions to the scientific understanding of dietary supplements. Dr. Bendich holds academic appointments as adjunct professor in the Department of Preventive Medicine and Community Health at UMDNJ and has an adjunct appointment at the Institute of Nutrition, Columbia University P&S, and is an Adjunct Research Professor, Rutgers University, Newark Campus. She is listed in Who's Who in American Women.

CPSIA information can be obtained at www.ICGtesting.com
Printed in the USA
LVOW070149231211

260828LV00003B/44/P